Diagnostic Electron Microscopy of Tumours

Also by the same author:

Ultrastructural Pathology of the Cell

Diagnostic Electron Microscopy of Tumours

Feroze N. Ghadially

MD, PhD, DSc(Lond), FRCPath, FRCP(C)
Professor and Joint Head of Pathology,
University of Saskatchewan, Saskatoon, Canada
Formerly Reader in Neoplastic Diseases and
Senior Lecturer in Experimental Pathology,
University of Sheffield, England

Butterworths
London   Boston
Sydney   Wellington   Durban   Toronto

United Kingdom/London
Butterworth & Co (Publishers) Ltd
88 Kingsway, WC2B 6AB

Australia/Sydney
Butterworths Pty Ltd
586 Pacific Highway, Chatswood, NSW 2067
Also at Melbourne, Brisbane, Adelaide and Perth

Canada/Toronto
Butterworth & Co (Canada) Ltd
2265 Midland Avenue, Scarborough, Ontario, M1P 4S1

New Zealand/Wellington
Butterworths of New Zealand Ltd
T & W Young Building, 77–85 Customhouse Quay, 1,
CPO Box 472

South Africa/Durban
Butterworth & Co (South Africa) (Pty) Ltd
152–154 Gale Street

USA/Boston
Butterworth (Publishers) Inc
10 Tower Office Park, Woburn, Massachusetts 01801

First published 1980
Reprinted 1980
Reprinted 1982
© Butterworth & Co (Publishers) Ltd, 1980

British Library Cataloguing in Publication Data

Ghadially, Feroze Novroji
    Diagnostic electron microscopy of tumours.
    1. Tumours – Diagnosis   2. Diagnosis, Electron
    microscopic
    I. Title
    616.9'92'0758   RC255   79 42839
    ISBN 0-407-00156-5

Typeset by Butterworth Litho Preparation Department
Printed and bound in Great Britain by
William Clowes (Beccles) Ltd

Preface

This book is addressed primarily to histopathologists and pathology residents who wish to examine tumour biopsies with the electron microscope or would like to be more conversant with such matters so that they can understand and evaluate electron micrographs and reports issued by electron microscopists. It is hoped that this book will also be of some value to physicians and surgeons, for electron micrographs are now beginning to be used in ever-increasing numbers at clinico-pathological conferences and seminars to augment and clarify histopathological findings.

In the majority of cases the histogenesis and classification of tumours can be unequivocally established by light microscopy, but in some instances the diagnosis remains ambiguous even after special staining techniques have been employed. It is in such cases that the electron microscopic study of the lesion may be helpful. The reason for this is that one can see with the electron microscope details of intracellular structure and intercellular relationships which are difficult or impossible to visualize with the light microscope. This provides fresh data by which one may be able to establish the histogenesis of a tumour which had proved impossible to diagnose by light microscopy.

It is for such reasons that the electron microscope is becoming a useful adjunct in the diagnosis of tumours, but it must be stressed that the electron microscope is no substitute for the light microscope, which still remains the supreme tool for the diagnosis of a majority of tumours. The two techniques are complementary, rather than rivals.

The purpose of this book is to lay before the reader the principles and thinking behind the ultrastructural examination of tumours. I hope also to provide sufficient factual data for the evaluation of a majority of tumour biopsies with the electron microscope. It is beyond the scope of this brief text to describe the ultrastructure of every tumour or discuss the histogenesis of rare and controversial neoplasms.

Ultrastructural study of a tumour biopsy is usually undertaken to answer quite specific questions that may have remained unresolved by light microscopy. For this reason I have included chapters asking specific questions such as: (1) Is it malignant? (2) Is it a carcinoma or sarcoma? and (3) Is it a squamous cell carcinoma or an adenocarcinoma?

However, not all the necessary information can be conveyed in such a format, so additional chapters dealing with other matters such as differences between normal and neoplastic cells and descriptions of some rare but ultrastructurally interesting tumours have also been included.

It is not my purpose to extol the virtues or usefulness of ultrastructural investigation of tumours, for this has been done again and again in every guise and form. If proof is sought in the form of actual instances where ultrastructural investigations have helped, then see: Rosai and Rodriguez (1968); Zimmerman *et al.* (1972); Laschi (1974); Gyorkey *et al.* (1975); Lagacé (1975); Bonikos, Bensch and Kempson (1976); Johannessen (1977); Hirano (1978); Regezi and Batsakis (1978); and Battifora and Applebaum (1979).

Also, I do not wish to dwell upon various popular preoccupations of our times such as 'cost effectiveness of the technique' and 'value to patient care'. I am confident that, with the passage of time, this growing field of endeavour will more than prove its worth, for many interesting ultrastructural findings yet remain to be correlated with tumour biology and behaviour. I feel that an important task for a text like this is to highlight these hopeful areas, even though some of them may appear far-fetched. It is hoped that this will provoke argument, study and research. Finally, I should point out that this is not a 'cook-book' either. However, the text commences with a brief analysis of the methods of tissue collection and preparation and other technical matters relevant to the problem of tumour diagnosis with the electron microscope.

References

BATTIFORA, H. and APPLEBAUM, E. L. (1979). Electron microscopy in the diagnosis of head and neck tumors. *Head and Neck Surg.*, 1, 202

BONIKOS, D. S., BENSCH, K. G. and KEMPSON, R. L. (1976). The contribution of electron microscopy to the differential diagnosis of tumours. *Beitr. Path. Anat.*, 158, 417

GYORKEY, F., MIN, K-W., KRISKO, I. and GYORKEY, P. (1975). The usefulness of electron microscopy in the diagnosis of human tumours. *Hum. Path.*, 6, 421

HIRANO, A. (1978). Some contributions of electron microscopy to the diagnosis of brain tumours. *Acta Neuropath.*, 43, 119

JOHANNESSEN, J. V. (1977). Use of paraffin material for electron microscopy. *Path. Ann.*, 12, 189

LAGACÉ, R. (1975). La microscopie électronique appliquée au diagnostic différentiel et à l'étude de l'histogenèse des tumeurs des tissus mous. *La Vie Méd. Canada Francais*, 4, 1102

LASCHI, R. (1974). The clinical value of electron microscopy. *Gaz. Inglese*, 3, 83

REGEZI, J. A. and BATSAKIS, J. C. (1978). Diagnostic electron microscopy of head and neck tumors. *Archs Path. Lab. Med.*, 102, 8

ROSAI, J. and RODRIGUEZ, H. A. (1968). Application of electron microscopy to the differential diagnosis of tumors. *Am. J. Clin. Path.*, 50, 555

ZIMMERMAN, L. E., FONT, R. L., TSO, M. O. M. and FINE, B. S. (1972). Application of electron microscopy to histopathologic diagnosis. *Trans. Am. Acad. Ophthal. Oto-lar.*, 76, 101

Acknowledgements

It is my pleasant duty to acknowledge the help given by my friends and colleagues and also the skill and dedication of my co-workers and technicians.

(1) Dr G. W. Cates, Dr O. G. Dodge, Dr T. E. Larsen, Dr J. W. Newstead and Dr L. F. Skinnider read through the typescript and offered many useful criticisms and suggestions. I am grateful to them for sharing their expertise and experience, for this has been most helpful in writing this book. Most of their suggestions have been incorporated; any errors are my responsibility entirely.

(2) I am grateful to (a) Dr A. H. Cameron for providing me with numerous blocks from cases of Ewing's sarcoma, rhabdomyosarcoma, neuroblastoma and granular cell myoblastoma; (b) Dr Imamura for a block from a case of Hand—Schüller—Christian disease; and (c) Dr Schnitka for blocks of tissue from an adrenal cortical adenoma. Electron micrographs obtained from such blocks are acknowledged in the legends, as also are electron micrographs obtained in collaboration with my co-workers.

(3) My thanks are also due to Mrs M Boyle, Mrs C. E. Dick, Mr J-M. A. Lalonde and Mr N. K. Yong for collecting and processing tissues, cutting ultrathin sections and preparing innumerable prints from which a few were selected for publication in this book. In the latter task Mr J. Junor and Mr R. Van den Beuken also assisted, particularly when special techniques were required to obtain prints from a less than perfect negative.

(4) The task of searching the massive literature on the ultrastructure of tumours, classifying and filing reprints and Xeroxed copies of papers, preparing reference lists and correcting and organizing the text into a publishable format was executed by my wife, Mrs E. Ghadially. The expert assistance of our library staff, Mrs L. Church and Mrs S. Sutherland, in running Medline and Medlar searches on innumerable subjects is gratefully acknowledged. The text was typed by Mrs E. Ghadially, Mrs M. Hopewell, Mrs K. Kalyn and Miss J. Klassen. Their skill at promptly converting an almost illegible manuscript into well-laid-out error-free sheets was a major factor in accelerating the production of this work.

(5) The task of producing this work has been greatly facilitated by the skill and knowledge of the editorial staff of Butterworths.

(6) Of the 195 electron micrographs published in this work, 35 come from external sources. For these illustrations I am indebted to the following authors and journals.

BECKER, N. H. and SOIFER, I. (1971). *Cancer*, 27, 712: Figs. 179, 180

DJALDETTI, M. (unpublished): Fig. 160

DJALDETTI, M., LANDAU, M., MANDEL, E. M., HARZAAV, L. and LEWINSKI, U. (1974). *Blut*, 29, 210: Fig. 159

ERLANDSON, R. A. (unpublished): Fig. 176

ERLANDSON, R. A. and TANDLER, B. (1972). *Archives of Pathology*, 93, 130: Figs 177, 178

JOHANNESSEN, J. V. (unpublished): Figs. 189, 190

KLEIN, B., LEWINSKI, U., SHABTAI, S., FREIDIN, N. and DJALDETTI, M. (1977). *Blut*, 35, 11: Figs. 167, 168

LAMBERTENGHI-DELILIERS, G., POZZOLI, E., ZANON, P. and MAIOLO, A. T. (1978). *Journal of Submicroscopic Cytology*, 10, 239: Figs. 153, 154, 155, 156

MOLLO, F. (unpublished): Figs. 187, 188

MUKHERJEE, T. M. (unpublished): Figs. 181, 182

NEWSTEAD, J. D. (unpublished): Figs. 6, 7

SENOO, A. (unpublished): Fig. 166

SHIPKEY, F. H. (unpublished): Fig. 192

SHIPKEY, F. H., LIEBERMAN, P. H., FOOTE, F. W. and STEWART, F. W. (1964). *Cancer*, 17, 821: Fig. 191

SKINNIDER, L. F. (unpublished): Fig. 137, 138

TANDLER, B. (unpublished): Fig. 94

TANDLER, B. (1966). *Archives of Otolargngology*, 84, 90: Fig. 84

TANDLER, B., HUTTER, R. V. P. and ERLANDSON, R. A. (1970). *Laboratory Investigation*, 23, 567: Figs. 85, 86, 87

TANDLER, R. and ROSSI, E. P. (1977). *Journal of Oral Pathology*, 6, 401: Fig. 93

VASUDEV, K. S. and HARRIS, M. (1978). *Archives of Pathology and Laboratory Medicine*, 102, 185: Figs. 112, 113, 114

(7) I am also grateful to the following journals and publishers for permission to use illustrations from past publications of which I am an author or co-author.

GHADIALLY, F. N. (1975). *Ultrastructural Pathology of the Cell*, London: Butterworths: Figs. 3, 4, 12, 20, 26, 27, 28, 33, 34, 35, 58, 59, 60, 61, 62, 63, 64, 65, 83, 98, 99, 139, 140, 141, 165, 169, 184, 185, 186, 193

GHADIALLY, F. N., LALONDE, J-M. A. and DICK, C. E. (1978). *Experientia*, 34, 1212: Fig. 36

GHADIALLY, F. N., LOWES, N. R. and MESFIN, G. M. (1977). *Journal of Pathology*, 122, 157: Figs. 96, 164

GHADIALLY, F. N. and MEHTA, P. N. (1970). *Cancer*, 25, 291: Fig. 29

GHADIALLY, F. N. and PARRY, E. W. (1966). *Cancer*, 19, 1989: Figs. 19, 32

GHADIALLY, F. N. and ROY, S. (1969). *Ultrastructure of Synovial Joints in Health and Disease*. London: Butterworths: Fig. 161

GHADIALLY, F. N. and SKINNIDER, L. F. (1976). *Experientia*, 32, 1061: Fig. 152

SKINNIDER, L. F. and GHADIALLY, F. N. (1973). *Archives of Pathology*, 95, 139: Fig. 170

SKINNIDER, L. F. and GHADIALLY, F. N. (1977). *British Journal of Cancer*, 35, 657: Fig. 151

Contents

Part 1

Ultrastructural techniques

1
Collecting and processing tissues for diagnostic electron microscopy

The methods of collecting and processing tissues for electron microscopy have been described in many books, as also have the techniques of ultramicrotomy and staining sections (Pease, 1964; Kay, 1965; Meek, 1970; Mercer and Birbeck, 1972; Weakley, 1972; Griffin, 1972; Glauert, 1974). It is not the purpose of this chapter to reiterate in a brief and inadequate manner that which is already well known and well documented. We will concentrate on practical matters of special interest to the diagnostic electron microscopist, for his needs and problems are somewhat different from those of the research worker using the electron microscope. This difference may be summarized by saying that while only the best in tissue preservation is good enough for the latter, this level of perfection is neither essential nor usually attainable in diagnostic electron microscopy. It is fortunate, therefore, that useful information may be obtained from specimens which have not been processed according to the accepted ideals or which have been retrieved from formalin or from a paraffin block.

This should not be construed as a licence for slipshod work. One should retain the traditional enthusiasm for prompt collection and proper fixation of tissues, for, as Johannessen (1977) so rightly points out: 'Improper tissue preparation greatly augments the possibility of missing the correct diagnosis as well as the possibility of making a wrong one.' Further, nothing can be more frustrating and disheartening than to find some rare tumour specimen which one would like to study in detail marred by poor fixation or improper handling. Let us then look at the ideals established by electron microscopists and see what penalties one has to pay if these ideals are not met.

Changes produced by delays in specimen collection

It is widely held (and quite rightly) that the delay between removal of the tissue and fixation should

be kept to a minimum (i.e. a few seconds or at most a minute or two). The reason for this is that morphological changes, largely due to anoxia, commence quite shortly after cessation of the circulation (e.g. after death of the individual) or severance (e.g. during surgery) of the blood supply. Experimentalists have gone to great lengths to cut this 'delay time' down to virtually zero seconds by perfusing fixatives into anaesthetized animals. This, of course, is hardly feasible in the human situation. A more widely practised method is to fix small pieces of tissue (less than 1 mm^3) immediately on removal from the body. In the case of a kidney or bone marrow biopsy, one can easily cut the delay time down to a few minutes, but when the surgeon has to put a tourniquet around a limb or when he has been clamping vessels before he exposes the tumour, the period of anoxia can be quite long.

Besides such delays there are also the delays due to the fact that the surgeon can hardly be expected to break off from operating to fix tissues, while the pathologist cannot possibly be present at every operation. The general practice is for the surgeon to give the tissue to a nurse, who passes the tissue to a trained electron microscopy technician waiting outside the operating theatre, or to a carrier who rushes the tissue to the laboratory. With such a multiplicity of individuals in the tissue collection chain, misunderstandings, complications and delays are almost inevitable.

What, then, are the penalties of such delays and how do they affect our chances of accurately diagnosing a tumour? The sequence of morphological changes that occur as a result of anoxia in normal tissues (e.g. liver or kidney) maintained at body temperature may be roughly summarized as follows. In about 15–90 s the intramitochondrial dense granules are likely to be reduced in number or disappear. By about 15–30 min the mitochondria are likely to be swollen and the rough endoplasmic reticulum may be dilated and/or vesiculated. By about 30—45 min margination and aggregation of chromatin is likely to be detectable in the nucleus. By about this time (45 min onwards) the mitochondria will begin to show woolly densities in their interior. This, incidentally, is considered to be a sign of irreversible cell injury or cell death, the earlier changes such as mitochondrial swelling and dilatations of the endoplasmic reticulum being reversible. It is worth noting that there are tissue variations. Relatively 'moist' tissues, particularly if they have a high content of lytic enzymes (e.g. kidney, liver and pancreas), deteriorate more rapidly than say, for example, skin. It would appear that similar changes also occur in tumour tissue (*Figure 1*), although this point does not seem to have been specifically investigated.

Changes of the kind described above, of course, offend the perfectionist in us but they pose no serious problems in arriving at a correct diagnosis. Various published illustrations lead one to conclude that no serious alteration (from the diagnostic point) occurs even after a 2 h delay in fixation. In kidney or liver (normal) kept at 20° C for 24 h the lysosomes appear intact and acid hydrolases are still demonstrable within them (Ito, 1962; Ericsson, Biberfeld and Selejelid, 1967), indicating that the stage of overt autolysis has not been reached. In contrast to this, serious autolytic changes will occur if the tissue is kept for such long periods at 37° C (Trump, Goldblatt and Stowell, 1962, 1965; Bassi and Bernelli-Zazzera, 1963; Latta *et al.*, 1965; Osvaldo *et al.*, 1965).

Thus, if for any reason the tissue cannot be fixed immediately, it should be stored at 4° C, but it should, of course, never be frozen* or allowed to dry.

Method of tissue processing employed in our laboratory

For various reasons (discussed later) fixation with glutaraldehyde followed by osmium is the method of choice for diagnostic electron microscopy. The method of tissue preparation employed in our laboratory may be briefly summarized as follows. Small pieces of tissue about 1 mm^3 are fixed as soon as possible in 2 per cent glutaraldehyde in 0.1 M cacodylate buffer (pH 7.3) for 1 h. After two 2 min

rinses in cacodylate buffer the tissue is post-fixed in 2 per cent osmium buffered in 0.1 M cacodylate (pH 7.3) for 1 h. The tissue pieces are then dehydrated in increasing concentrations of ethanol cleared in propylene oxide and embedded in Epon.

Semi-thin sections cut from these blocks (stained with toluidine blue) are examined with the light microscope. Thin sections obtained from selected blocks are mounted on copper grids, stained with uranyl acetate and lead citrate, and examined with the Zeiss EM-9S electron microscope.

Almost all the illustrations stemming from our laboratory and published in this book were obtained from tumours prepared in this fashion; the exceptions are noted in the legends.

Choice of fixatives

The list of fixatives and recipes is a very long one, but this need not concern us too much, because most of the proposed formulae offer little advantage over the standard method of fixation described earlier. For various reasons fixation with glutaraldehyde followed by osmium is the method of choice for diagnostic electron microscopy, and fixation in osmium alone is not recommended. It is essential to know the reasons why this is so, and what artefacts to expect.

Osmium is an excellent fixative, and since it fixes by combining with lipids,† it preserves membranous structures exceptionally well. This, combined with the fact that some proteinaceous material leaches out, results in aesthetically pleasing electron micrographs, for sharp black lines are seen against a fairly light background. However, the fact that proteinaceous material is not fixed and immobilized by osmium does create some problems. For example, zymogen granules lose up to 70 per cent of their enzymic protein content during osmium fixation; they then present as quite pale structures or are grossly distorted and disrupted (Erlandson and Tandler, 1972). This is not too helpful when one is trying to diagnose an acinic cell carcinoma (Chapter 17).

In contrast to this is glutaraldehyde, which fixes by cross-linking proteins so that zymogen granules

---

*This happens sometimes in the pathology laboratory where the specimen is frozen for quick sectioning and then, when the diagnosis is difficult a piece is taken for electron microscopy.

†The primary site of reaction of osmium is with C = C double bonds of unsaturated fatty acids; 1 molecule of OsO$_4$ reacts with each double bond (Stoeckenius and Mahr, 1965).

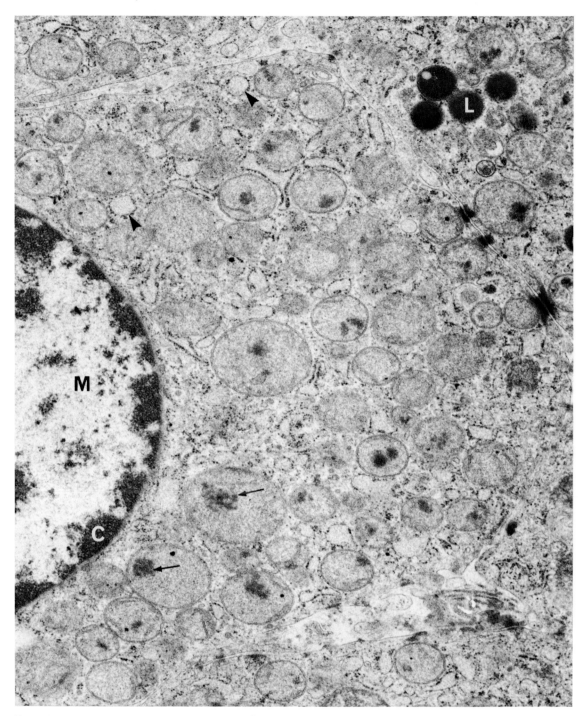

Figure 1 *Hepatoblastoma. A retroperitoneal mass (575 g) excised from a 1-year-old male. Delay between cutting off of the blood supply and fixation was probably of the order of 1 h. Anoxia leading to irreversible cell injury is evidenced by the flocculent or woolly densities (arrows) in mito-chondria. Note also the vesiculated rough endoplasmic reticulum (arrowheads) and aggregation and margination of the chromatin (C) leaving behind an unusually pale nuclear matrix (M). The lysosomes (L) appear quite intact and well preserved.* ×21 000

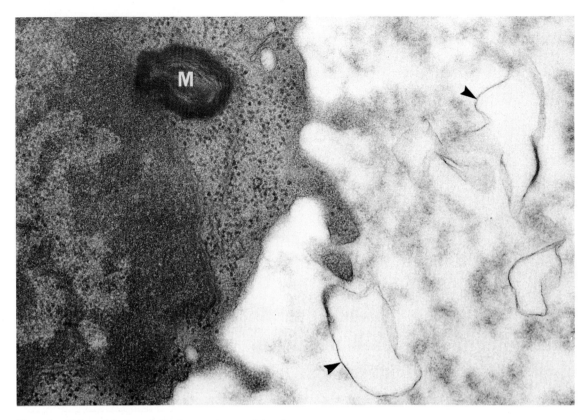

Figure 2 *Hairy cell leukaemia (buffy coat from peripheral blood). Specimen remained in glutaraldehyde for 4 days. Note the dense almost black appearance of the leukaemic cell, which contains a myelin figure (M). Myelinoid membranes (arrowheads) are also seen outside the cell.* ×60 000

are well preserved and present as characteristic homogeneously electron-dense granules which are easy to identify. However, during glutaraldehyde fixation lipids tend to leach out and become hydrated and form myelinoid membranes and figures, which (being lipid) are subsequently fixed by osmium (used as a post-fixative*) and present as electron-dense membranous structures (*Figure 2*) within and outside cells. These might be mistaken by the novice for pathological lesions (particularly when myelin figures occur in mitochondria) but otherwise constitute no great problem. Prolonged fixation (many hours or days) in glutaraldehyde should be avoided or else the cells will have a very dark almost black

appearance (*Figure 2*) and intracellular details, although well preserved, will be difficult or impossible to demonstrate in electron micrographs. There is little point in using a concentration of glutaraldehyde greater than 2 per cent or in prolonging fixation beyond 1 h† if blocks of tissue less than 1 mm³ are employed.

The pattern of heterochromatin familiar to light microscopists is best visualized after glutaraldehyde fixation followed by post-fixation in osmium and double staining with lead and uranium. In tissues

*If post-fixation in osmium is omitted, the membranes appear as clear electron-lucent lines against a dark background.

†If tissues have to be stored at this stage (i.e. after 1 h in glutaraldehyde), it is best to store them in buffer at 4°C. This is routine practice in many laboratories where tissues are held in buffer until histological investigations are completed and a decision made as to whether an electron microscopic study is needed. This is also a good way to send tissues by post.

fixed in osmium (collidine or veronal acetate-buffered) and stained with lead, nuclei have a somewhat homogeneous appearance and condensations of chromatin with the patterns familiar to light microscopists are either absent or barely discernable.*

This difference is attributable to the staining techniques (*Figures 3* and *4*) employed and also to the

*The differences in heterochromatin pattern engendered by preparative procedures are best demonstrated in plasma cells, where the nucleus contains heterochromatin masses arranged in the familiar cart-wheel or clock-face pattern. In order to avoid duplication, illustrations supporting the statements in this paragraph are presented in Chapter 14, which deals with normal and neoplastic plasma cells. At this stage the reader may like to look at *Figures 161* and *162.*

fixative and buffer used. It is clear that lead is a poor stain for chromatin, while uranium, particularly alcoholic uranium, stains chromatin intensely.

(Uranium can combine with DNA in amounts sufficient to increase the dry weight by a factor of almost 2 (Huxley and Zubay, 1961)). In my experience, tissues fixed in cacodylate-buffered osmium and stained with uranium and lead give a good visualization of the familiar chromatin pattern only a little less compact and dense than that obtained from glutaraldehyde fixation and double staining with uranium and lead.

Yet another point in favour of glutaraldehyde fixation is that it preserves microtubules, while the results with osmium are variable. Some microtubules,

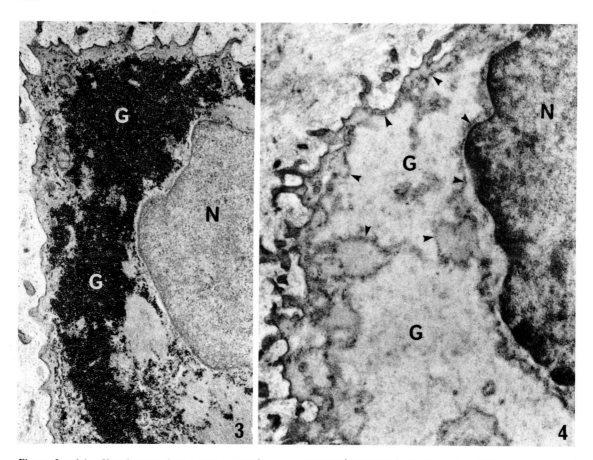

Figures 3 and 4 *Chondrocytes from osmium-fixed (cacodylate buffer) articular cartilage. Sections were cut from a single block; some were stained with lead and others with uranium. In the lead-stained section (Figure 3) large collections of intensely stained monoparticulate glycogen (G) are evident but the characteristic heterochromatin pattern is not revealed in the nucleus (N). Conversely, in the uranium-stained section (Figure 4) the heterochromatin pattern is easily seen in the nucleus (N) but only 'lakes' of virtually unstained glycogen (G) are present. The boundary of one of these 'lakes' is indicated by arrowheads. ×21 000; ×21 000 (From Ghadially, 1975)*

such as the nine peripheral pairs of microtubules in cilia, are well preserved with osmium but the central ones are at times altered or lost. The microtubules in the mitotic spindle can sometimes be seen in osmium-fixed material but those in platelets invariably disappear. If the object is to demonstrate microtubules, then glutaraldehyde fixation must be considered absolutely essential. In this respect, glutaraldehyde at room temperature is preferable to glutaraldehyde at 4° C, and glutaraldehyde at 37° C is even better.

One of the well-known rules of ideal specimen preservation for electron microscopy has been to use ice-cold fixatives, this being achieved by keeping the tube of fixative in a beaker full of crushed ice. The idea behind this is to arrest enzyme activity rapidly by immersion of the tissue in the cold fixative. Such sophistication, while laudable for certain types of studies, is somewhat superfluous for diagnostic electron microscopy and, as we have seen, is not ideal for preserving microtubules.

In my laboratory we no longer bother about the temperature of the glutaraldehyde. It is removed from the refrigerator where it is stored, and by the time it is used the temperature is somewhere between ice-cold and room temperature.

Finally, it should be noted that osmium tetraoxide is quite a noxious substance to handle.* Hence, it is safer to distribute glutaraldehyde in the hospital or elsewhere but keep the osmium in the laboratory, accessible only to skilled electron microscopy technicians who know how to handle it.

Importance of using small blocks of tissues

Both glutaraldehyde and osmium penetrate tissues very slowly (about 0.4—0.6 mm in 1 h). Hence, it follows that if large blocks of tissues are used, quite marked anoxic and autolytic changes will occur in the central regions of the specimen. Using ice-cold fixative helps to hold back such changes until the fixative arrives and fixes the central regions. The need for small blocks then is obvious, but a point that is at times not understood is that this cutting up has to be carried out immediately and not at some later time in the laboratory. One can also use slices or ribbons of tissue (instead of blocks) as long as they are no more than 1 mm thick. The 'cutting

up' must be carried out in a drop or two of the fixative, so as to avoid drying and reduce mechanical damage. We do this on a card with a new razor blade; both are discarded after the pieces of tissue are transferred to the bottle containing the fixative.

The importance of using small blocks of tissue has been repeatedly (and quite rightly) stressed in the literature, but the dangers of going to the opposite extreme have not been brought out. The peripheral parts of any block of tissue show some evidence of mechanical damage; the degree depends on the friability of the tissue and the skill of the operator in cutting up the material. With a 1 mm^3 block there is usually ample undamaged tissue available for study, but in very minute blocks the entire specimen is likely to be beset by cracks, tears and ruptured cells.

Search for a fixative suitable for both light and electron microscopy

The advantages of having one fixative 'ideal' for both light and electron microscopy are obvious, but this is not easily achieved. Glutaraldehyde is too expensive for general use and it alters the cutting and staining properties in a way unacceptable to light microscopists.† On the other hand, unbuffered commercially available formalin causes quite marked disruption of intracellular architecture. This is thought to be due to its methanol content, which probably acts as a coagulative fixative and a protein denaturant (Pease, 1964; Lynn, Martin and Race, 1966; Carson, Lynn and Martin, 1972).

Paraformaldehyde in suitable buffers has been recommended (Pease, 1964; Lynn, Martin and Race, 1966; Carson, Lynn and Martin, 1972) but it is expensive and difficult to prepare, and does not store well. It is beginning to be realized (Carson, Martin and Lynn, 1973; McDowell and Trump, 1976) that formaldehyde is not quite as bad as one had imagined and that, in fact, formaldehyde in a modified Millonig's phosphate buffer gives surprisingly good

---

*The toxicity of buffers such as veronal acetate and cacodylate should also be borne in mind.

†Glutaraldehyde penetrates tissues more slowly than formaldehyde; hence, the central areas of the much larger blocks used for light microscopy remain unfixed for prolonged periods, allowing autolysis to occur (Yanoff, Zimmerman and Fine, 1965; Chambers, Bowling and Grimley, 1968). Other disadvantages include (1) tissue often too brittle to cut properly; (2) enhanced eosinophilia, which gives the sections an overstained appearance; and (3) the PAS reaction tends to be obscured.

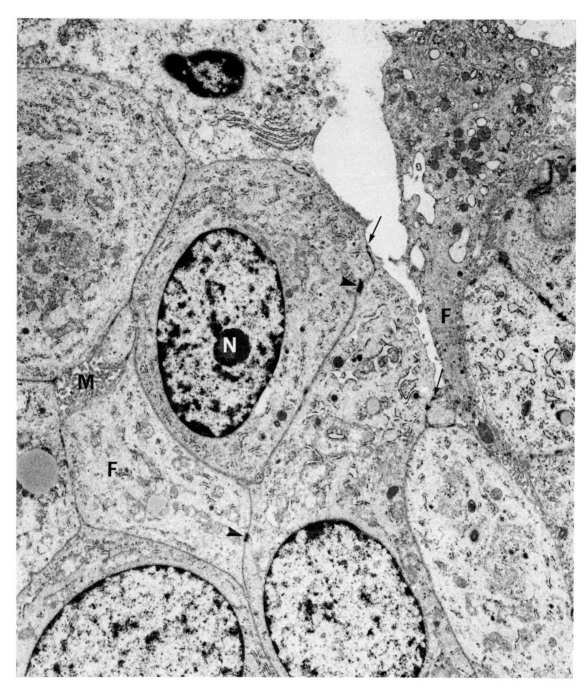

Figure 5 *Tissue from a recurrent umbilical hernia, variously diagnosed as a 'weird serosal (mesothelial) hyperplasia' or a 'mesothelioma almost certainly benign', on the basis of histology and a 6 year clinical history. Tissue was sent to us for electron microscopic examination after it had been in buffered formalin (brown and opaque) for about 2 months. The rounded nuclei, small nucleolus (N) and paucity of polyribosomes are in keeping with the virtual absence of mitoses evidenced by light microscopy and the clinical history of slow growth. The tight junctions (arrows), desmosome-like junctions (arrowheads), intercellular space lined by microvilli (M) and cells containing rough endoplasmic reticulum and collections of intracytoplasmic filaments (F) (too fine to be resolved at this low magnification but giving the cytoplasm a homogeneous appearance) are in keeping with the idea that this is a lesion of mesothelial cells. ×9000*

results, at least as good as those given by paraformaldehyde. What is more, the preservation of cell architecture is quite adequate for diagnostic purposes even when tissues have been stored in phosphate-buffered formaldehyde for many months (*Figure 5*).

If such a fixative is routinely used in the histology laboratory, then the electron microscopist can retrieve material by taking thin slices (less than 1 mm thick) from the well-fixed surface of the specimen. Such slices are diced into small pieces, rinsed in buffer, post-fixed in osmium and then processed in the usual way for electron microscopy.

Numerous attempts have been made to obtain the 'ideal' fixative by including both formaldehyde (superior penetrating power) and glutaraldehyde (superior cross-linking properties) in the fixative solution (Bowes and Carter, 1965; Karnovsky, 1965; Yanoff, 1973; Romet and Mathiessen, 1975). A recent innovation in this line is a mixture containing 4 per cent formaldehyde and 1 per cent glutaraldehyde in phosphate buffer (Penttila, McDowell and Trump, 1975), which is said to produce high-quality sections for both light and electron microscopy.

Fast methods of processing tissues

Traditional methods of preparing tissues for electron microscopy take about 4 or 5 days. If establishing the histogenesis of a tumour is a matter of some urgency, the processing can be speeded up by various manoeuvres, such as: (1) cutting down the time spent in the intermediate stages of dehydration but preferably not in the final stage in absolute alcohol; (2) reducing infiltration time; and (3) accelerating polymerization of the plastic by using higher temperatures. For details about such methods the reader is referred to Johannessen (1973), who describes a method whereby electron micrographs can be obtained within 24 h of receiving a specimen (see also Bencosme and Tsutsumi, 1970). Rowden and Lewis (1974) describe an even more rapid method whereby sections are ready to examine in the electron microscope in about 3 h. Fast processing is materially assisted by using blocks of tissue smaller than usually employed, but great care must be taken in cutting up the specimen, to minimize mechanical disruption of the tissue. The traditional slower methods of tissue preparation tend to be less demanding technically, for the timing of each stage is less critical.

Reprocessing paraffin-embedded tissue for electron microscopy

The technical quality of reprocessed paraffin-embedded tissues is usually very poor, but even so on more than one occasion conclusive diagnostic information has been obtained from such 'rescued' material (Johannessen, 1977),* and there are instances where this technique offers advantages over tissues routinely collected for electron microscopy.

The decision to retrieve and reprocess tissue from a paraffin block stems from various motives, such as: (1) too late a realization that electron microscopy could have assisted in the diagnosis of that particular tumour; (2) a desire to take a closer look at some cells, inclusions or unexplainable feature unexpectedly revealed by light microscopy; and (3) to locate objects (i.e. cells, inclusions, etc.) which are present in such small numbers in the specimen that the chance of 'catching' one in the minute randomly collected samples used for electron microscopy are remote.

An example of the latter situation is seen in the diagnosis of rhabdomyosarcoma. In the minute blocks of tissue collected for electron microscopy one may at times seek in vain for a cell that is unequivocally acceptable as a rhabdomyoblast (Chapter 10), yet there may be cells in the much larger blocks of tissue collected for light microscopy which look suspiciously like rhabdomyoblasts. In such instances one can dissect out the relevant portion from the paraffin block and at times succeed in demonstrating rhabdomyoblasts containing myofibrils, for, amazingly enough, they can survive such treatment. Desmosomes, tonofilaments, melanin granules, APUD granules, zymogen granules, virus particles and quite a few other structures are also recognizable in such retrieved material.

The technique of retrieving and reprocessing tissues for electron microscopy is quite simple. The requisite piece containing the area of interest is dissected out from the block and deparaffinized with the aid of solvents such as xylene or chloroform. The tissue is then rehydrated, cut into 1 mm cubes, rinsed in buffer, osmicated, dehydrated and embedded in the plastic of one's choice and sectioned and stained in the usual fashion.

*This excellent review, entitled 'Use of paraffin material for electron microscopy', gives technical details and information about cases where this technique has been useful in establishing a diagnosis.

Semi-thin sections

'Semi-thin sections' is an appropriate term used by many workers to describe the 0.5—1 µm thick sections obtained from tissues embedded in plastic for electron microscopy. Some workers, however, prefer to call them 'thick sections', which is rather confusing. The term 'thick sections' should be reserved for paraffin sections, which are at least five times as thick, and the term 'thin sections' or 'ultrathin sections' for the 60—80 nm thick sections commonly used for electron microscopy.

Semi-thin sections stained with metachromatic dyes (usually toluidine blue) show intracellular details far more clearly than can be visualized in paraffin sections. This advantage stems from the thinner size and the superior method of tissue processing employed. The obvious disadvantages are the small size of these sections and the difficulty of using conventional histopathological staining methods and histochemical techniques. This varies with the type of plastic used for embedding (Senoo, Watanabe and Doi, 1977). With Epon-embedded material the number of stains that can be usefully employed is limited. However, numerous papers have appeared showing that one can stain Epon-embedded material with haematoxylin and eosin and by a few other histopathological staining methods (Mayor, Hampton and Rosario, 1961; Schantz, 1965; Aparicio and Marsden, 1969; Pool, 1969; Shires, Johnson and Richter, 1969; Chang, 1972; Snodgress et al., 1972; Stoeckel et al., 1972).

Staining

Double staining with uranium and lead is quite essential. The former is needed for staining chromatin, while the latter is necessary for staining glycogen.

Uranium stains glycogen very faintly or not at all (*Figure 4*). The appearance presented by glycogen particles and deposits depends to some extent on the method of tissue fixation and preparation employed, for this determines the proportion of glycogen preserved in the tissue and that lost during processing. The appearance seen is also dependent on the method by which the sections are stained. A spectrum of appearances is seen, but the two extremes of the scale are represented by lead staining, where the glycogen particles appear highly electron-dense, (*Figure 3*) and by uranium staining, where solitary glycogen particles appear as 'holes' or very faintly

stained particles, difficult to discern. In uranium-stained material collections of glycogen particles may present as lucent or faintly stained areas (glycogen lakes) within the cytoplasm (*Figure 4*).

A procedure which has gained much popularity in recent times is *en bloc* staining with unbuffered aqueous uranium acetate after fixation but prior to dehydration. This gives good visualization of general details and is particularly useful for the demonstration of the structure of cell membranes and cell junctions. The routine application of this technique is, however, hampered by the fact that much glycogen is extracted and what remains shows marked morphological alterations (Vye and Fischman, 1970).

References

APARICIO, S. R. and MARSDEN, P. (1969). Application of standard microanatomical staining methods to epoxy resin-embedded sections. *J. Clin. Path.*, **22**, 589

BASSI, M. and BERNELLI-ZAZZERA, A. (1963). Ultrastructural cytoplasmic changes of liver cells after reversible and irreversible ischemia. *Expl Mol. Path.*, **3**, 332

BENCOSME, S. A. and TSUTSUMI, V. (1970). A fast method for processing biologic material for electron microscopy. *Lab. Invest.*, **23**, 447

BOWES, J. A. and CARTER, C. W. (1965). Cross-linking of collagen. *J. Appl. Chem.*, **15**, 296

CARSON, F., LYNN, J. A. and MARTIN, J. H. (1972). Ultrastructural effect of various buffers, osmolality and temperature on paraformaldehyde fixation of the formed elements of blood and bone marrow. *Tex. Rep. Biol. Med.*, **30**, 125

CARSON, F. L., MARTIN, J. H. and LYNN, J. A. (1973). Formalin fixation for electron microscopy; a re-evaluation. *Am. J. Clin. Path.*, **59**, 365

CHAMBERS, R. W., BOWLING, M. C. and GRIMLEY, P. M. (1968). Glutaraldehyde fixation in routine histopathology. *Archs Path.*, **85**, 18

CHANG, S. C. (1972). Hematoxylin-eosin staining of plastic embedded tissue sections. *Archs Path.*, **93**, 344

ERICSSON, J. L. E., BIBERFELD, P. and SELEJELID, R. (1967). Electron microscopic and cytochemical studies of acid phosphatase and aryl sulfatase during autolysis. *Acta Path. Microbiol. Scand.*, **70**, 215

ERLANDSON, R. A. and TANDLER, B. (1972). Ultrastructure of acinic cell carcinoma of the parotid gland. *Archs Path.*, **93**, 130

GHADIALLY, F. N. (1975). *Ultrastructural Pathology of the Cell.* London: Butterworths

GLAUERT, A. M. (1974). *Practical Methods of Electron Microscopy*, Vol. 3. Amsterdam/New York: North-Holland/American Elsevier

GRIFFIN, R. L. (1972). *Ultramicrotomy.* Baltimore: Williams and Wilkins

HUXLEY, H. E. and ZUBAY, G. (1961). Preferential staining of nucleic acid-containing structures for electron microscopy. *J. Biophys. Biochem. Cytol.*, **11**, 273

ITO, S. (1962). Light and electron microscopic study of membranous cytoplasmic organelles. In *The Interpretation of Ultrastructure,* ed. R. J. C. Harris, Symposia of the International Society for Cell Biology, Vol. 1, p. 129. New York: Academic Press

JOHANNESSEN, J. V. (1973). Rapid processing of kidney biopsies for electron microscopy. *Kidney Int.,* 3, 46

JOHANNESSEN, J. V. (1977). Use of paraffin material for electron microscopy. *Path. Ann.,* 12, 189

KARNOVSKY, M. J. (1965). A formaldehyde-glutaraldehyde fixative of high osmolality for use in electron microscopy. *J. Cell. Biol.,* 27, 137A

KAY, D. H. (1965). *Techniques in Electron Microscopy,* 2nd edn. Oxford: Blackwell Scientific

LATTA, H., OSVALDO, L., JACKSON, J. D. and COOK, M. L. (1965). Changes in renal cortical tubules during autolysis. *Lab. Invest.,* 14, 635

LYNN, J. A., MARTIN, J. H. and RACE, G. J. (1966). Recent improvement of histologic techniques for the combined light and electron microscopic examination of surgical specimens. *Am. J. Clin. Path.,* 75, 704

McDOWELL, E. M. and TRUMP, B. F. (1976). Histologic fixatives suitable for diagnostic light and electron microscopy. *Archs Path. Lab. Med.,* 100, 405

MAYOR, H. D., HAMPTON, J. C. and ROSARIO, B. (1961). A simple method for removing the resin from epoxy-embedded tissue. *J. Biophys. Biochem. Cytol.,* 9, 909

MEEK, G. A. (1970). *Practical Electron Microscopy for Biologists.* New York: Wiley—Interscience

MERCER, E. H. and BIRBECK, M. S. C. (1972). *Electron Microscopy, A Handbook for Biologists,* 3rd edn. Oxford: Blackwell Scientific

OSVALDO, L., JACKSON, J. D., COOK, M. L. and LATTA, H. (1965). Reactions of kidney cells during autolysis. Light microscopic observations. *Lab. Invest.,* 14, 603

PEASE, D. C. (1964). *Hisological Techniques for Electron Microscopy,* 2nd edn. New York: Academic Press

PENTTILA, A., McDOWELL, E. M. and TRUMP, B. F. (1975). Effects of fixation and post fixation treatments on volume of injured cells. *J. Histochem. Cytochem.,* 23, 251

POOL, C. R. (1969). Hematoxylin-eosin staining of OsO_4-fixed Epon embedded tissue: prestaining oxidation by acidified H_2O_2. *Stain Technol.,* 44, 75

ROMET, P. and MATTHIESSEN, M. E. (1975). Fixation of fetal pig liver. *J. Ultrastruct. Res.,* 50, 363

ROWDEN, G. and LEWIS, M. G. (1974). Experience with a three-hour electron microscopy biopsy service. *J. Clin. Path.,* 27, 505

SCHANTZ, A. (1965). Iron-hematoxylin and safranin O as a polychrome stain for Epon sections. *Stain Technol.,* 40, 279

SENOO, A., WATANABE, H. and DOI, Y. (1977). Colour photographs by JB-4 methylmethacrylate divinylbenzene (JMD) embedding method. *Rinshokeusa,* 21, 15

SHIRES, T. K., JOHNSON, M. and RICHTER, K. M. (1969). Hematoxylin staining of tissue embedded in epoxy resins. *Stain Technol.,* 44, 21

SNODGRESS, A. B., DORSEY, C. H., BAILEY, G. W. and DICKSON, L. G. (1972). Conventional histopathologic staining methods compatible with Epon embedded, osmicated tissue. *Lab. Invest.,* 26, 329

STOECKEL, M. E., PORTE, A., DELLMANN, H. D. and GERTNER, C. (1972). Selective staining of neurosecretory material in semi-thin epoxy sections by Gomori's aldehyde fuchsin. *Stain Technol.,* 47, 81

STOECKENIUS, W. and MAHR, S. C. (1965). Studies on the reaction of osmium tetroxide with lipids and related compounds. *Lab. Invest.,* 14, 458

TRUMP, B. F., GOLDBLATT, P. J. and STOWELL, R. E. (1962). An electron microscopic study of early cytoplasmic alterations in hepatic parenchymal cells of mouse liver during necrosis in vitro (autolysis). *Lab. Invest.,* 11, 986

TRUMP, B. F., GOLDBLATT, P. J. and STOWELL, R. E. (1965). Studies on necrosis of mouse liver in vitro. Ultrastructural alterations in the mitochondria of hepatic parenchymal cells. *Lab. Invest.,* 14, 343

VYE, M. V. and FISCHMAN, D. A. (1970). The morphological alteration of particulate glycogen by *en bloc* staining with uranyl acetate. *J. Ultrastruct. Res.,* 33, 278

WEAKLEY, B. S. (1972). *A Beginner's Handbook in Biological Electron Microscopy.* Edinburgh London: Churchill Livingstone

YANOFF, M. (1973). Formaldehyde-glutaraldehyde fixation. *Am. J. Ophthal.,* 76, 303

YANOFF, M., ZIMMERMAN, L. E. and FINE, B. S. (1965). Glutaraldehyde fixation of whole eyes. *Am. J. Clin. Path.,* 44, 167

2
Choosing an electron microscope

There is little doubt that the high cost of electron microscopes and exaggerated notions about the complexities and difficulties of operating and maintaining them have deterred many from embarking on diagnostic electron microscopy. Such fears are, perhaps, justified if one is thinking about a 'state of the art' high-performance instrument (resolution better than 0.2 nm, cost $ 125 000–$250 000) fitted with numerous frills and facilities rarely if ever needed by the pathologist.

Diagnostic electron microscopy and, indeed, even most research studies on pathological tissues of man and experimental animals require nothing more than the ability to look at and photograph ultrathin sectioned material at quite low or modest magnifications. For this a medium-performance instrument (resolution around 0.7 nm, cost $50 000–$70 000) is the instrument of choice and not just a poor substitute. The reasons for this are as follows.*

In ultrathin sections of plastic-embedded material the best resolution attainable is about 2 nm† (Meek, 1970). Thus, the medium-performance instrument with its 0.7 nm resolution is more than adequate for our needs. Certainly the better than 0.2 nm resolving power of the high-performance instrument can offer no additional advantage for the specimen sets the limit to the resolution.ƒ

The human eye can at close distance separate individual lines of a ruled grating 0.075 mm apart (Meek, 1970). However, this is a very taxing performance and requires optimum contrast and lighting conditions to attain. A more realistic figure for the resolving power of the human eye is about 0.25 mm, because this can be attained without much strain under normal situations (Meek, 1970).

As noted earlier the resolving power attainable in ultrathin sections is about 2 nm. It follows, then, that in a print (electron micrograph) at × 100 000 (where 2 nm is magnified to 0.2 mm) one should be able to, and in fact can, discern objects or distances between objects 2 nm or greater. The corollary to this is that if nothing less than 2 nm is resolved, however high the magnification, then any enlargement much above ×100 000 will be 'empty magnification' — that is to say, an increase in size without more resolution or information. Now one can comfortably obtain a print at ×100 000 magnification by using an electron optical magnification (i.e. magnification in the negative) of ×20 000–×40 000 followed by an optical enlargement (i.e. with a photographic enlarger) of ×5–×2.5, and this is well within the capability of the medium-performance electron microscope.

It is said* that one should keep the electron optical magnification high and the optical enlargement low, for if the latter is more than about ×6 or at the most ×8, this might lead to a situation of 'empty magnification'.† The limiting factors here are thought to be the thickness of the photographic emulsion (the thinner the better) and grain size (depends mainly on film speed and development) in the negative. Experience, however, shows that more often the limit on enlargement is set by the fact that few negatives are perfectly focused and sharp enough

---

*In this discussion I am omitting from consideration special studies such as virological studies carried out on negatively stained preparations or the developing field of electron probe X-ray analysis (Ghadially, 1979), which has a great future in research and diagnostic pathology. For such studies the more sophisticated state of the art microscope is necessary.

†Ottensmeyer and Pear (1975) are more pessimistic. They state 'images of sections of biological tissue rarely show biologically significant resolution of 30Å or better.'

ƒIt is also regrettably true that a majority of high-resolution instruments are not, in fact, operated at anywhere near their capacity or performance for reasons connected with poor maintenance and lack of operator skills.

---

*I have no serious quarrels with this statement. My own personal preference is to produce negatives which do not as a rule need to be enlarged more than ×5, but any 'half-decent' negative should be able to stand a ×10 enlargement.

†There is nothing wrong or wicked about 'empty magnification' as long as we know what we are doing and do not delude ourselves, for there are times when a larger print may be deemed essential for publication purposes or for exhibition at a scientific meeting.

to stand much enlargement. The amazing amount of detail that is available in a perfectly focused negative taken (by Dr Newstead) at quite low magnification is demonstrated in *Figures 6* and *7*.

Figure 6 shows fragments of isolated myelin sheath in a subcellular fraction of brain photographed at the electron optical magnification of ×2500 and an optical enlargement of ×6. *Figure 7* was produced

Such considerations, combined with the extra cost, effort and technical expertise needed to keep more sophisticated instruments operational, should convince one that the medium-performance instrument is ideal for our true needs. I therefore concur with Meek (1970) when he states that 'extreme resolving power is seldom either possible or necessary', and that 'instruments capable of extreme resolution

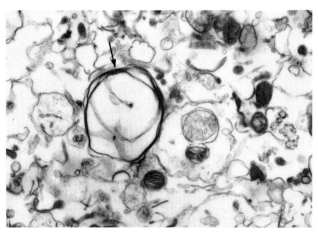

Figure 6   *Isolated myelin from a synaptosome pellet. Arrow indicates portion of the myelin sheath which is shown much enlarged in Figure 7. Electron optical enlargement ×2500. Optical enlargement ×6. Final magnification ×15 000 (J. D. Newstead, unpublished electron micrograph)*

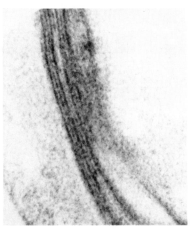

Figure 7   *Isolated myelin from a synaptosome pellet. Same negative as in Figure 6. The area indicated by arrow in Figure 6 is shown much enlarged here. Note the demonstration of the trilaminar membrane structure within the myelin. Electron optical magnification ×2500. Optical enlargement ×64. Final magnification ×160 000 (J. D. Newstead, unpublished electron micrograph)*

by enlarging a part of the same negative ×64. This clearly demonstrates that the trilaminar membrane structure and the intermediate line are recorded even in a negative taken at so low a magnification. While one would not wish to suggest that this kind of performance is recommended procedure, it does show that the top magnification available with a medium-performance microscope is, if anything, too much and not too little for our needs.

A glance at the magnification of electron micrographs published in books and pathology journals will convince the reader that most biological work is done at quite low magnifications and that electron micrographs published at a magnification of ×100 000 or more are quite rare. Thus, most electron microscopic negatives are taken at a magnification between ×1500 and ×15 000; only rarely does one take an electron micrograph at ×20 000 or ×30 000.

are sought more as a matter of laboratory prestige than a necessity'.

Having had some experience with a couple of high-performance instruments (expensive white elephants would be a better description), I decided to give a medium-performance instrument a try. All electron micrographs published in this book and stemming from my present laboratory were obtained with the Zeiss EM-9S: a single-condenser microscope which has a resolution of 0.75 nm and a top magnification of ×60 000 (purchased in 1969 for $33 000). Over 24 000 electron micrographs have been taken with this instrument, of which some 1000 or more have been published in various journals and books. At the moment of writing, this microscope is used routinely by six operators of varying skills.

This microscope is serviced once a year. We do

not clean the apertures; they are replaced once a year. Breakdown and emergency service calls are rare, and the day-to-day maintenance and alignment requirements are virtually nil. It takes only a few minutes to correct astigmatism or locate a 'lost beam'. Changing films (60, 2¼ × 2¼ in films at each loading) and replacing burnt-out filaments takes so little time that I prefer to do this myself rather than ask a technician to do it. The instrument is so well automated that people can be trained to use it in a day or two. It is unfortunate that varying mixtures of high-pressure salesmanship, ignorance and vanity

have militated against a more widespread use of such instruments.

References

GHADIALLY, F. N. (1979). Invited review: the techniques and scope of electron-probe x-ray analysis in pathology. *Pathology*, 11, 95

MEEK, G. A. (1970). *Practical Electron Microscopy for Biologists*. New York: Wiley—Interscience

OTTENSMEYER, F. P. and PEAR, M. (1975). Contrast in unstained sections: A comparison of bright and dark field electron microscopy. *J. Ultrastruct. Res.*, 51, 253

Part 2

Ultrastructural assessment of behaviour and growth rate of tumours

3
Is it malignant?

It had been hoped that the electron microscope would reveal a specific morphological alteration which could be regarded as the hall-mark of malignancy, but such a hope has not fructified. The criteria by which we try to assess the degree of malignancy or innocence of a neoplasm with the electron microscope remain virtually the same as those used in light microscopy. Our diagnostic criteria may be divided into three categories: (1) cytological changes; (2) disordered intercellular relationships; and (3) evidence of infiltration.

Cytological changes

Light microscopists have long recognized that tumour cells, as a class, differ from normal cells in a variety of ways, and that although no single change is pathognomic, the spectrum of changes taken together can be a fairly reliable indicator of malignancy. The electron microscope adds a new dimension to the study of such long-familiar changes and also shows a few others that cannot be discerned with the light microscope. Such knowledge is essential for studying tumours with the electron microscope. A brief account of this is presented in Chapter 4. More details may be found elsewhere (Bernhard and Granboulan, 1963; Bernhard, 1969; Ghadially, 1975).

Intercellular relationships

Changes in intercellular relationships can be better appreciated by electron microscopy than by light microscopy. Electron microscopy has much to offer here, for alterations in cell junctions are a characteristic and constant feature of carcinomas, and, as we will see later (Chapters 5 and 6), these and associated changes of surface specialization are of value in distinguishing carcinoma from sarcoma and determining whether a tumour shows adenomatous

or squamous differentiation. However, such changes found in obviously malignant lesions are of little value in determining unequivocally the malignancy or innocence of a doubtful lesion.

Infiltration

The extent and depth of the infiltrative process can hardly be appreciated in the less than 1 mm^2 sections, intersected by grid bars, employed in electron microscopy; hence, light microscopy remains the method of choice for studying this important criterion of malignancy.

One might imagine that the earliest sign of invasion (e.g. extension of tumour cells through breaks in the basal lamina) might be more clearly revealed by the electron microscope and that this might permit recognition of an early malignant change. However, it is now clear that small breaks in the basal lamina can in rare instances be found even in normal epithelia, and one may also find a cell process traversing a gap in the basal lamina. In both inflammatory and neoplastic states these features are more marked and more frequently encountered (Frithiof, 1969). Conversely, the lamina may be thickened and/or reduplicated in some benign or not too aggressive tumours (*Figure 8*), and it can also be quite prominent and well developed near the infiltrating margin of even highly malignant anaplastic carcinomas (*Figure 9*).

Thus, it would appear that the electron microscope is of little value in distinguishing early infiltration due to neoplasia from that due to other conditions, and one is tempted to conclude that in the present state of our knowledge the electron microscope is unlikely to provide an unequivocal answer in cases where the innocence or malignancy of a lesion remains in doubt after careful light microscopic investigation. Even so, the study of the basal lamina may not be entirely unrewarding, for evidence is accumulating which suggests that a

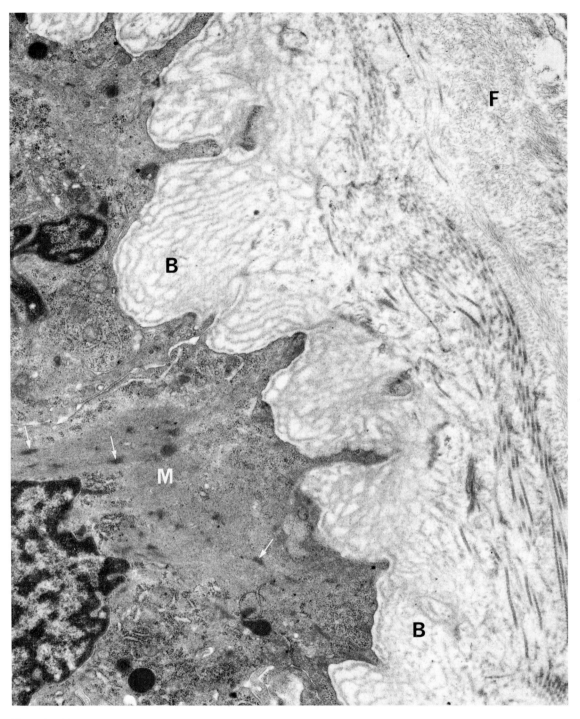

Figure 8 *Fibroadenoma of the breast. A reduplicated basal lamina (B) is seen between the myoepithelial cells which lie at the outskirts of the adenomatus elements (not included in the picture) and the fibrous (F) component of the tumour. The myofilaments (M) in the myoepithelial cell are too fine to be resolved at this magnification but the focal densities (arrows) along their course are easily discerned. ×19 000*

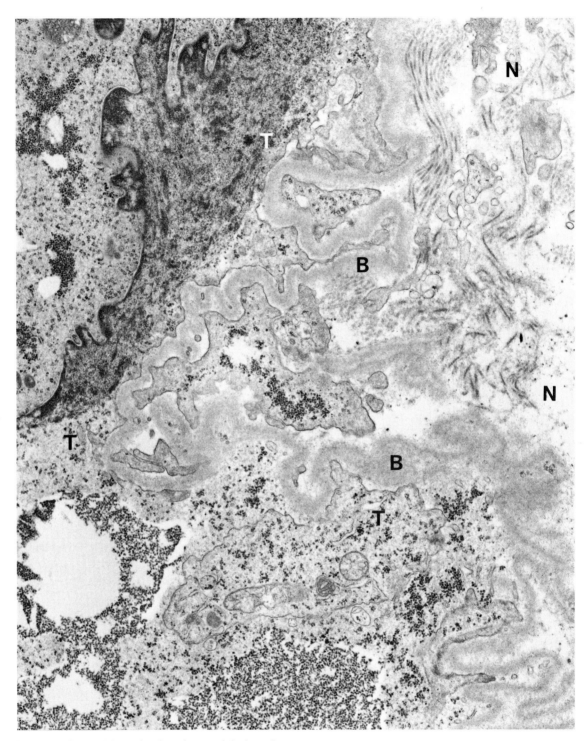

Figure 9 *Poorly differentiated carcinoma of the bronchus.*
A prominent basal lamina (B) is seen at the interface
between the tumour (T) and normal (N) tissue. ×20 000

reduplicated basal lamina may be an indicator of innocence or a relatively low degree of clinical malignancy (Gould and Battifora, 1976). This might yet prove to be a useful ultrastructural diagnostic criterion.

References

BERNHARD, W. (1969). Ultrastructure of the cancer cell. In *Handbook of Molecular Cytology,* eds. A. Lima-De-Faria. Amsterdam: North-Holland

BERNHARD, W. and GRANBOULAN, N. (1963). The fine structure of the cancer cell nucleus. *Expl Cell Res*. Suppl. 9, 19

FRITHIOF, L. (1969). Ultrastructure of the basement membrane in normal and hyperplastic human oral epithelium compared with that in preinvasive and invasive carcinoma. *Acta Path. Microbiol. Scand.,* Suppl., 200, 1

GHADIALLY, F. N. (1975). *Ultrastructural Pathology of the Cell*. London: Butterworths

GOULD, V. E. and BATTIFORA, H. (1976). Origin and significance of the basal lamina and some interstitial fibrillar components in epithelial neoplasma. *Path. Ann.,* 11, 353

4
Differences between normal and neoplastic cells

The differences between the major organelles of normal and neoplastic cells form the topic of this chapter. Other organelles and inclusions will be dealt with later. For example, melanosomes will be dealt with when we deal with melanomas (Chapter 7) and cell junctions when we deal with carcinomas and sarcomas (Chapter 5).

Nucleus

Size and shape

The increased size and the irregularities of shape of neoplastic cell nuclei have long been known to light microscopists. The electron microscope reveals even more dramatically the extremes of complex and bizarre forms that the nuclei of tumour cells can assume (*Figure 10*). At times the nucleus is so extensively segmented and beset by invaginations that it assumes an almost sponge-like character. Therefore, when one examines a tumour biopsy, it is worth comparing in one's mind the form of the nuclei in the specimen with what one would expect to find in the parent cell of origin, for irregularity of nuclear shape is a common feature of neoplasia and some of the most irregular nuclei occur in highly malignant tumours.

However, as is well known, the nuclei of some malignant tumours can be quite small and may show little or no irregularity of form even with the electron microscope. One may also sometimes find a few irregular nuclei even in normal tissues or a benign tumour. The most florid example of this I have seen was in a fibroadenoma of the breast, where a few neoplastic fibroblast nuclei were enlarged and had a surprisingly bizarre shape (*Figure 11*). The patient had been taking contraceptive pills for many years and was 3 months pregnant, so perhaps hormonal changes were responsible for this phenomenon. Such exceptions, however, are rare and do not detract from the generalization that nuclei of malignant cells are, as a rule, markedly irregular in form as compared with normal nuclei.

Chromatin

DNA occurs in the nucleus combined with histones and other proteins. This combination constitutes chromatin. The idea that the essential malignant change is a specific alteration or lesion in the DNA molecule is deeply rooted in our philosophy, but this idea can hardly be pursued in ultrathin sections of plastic-embedded tissue, where the attainable resolution is about 2 nm (see Chapter 2) and the filaments are so tightly coiled as to present as granules rather than filaments.

Two forms of chromatin are known to occur in the interphase nucleus: (1) a condensed, presumably inactive form called heterochromatin, which is basophilic with the light microscope and presents as collections of rounded or irregular-shaped electron-dense granules in ultrathin sections; and (2) an active form called euchromatin, which is dispersed in the nuclear matrix. This presents as feebly stained areas with basic dyes. Euchromatin cannot be confidently identified in electron micrographs either.

Heterochromatin occurs as aggregates in certain preferred sites in the nucleus, and it is this phenomenon which produces the familiar chromatin pattern (e.g. the clock-face or cart-wheel pattern seen in plasma cell nuclei).

It is now clear that not only the distribution but also the proportion of heterochromatin to euchromatin varies from one cell type to another. Since it is well established that the average amount of DNA in the somatic cell nuclei from various tissues of a given species is constant, one can argue that in nuclei poorly endowed with heterochromatin there will be more of the metabolically active euchromatin (Fawcett, 1967). Thus, one may expect that metabolically active cells will have a paler-staining nucleus with fewer and smaller heterochromatin masses. This thesis is borne out by the fact that stem cells or blast

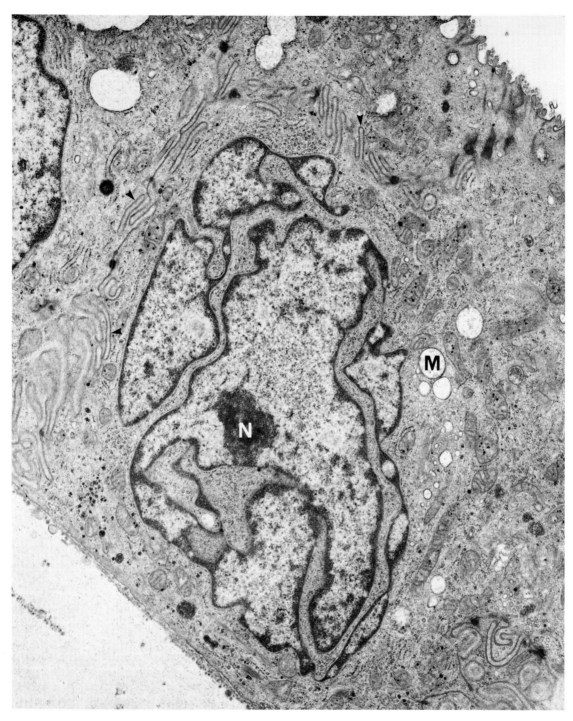

Figure 10   *Adenocarcinoma of the appendix which had produced pseudomyxoma peritonei. Note the bizarre nucleus beset by deep invaginations. Other features of interest include a marginated nucleolus (N), interdigitations of cell membranes (arrowheads) and mucous droplets (M).* ×*16 000*

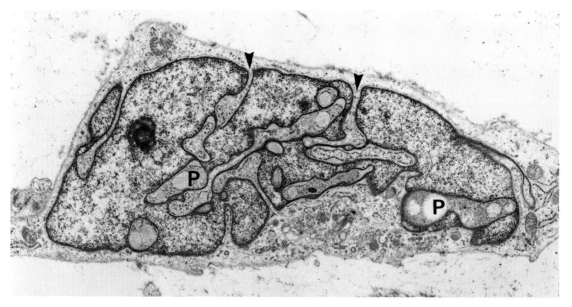

Figure 11   *Fibroadenoma of breast. A neoplastic fibroblast from the fibrous component of the tumour, showing meandering invaginations (arrowheads) which when transected present as pseudoinclusions (P) in the nucleus. ×12 000 (Ghadially and Lalonde, unpublished electron micrograph)*

cells have paler nuclei, and that in a maturing series of cells such as the red blood cells an increasing concentration of heterochromatin masses becomes evident as the cell matures and becomes metabolically less active.

The well-known hyperchromasia of the neoplastic nucleus is now attributed to polyploidy. With the electron microscope these hyperchromatic nuclei are seen to contain larger and/or more numerous heterochromatin masses. However, in tumours one also finds quite pale nuclei with a paucity of heterochromatin and, hence, presumably an excess of the more active euchromatin (*Figure 12*). This point, evident also with light microscopy, has perhaps not been sufficiently stressed despite early recognition of this phenomenon by light microscopists (Caspersson and Santesson, 1942; Montella, 1954), who referred to tumour cells with hyperchromatic nuclei and a not particularly enlarged nucleolus as type A cells and to cells with a pale nucleus and enlarged nucleolus as type B cells.

The significance of type A and B cells has not been probed, but applying the ideas discussed earlier, one is tempted to speculate that, while the hyper-chromatic nucleus may be of diagnostic import (as an indicator of polyploidy), it is the cell with the pale nucleus (an indicator of an increased amount of functionally active euchromatin) and an enlarged nucleolus (an indicator of active synthesis of ribosomal RNA and, hence, ribosomes and protein) which is more important from the point of view of active cell proliferation and, hence, growth of the tumour.

Neoplasms of plasma cells (see illustrations in Chapter 14) afford further support for such a thesis, for in benign plasmacytomas the characteristic heterochromatin pattern of the plasma cell nucleus is more or less retained but in malignant versions such as multiple myeloma and plasma cell leukaemia this pattern is lost and, indeed, in many cases the nucleus is large and pale, for it contains only scant small aggregates of heterochromatin.

Interchromatin and perichromatin granules

Interchromatin and perichromatin granules are too small to be resolved by the light microscope, but they are readily recognized by electron microscopy. Knowledge about their occurrence and distribution

25

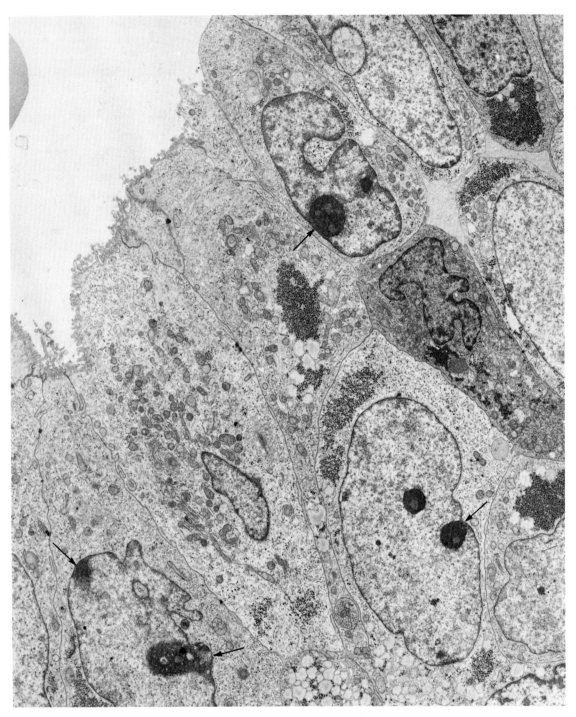

Figure 12   *A fragment of adenocarcinoma found in ascitic fluid. Most of the nucleoli seen in this electron micrograph are marginated (arrows). Note also the irregularity of nuclear shape and the variability of heterochromatin content. The two nuclei at the top right-hand corner of the electron micrograph contain abundant heterochromatin and would thus appear hyperchromatic at light microscopy, while the remainder are poor in heterochromatin content and would present a paler appearance. ×6000 (From Ghadially, 1975)*

26

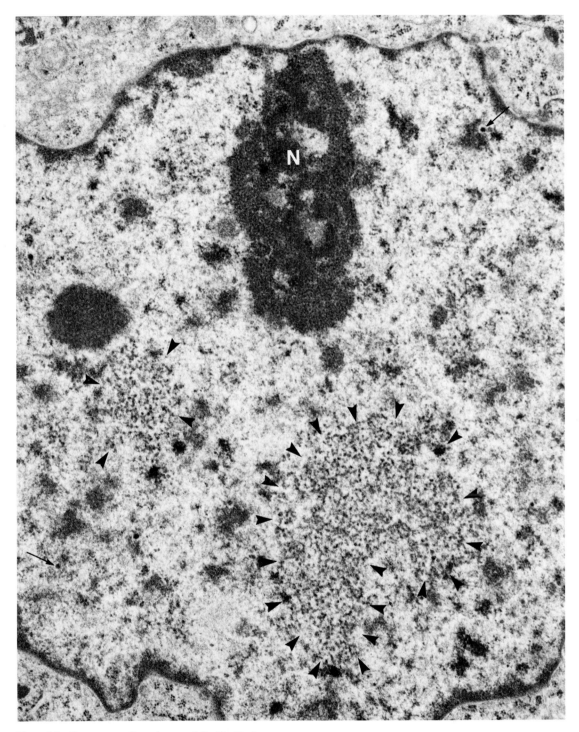

Figure 13 *Squamous cell carcinoma of the lip. Nucleus showing collections (demarcated by arrowheads) of interchromatin granules and a few perichromatin granules (arrows) with a halo around them. Note also the enlarged marginated nucleolus (N). ×32 000*

in the nuclei of various cell types and tumours is incomplete, but this is an interesting topic worthy of a brief review.

Perichromatin granules, as their name implies, usually lie on the borders of chromatin areas. These electron-dense, solitary, spherical granules are separated from the adjacent chromatin by an electron-lucent halo. The granule itself measures 30—35 nm in diameter; the over-all diameter, including the halo, is about 75 nm (Watson, 1962; Bernhard and Granboulan, 1963). It has been estimated that the hepatocyte nucleus contains 500—2000 such granules.

Interchromatin granules are highly electron-dense. They have an angular shape and vary in size from 15 to 50 nm (Granboulan and Bernhard, 1961; Bernhard and Granboulan, 1963; Jezequel and Marinozzi, 1963; Swift, 1963). They usually occur in clusters in the nuclear matrix, but single granules or short linear arrays of granules are also fairly common.

The function and chemical composition of inter-chromatin and perichromatin granules has not been clearly established. It has been suggested (Watson, 1962; Bernhard and Granboulan, 1963) that both RNA and DNA may be present in the perichromatin granules and that both types of granules should be regarded as nuclear ribosomes. More recently it has been suggested that perichromatin granules probably contain messenger RNA (Bouteille, 1972).

An abundance of interchromatin granules is seen in various tumours (*Figure 13*). According to Bernhard and Granboulan (1963), interchromatin granules are seen more frequently in tumour cells, and Reddy and Svoboda (1968) have observed that: 'In chronic studies of carcinogenesis in rat liver the most consistent ultrastructural alteration is an apparent increase in interchromatinic granules.' An abundance of perichromatin granules has been noted in some tumours; for example, scirrhous carcinomas of the breast (Murad and Scarpelli, 1967). I, too, have frequently been impressed by the abundance of either interchromatin or perichromatin granules in neoplastic nuclei. My impression is that in a given tumour one either finds numerous interchromatin granules or quite prominent perichromatin granules, but an abundance of both these types of granules does not occur in the same tumour (*Figure 14*).

Recent studies indicate that an increase in the number of perichromatin granules may be an indicator of aberrations in protein-synthetic activity, for this change is noted after administration of drugs such as cycloheximide (an inhibitor of protein synthesis) and galactoflavin (induces riboflavin deficiency) and exposing cells to subnormal temperature (Heine *et al.*, 1971; Daskal *et al.*, 1975; Norton *et al.*, 1977).

One now wonders whether the prominence of perichromatin granules in some tumours is an indicator of naturally occurring aberrations of protein synthesis or whether they reflect the effectiveness of some therapeutic measure in inhibiting protein synthesis. I have at times seen quite prominent perichromatin granules in residual tumour after therapy. However, studies on animal and human tumours before and after various types of therapy are needed before one can evaluate such sporadic observations. At the moment we do not know much about the size and distribution of these granules in various normal and neoplastic cell types. It would appear that most workers on tumour ultrastructure have ignored these granules, while a few have mistaken them for virus particles.

Nuclear envelope and pores

A classic light microscopic feature of the neoplastic nucleus on which we place much importance when examining cytological smears is the so-called 'thickening of the nuclear membrane'. However, it is now abundantly clear from ultrastructural studies that: (1) the nucleus is not enclosed by a 'nuclear membrane' but by a double membraned envelope; (2) the nuclear envelope is too fine to be resolved and visualized by the light microscope; and (3) there is no thickening of the nuclear envelope as a whole or of its membranes in the neoplastic nucleus.

What appears at light microscopy as a 'nuclear membrane' is in fact the rim of peripheral or marginal heterochromatin which lies adjacent to the inner membrane of the nuclear envelope and the so-called 'thickening' reflects the increase in width of this marginated chromatin. Thus, the 'thickened membrane' phenomenon is part and parcel of the hyperchromasia, polyploidy and increased heterochromatin content of some neoplastic nuclei.

As is now well known, the two membranes of the nuclear envelope fuse in places to produce the nuclear pores which are pathways of nucleocytoplasmic exchanges. Numerous studies (for a review and references see Ghadially, 1975) now attest to the fact that in situations where there is an increase in metabolic activity there is a concurrent increase in the size and number of nuclear pores, while a re-

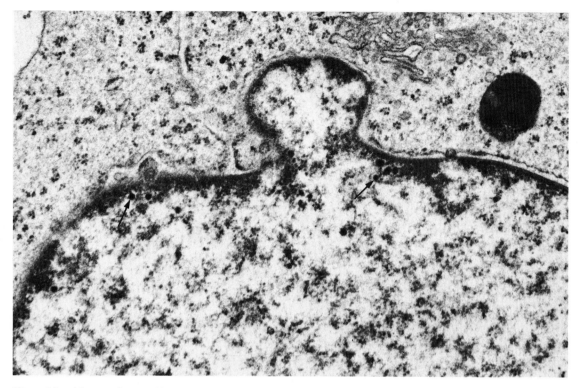

Figure 14 *Adenocarcinoma of lung. Nucleus showing prominent perichromatin granules (arrows).* ×36 000

duction in number and size characterizes diminished metabolic activity. However, we are quite ignorant about the state of nuclear pores in neoplastic nuclei. In routine preparations, at least, no consistent alterations in size or number of pores is evident. Some elegant methods of studying nuclear pores in isolated nuclear envelopes and in freeze-fractured material are now available but they have rarely been employed to compare nuclear pores of normal and neoplastic nuclei. What little evidence there is suggests that there is an increase in the number of nuclear pores in some neoplastic nuclei (e.g. Rejthar and Blumajer, 1974; Švejda, Vrba and Blumajer, 1975). This could be quite a rewarding field for future investigations.

Nuclear fibrous lamina

The nuclear fibrous lamina presents as a band of fine-textured medium-density material adjacent to the inner membrane of the nuclear envelope. At first it was thought that this lamina occurred only in the cells of some invertebrates, but Fawcett (1966) and Patrizi and Poger (1967) showed that a fibrous lamina (about 30 nm thick) does occur in certain vertebrate cells. Later studies suggest that the nuclei of most cells have a nuclear fibrous lamina, but this is usually quite thin (usually less than 15 nm) and, hence, passes unnoticed. Further, it has been shown that the nuclear fibrous lamina is not a static structure of fixed dimensions for a given cell type but that it is a dynamic component of the nucleus capable of undergoing hypertrophy and involution in physiologically and pathologically altered states (Ghadially, Oryschak and Mitchell, 1974).

A thickening of the nuclear fibrous lamina (up to 95 mm thick) has been noted in repair tissue filling surgically produced deep defects in articular cartilage (Ghadially, Fuller and Kirkaldy-Willis, 1971; Ghadially, Bhatnager and Fuller, 1972) and in the synovial intimal cells in cases of rheumatoid arthritis (Ghadially, Oryschak and Mitchell, 1974; Oryschak, Mitchell and Ghadially, 1976). We (Oryschak, Ghadially and Bhatnager, 1974) have also found that the nuclear fibrous lamina in the articular cartilage of 2-month-old rabbits is much thinner (less than 5 nm thick) than in mature animals (between 20 and 30 nm).

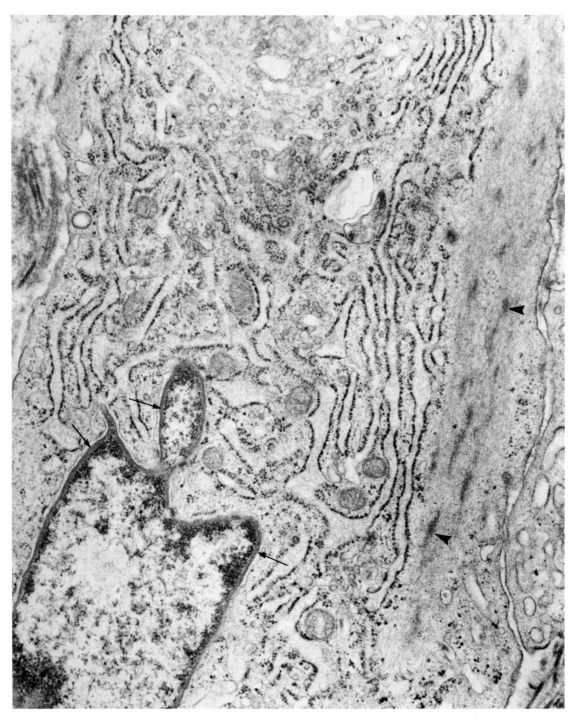

Figure 15   *Repair tissue from thigh. Myofibroblast showing myofilaments with focal densities (arrowheads), abundant rough endoplasmic reticulum and Golgi complex and a nucleus with a prominent nuclear fibrous lamina (arrows). ×31 000 (Ghadially and Lalonde, unpublished electron micrograph)*

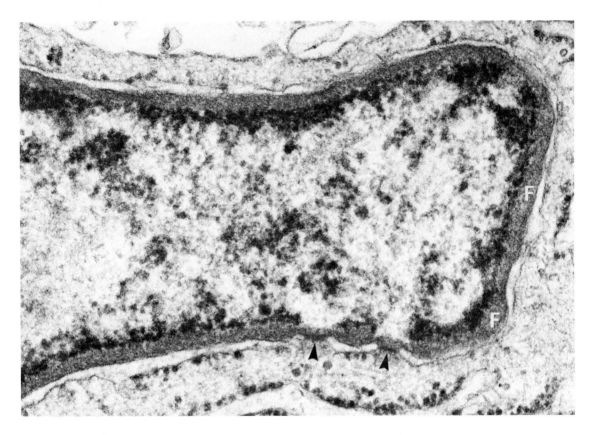

Figure 16 *Repair tissue from thigh. Same case as Figure 15. High-power view of a portion of the nucleus from a myofibroblast. Note the prominent nuclear fibrous lamina (F) and nuclear pores (arrowheads). ×90 000 (Ghadially and Lalonde, unpublished electron micrograph)*

Personal observations on tumours lead me to believe that the nuclear fibrous lamina must be very thin or absent in the nuclei of malignant tumours.

From data available to date it would appear that the fibrous lamina is not an indicator of rapidly growing cells, be they normal or neoplastic, but it may be an indicator of chronic inflammation and a repair reaction. Hence, this feature may be of some value in distinguishing such states, but clearly more observations about the state of the lamina in tumours are first needed.

Figures 15 and *16* illustrate prominent nuclear fibrous laminae found in myofibroblasts, from a lesion in the thigh of a 14-year-old boy that was clinically diagnosed as a sarcoma. Light microscopy did not support the idea that the lesion was malignant, but its precise nature remained obscure. Electron microscopy showed a fibrotic lesion in

which numerous myofibroblasts with a prominent nuclear fibrous lamina were found. Since myofibroblasts* have been seen in granulation and repair tissue, and since a thickened fibrous lamina is also seen in such states, we concluded that this was more likely to be a repair reaction to some unknown injury rather than a tumour.

Intranuclear inclusions

Inclusions are much more frequently seen in the nuclei of tumours than in normal cells. The true extent of this phenomenon and the nature of these inclusions are best appreciated by electron micro-

---

*A sarcoma of myofibroblasts is known to occur (see Chapter 10), but a nuclear fibrous lamina has not been described in such neoplastic myofibroblasts.

31

scopy, for many inclusions are too small to be visualized by the light microscope and even in the larger ones details of structures contained in the inclusion are rarely well visualized by the light microscope.

Little wonder, then, that in the past these inclusions have been mistaken for viral inclusions or the causative agent of neoplasia. A classic example of this is the Russell body, which Russell (1890) thought was a fungus and an aetiological agent of cancer. A reactive plasmacytosis is at times seen near tumours, and it is within the dilated cisternae of the plasma cell that Russell bodies usually occur. Sometimes, however, they are also found in the nucleus (*Figure 17*).

Electron microscopic studies have now made it amply clear that most nuclear inclusions contain cytoplasmic structures (organelles and inclusions such as lipid and glycogen) and are non-viral. It is also evident that a large majority of these inclusions are, in fact, pseudoinclusions (*Figure 18*), for the apparently included material does not lie free in the nuclear matrix but is separated from it by an invagination of the nuclear envelope. Virtually every cytoplasmic organelle and inclusion has, at one time or another, been found within such pseudoinclusions. True inclusions, where the included material lies free in the nuclear matrix, are quite rare (*Figure 19*).

The fact that pseudoinclusions are common in neoplastic nuclei is easily explained by the irregularity of shape and numerous invaginations found in such nuclei. Various theories have been proposed as to how cytoplasmic structures come to form true inclusions in the nucleus. In some instances it would appear that true inclusions derive by a dissolution of the invaginating membranes of the nuclear envelope surrounding a pseudoinclusion, but in other instances it would appear that organelles are accidentally

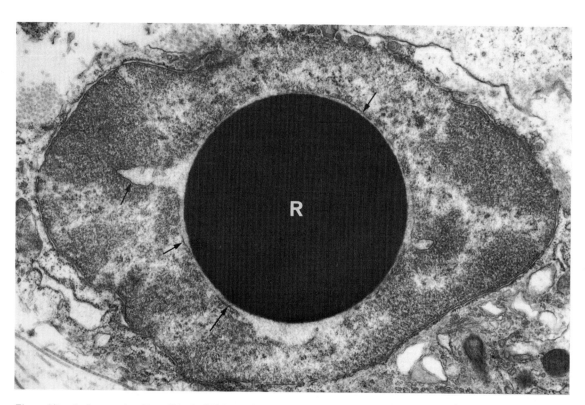

Figure 17 *An intranuclear Russell body (R) found in a plasma cell, in a stomach biopsy from a case of hairy cell leukaemia. These bodies are formed in the cisternae of the rough endoplasmic reticulum. From there they sometimes migrate into the nucleus as single membrane bound (arrows)* *(derived from the inner membrane of the nuclear envelope) pseudoinclusions. Later, dissolution of the membrane releases these bodies into the nuclear matrix. ×23 000 (From Ghadially and Lalonde, 1979)*

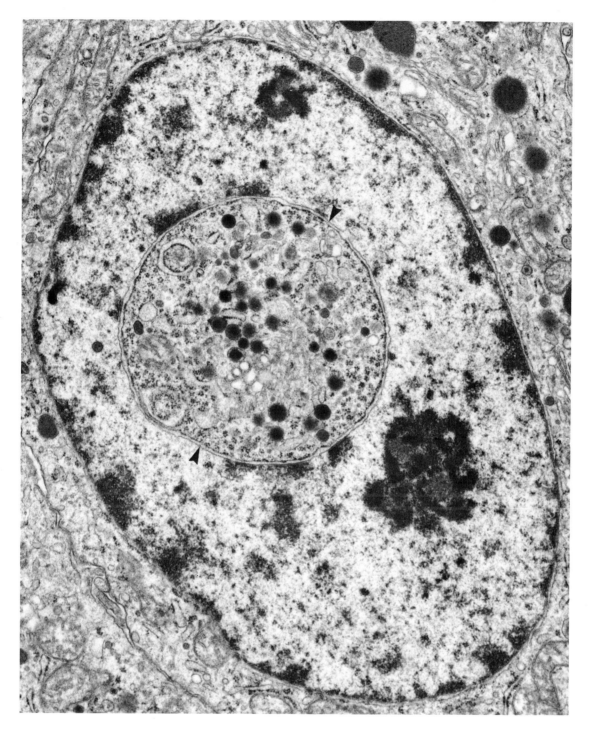

Figure 18 *Nucleus from a bronchial carcinoid showing a pseudoinclusion containing cytoplasmic structures, including numerous APUD granules. The characteristic double membrane (arrowheads) (derived from the inner and outer membranes of the nuclear envelope) demarcating the pseudoinclusion is clearly visualized.* ×26 000

included in the nucleus during mitosis.* In the case of materials such as lipid or glycogen (*Figure 19*) one has to consider the possibility that synthesis occurred within the nucleus. In the case of glycogen inclusions found in the nuclei of Novikoff ascites hepatoma cells there is good experimental evidence (using tritium-labelled D-glucose) that glycogen synthesis can occur in the nucleus.

It seems likely that the greater frequency of true inclusions in neoplastic nuclei reflects the frequent and abnormal mitoses in tumours, while the pseudo-inclusions reflect irregularity of form of the neoplastic nucleus.

Virus-like particles (called 'VLP') have at times been found in the nuclei of human tumours. Often the resemblance to virus particles is quite tenuous.

*It will be recalled that the nuclear membrane disintegrates and disappears during mitosis.

Even if one were to concede that these are virus particles, this does not mean that they are aetiologic agents of cancer. In order to avoid pitfalls, one should acquaint oneself with the appearance of intranuclear virus particles and their approximate sizes.

Nucleolus

Variations in size, shape and numbers

Nucleolar alterations are some of the most constant and diagnostically important accompaniments of the neoplastic state. Such alterations include: (1) increase in the size of the nucleolus; (2) increase in the number of nucleoli; and (3) variations and irregularity of size and shape.

With the electron microscope the nucleolus is seen to be composed of granular (15–20 nm in

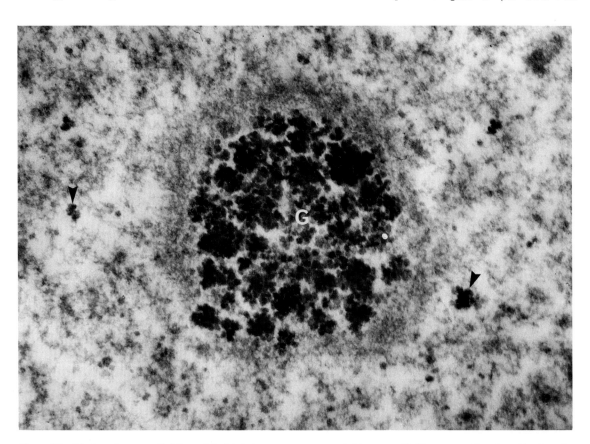

Figure 19 *Nucleus from a well-differentiated hepato-cellular carcinoma. Fixed in osmium (phosphate buffer), stained with lead only. A focal deposit of glycogen (G)* *surrounded by some fibrillary material and smaller deposits of glycogen (arrowheads) are seen scattered in the nuclear matrix. ×75 000 (From Ghadially and Parry, 1966)*

34

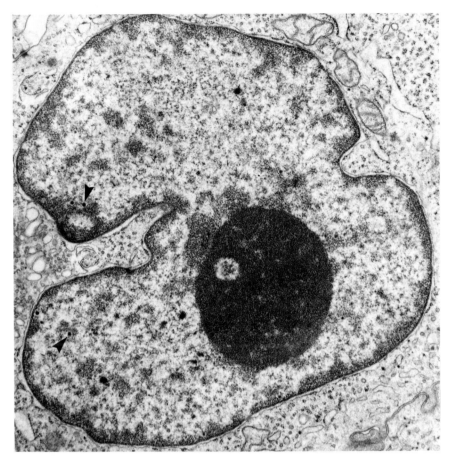

Figure 20 *A compact but enlarged nucleolus from a metastatic adenocarcinoma (primary site probably stomach or colon). Note also the perichromatin granules (arrowheads). ×16 500 (From Ghadially, 1975)*

diameter) and filamentous (5 nm diameter and 30–40 nm long) material. Two types of nucleoli are recognized; but with many intermediate forms and variations. On the one hand, we have 'open nucleoli', where a reticular nucleolonema (branching anastomosing thread-like structure) is evident, and on the other, 'compact nucleoli', where this thread-like structure is absent or so compacted as not to be evident. Both forms are seen in normal and neoplastic cells (*Figures 20* and *21*).

The prominence of the nucleolus in proliferating cells such as embryonic cells, stem cells, cells in tissue culture, tumour cells and cells producing a protein-rich secretory product (e.g. pancreatic acinar cells) has long suggested that the nucleolus plays a key role in protein synthesis (Caspersson and Schultz, 1940; Caspersson and Santesson, 1942; Caspersson, 1950). Since then evidence has accumulated which shows that this is because the nucleolus is the site of synthesis of the precursors of ribosomal RNA (Perry, 1964, 1966, 1969).

Enlargement of the nucleolus is a well-known feature of tumour cells (*Figures 20* and *21*). This phenomenon, first observed by Pianese (1896), has been demonstrated by MacCarty (1937) and by many others since to be true for a large number and variety of tumours. Although this enlargement can be quite impressive and is a fairly constant feature of the neoplastic state, it is by no means the hall-mark of malignancy. Thus, Stowell (1949)

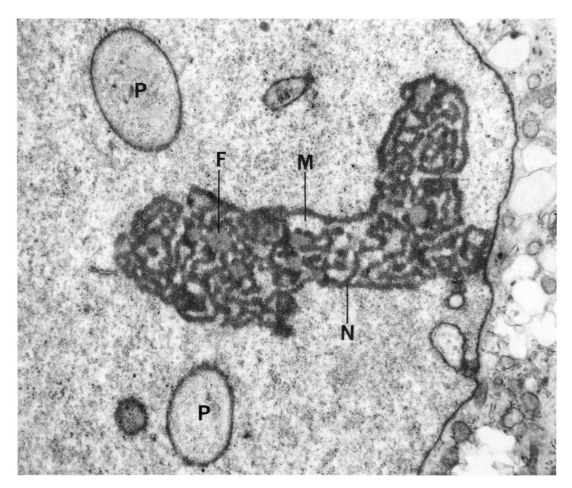

Figure 21 *Carcinoma of bronchus. An enlarged, irregular, marginated nucleolus found in a tumour cell. Note the reticular nucleolonema (N), fibrillar centres (F) and nuclear matrix (M) in the interstices of the nucleolonema. Pseudo-inclusions (P) are also present. × 22 000 (From Ghadially, 1975)*

showed that nucleoli larger than those occurring in malignant hepatoma can be found in regenerating rat liver after partial hepatectomy. Early nucleolar enlargement has been observed in the skin of mice painted with carcinogens, but here also it is largely related to the hyperplastic rather than the neoplastic state engendered by such treatment (Cowdry and Paletta, 1941; Cooper, 1956). Other similar non-specific nucleolar changes in malignancy include margination of the nucleolus, irregularity of shape and an increase in numbers of nucleoli. The latter is said to be related to the aneuploidy of cancer cells, but splitting of pre-existing nucleoli also seems to be involved.

Nucleolar margination

The nucleolus can move within the nucleus and, in states of active protein synthesis, it may come to lie against the nuclear membrane. (This phenomenon is referred to as nucleolar margination.) For example, intense protein-synthetic activity occurs in the regenerating liver of the rat after partial hepatectomy, and Swift (1959) has noted that some 50 per cent of the nucleoli move to the nuclear margin. It is therefore not surprising to find that nucleolar margination is frequently seen in a variety of tumours (*Figures 10, 12, 13* and *21*).

Although, as a general rule, there is a positive correlation between the degree of malignancy and the rate of growth of a tumour, this is not invariably so, and even some benign tumours are known to have a rapid growth phase. An example of this is the keratoacanthoma, a benign usually self-regressing tumour which mimics a carcinoma in both its histological appearance and its rapid growth rate (Ghadially, 1961, 1971; Ghadially, Barton and Kerridge, 1963). Such tumours can be produced experimentally (Ghadially, 1958), and nucleolar margination is frequently observed during the growth phase of this benign tumour (Ghadially, 1975).

Irregularities of nuclear shape, invaginations of the nuclear envelope and pseudoinclusions are common features of the neoplastic nucleus, and in some rapidly growing malignant tumours such deep invaginations are seen to make contact with or penetrate the nucleolus (*Figure 22*). This may be looked upon as another variety of nucleolar margination, for here, too, the nucleolus comes in intimate contact with the nuclear envelope.

The phenomenon of nucleolar margination has led many observers to speculate that such an arrangement facilitates nucleocytoplasmic exchanges. Thus, regarding nucleolar margination, Oberling and Bernhard (1961) state: 'One can assume that trans-portation of nucleolar products towards the cytoplasm is highly facilitated by this arrangement.'

In conclusion one may say that nucleolar margination and the other nucleolar changes described earlier are indicators of active protein synthesis and in a tumour this implies a fast-growing lesion, which is usually malignant.

Mitochondria

Although no constant or specific alteration of mitochondrial morphology characterizes the neoplastic state, one does find a host of changes which have interesting implications.

Energy production in normal and neoplastic tissues

It is now well established that the mitochondrion is the major source of cellular ATP. Since it supplies the cell with most of its usable energy, it is considered to be the power-house or power-plant of the cell (Siekevitz, 1957; Lehninger, 1960, 1961, 1965; Racker, 1968). In cell fractions prepared by homogenization of eukaryotic cells, enzymes of the Krebs

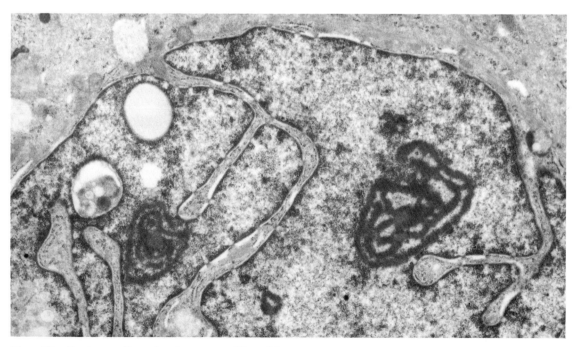

Figure 22 *Carcinoma of bronchus. Same case as Figure 21. Nucleus showing deep invaginations of the nuclear envelope contacting nucleoli with a reticular nucleolonema.* ×*15 000*

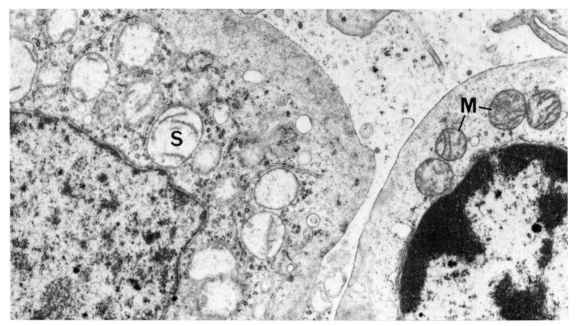

Figure 23   *Seminoma. The swollen mitochondria (S) in the tumour cell are well contrasted from the normal-looking mitochondria (M) in the lymphocyte. ×22 000*

cycle, oxidative phosphorylation and respiratory chain are found to be largely confined to the mitochondrial fraction, while the enzymes of anaerobic glycolysis occur in the unsedimented supernatant (cytoplasmic matrix or hyaloplasm).

Numerous studies have long established the fact that there is a positive correlation between the metabolic activity of a tissue and the number and size of mitochondria and also the size, surface area and concentration of cristae (for examples, attesting to this generalization see Rouiller, 1960; Novikoff, 1961; Lehninger, 1965; Fawcett, 1967; Ghadially, 1975). In malignant tumours we find an exception or an apparent exception to this rule, for here we have a metabolically active fast-growing tissue where the mitochondria are: (1) often too few; (2) more fragile than normal; and (3) pleomorphic in the sense that in a given tumour or even a tumour cell one may find large and small mitochondria with sparse or numerous cristae. One or more of these features is quite prominent in fast-growing malignant tumours but less apparent or absent in well-differentiated tumours and benign tumours.

The idea that mitochondria in tumours are defective is also supported by many biochemical studies. Thus, for example, it has been shown that

mitochondria isolated from hepatomas exhibit a lower respiratory capacity than mitochondria from normal liver (Kielley, 1952; Emmelot *et al.*, 1959; Devlin and Pruss, 1962; Fiala and Fiala, 1967; Arcos *et al.*, 1969; Sordahl *et al.*, 1969; Pedersen *et al.*, 1970).

The paradox of a fast-growing tissue with a paucity of mitochondria and/or defective mitochondria may be explained by recalling the historical work of Warburg (1956, 1962), which showed the predominance of glycolysis over respiration in the energy metabolism of tumours. Since the enzymes of anaerobic glycolysis occur in the cytoplasmic matrix, one may argue that a paucity of functioning mitochondrial mass would hardly embarrass the metabolic activity of a malignant tumour. Thus, in fact, there seems to be a good correlation between what is seen with the electron microscope and the respiratory biochemistry of neoplastic tissue.

Morphological changes in mitochondria

Normal-looking well-preserved mitochondria are infrequently seen in malignant neoplasms. The mitochondria are frequently swollen (*Figure 23*) and at times disrupted owing to a flooding of the matrix

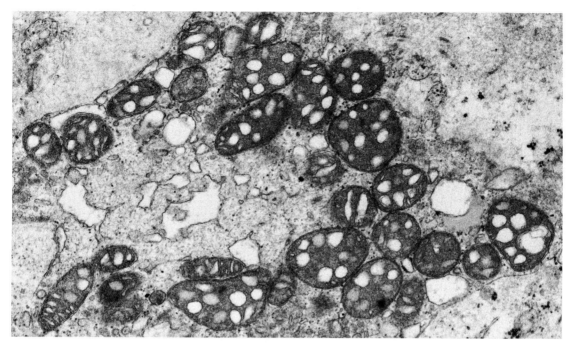

Figure 24   *Residual retroperitoneal leiomyosarcoma after radiation. Note mitochondria with swollen intracristal space and dense matrix. This is sometimes referrred to as the 'condensed configuration'.* ×28 000

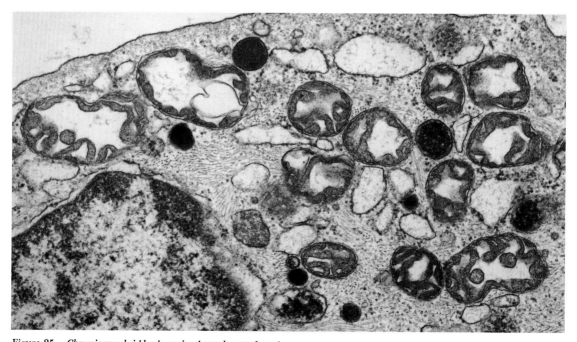

Figure 25   *Chronic myeloid leukaemia. A myelocyte found in the peripheral blood. The mitochondria show a more advanced stage of intracristal swelling than those shown in Figure 24.* ×41 000

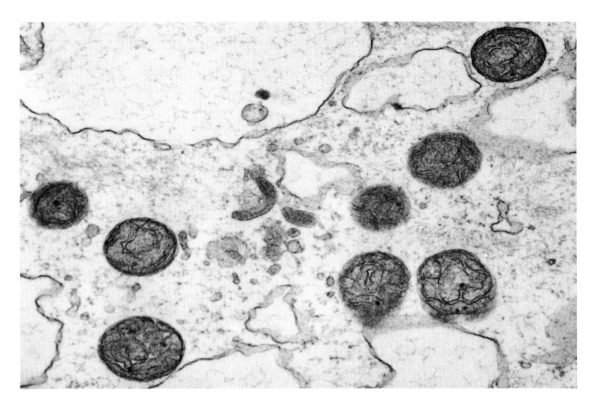

Figure 26 *Adenocarcinoma of the ovary. A tumour cell showing mitochondrial pyknosis. In some instances where the matrix is not too dense, disoriented and fused cristae are discernable.* ×*10 000 (From Ghadially, 1975)*

chamber with water. Less frequently it is the intra-cristal space which is flooded (*Figures 24* and *25*). This produces mitochondria with a dense matrix (at times referred to as the 'condensed configuration').

Changes of the type described above are probably multifactorial. They may be due to factors such as: (1) anoxia produced during surgery (e.g. application of a tourniquet or clamping of blood vessels before the tumour is removed); (2) cell injury and cloudy swelling due to vascular and/or metabolic disturbances (naturally occurring or produced by therapy) in the tumour; and (3) delayed or improper fixation of tissue (Chapter 1).

That this is not the whole story is attested by the fact that while the mitochondria in the tumour cells may be grossly swollen, those in accompanying non-neoplastic cells may be fairly well-preserved (*Figure 23*). Thus, once again we have to fall back on the idea that mitochondria in tumours are abnormal and unusually fragile.

Less common alterations of mitochondrial morphology seen in tumours include:* (1) pyknotic mitochondria (*Figure 26*), which are thought to indicate a regressive or involutionary mitochondrial change; and (2) rod-like, C-shaped or ring-shaped mitochondrial profiles with longitudinal instead of the usual transverse cristae (*Figures 27* and *28*). This transformation (i.e. transverse to longitudinal cristae) is thought to denote a deficiency of cytochrome oxidase in the mitochondrion.

Mitochondria in tumours of steroid producing cells

In most cells mitochondria with lamellar cristae are found, but in certain other cells, such as the steroid-secreting cells, the mitochondria have tubular cristae. This difference is carried over in tumours; hence, this is of diagnostic value in identifying tumours arising from steroid-secreting cells (Chapter 16).

*It should be noted that such mitochondrial changes have been seen in non-neoplastic states also.

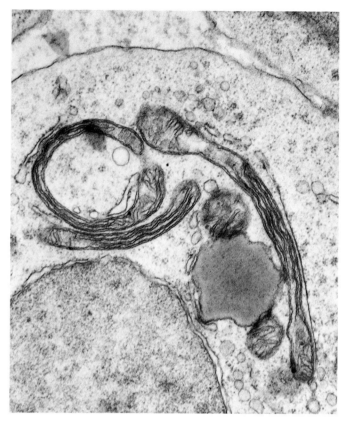

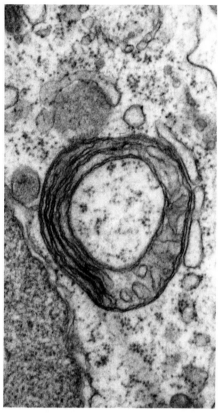

Figure 27 *Acute lymphoblastic leukaemia. A leukaemic cell showing mitochondria with longitudinal cristae and a few transverse cristae (partial transformation). One mitochondrion presents a C-shaped profile. ×26 000 (From Ghadially, 1975)*

Figure 28 *Acute lymphoblastic leukaemia. Same case as Figure 27. A leukaemic cell showing a ring-shaped mitochondrial profile with partial transformation of cristae. ×40 000 (From Ghadially, 1975)*

Mitochondria in oncocytomas

In oncocytomas the cytoplasm of the tumour cells is packed with innumerable mitochondria, but this does not argue against the concept expounded in this section, for it is thought that these mitochondria are biochemically defective and that this is an example of compensatory hyperplasia occurring at the organelle level (Chapter 9).

Rough endoplasmic reticulum

The main function of the rough endoplasmic reticulum with its attached polyribosomes is the production of secretory or export protein; the protein required for endogenous cellular needs is produced by the polyribosomes lying free in the cytoplasmic matrix.* Cells which produce a protein-rich secretion (e.g. hepatocytes, pancreatic acinar cells, plasma cells, fibroblasts and osteoblasts) have a well-developed rough endoplasmic reticulum, and to a greater or lesser extent rough endoplasmic reticulum persists in tumours arising from such cells (*Figure 29*). The comments that follow relate mainly to such cells and their tumours.

*This is a good generalization, but there are exceptions or apparent exceptions, the best-known being the acid hydrolases of the lysosome, which are synthesized by the polyribosomes of the rough endoplasmic reticulum. It is a moot point as to whether one considers the reaction between these enzymes (packaged in primary lysosomes) and phagocytosed material as occurring truly within or outside the cell.

41

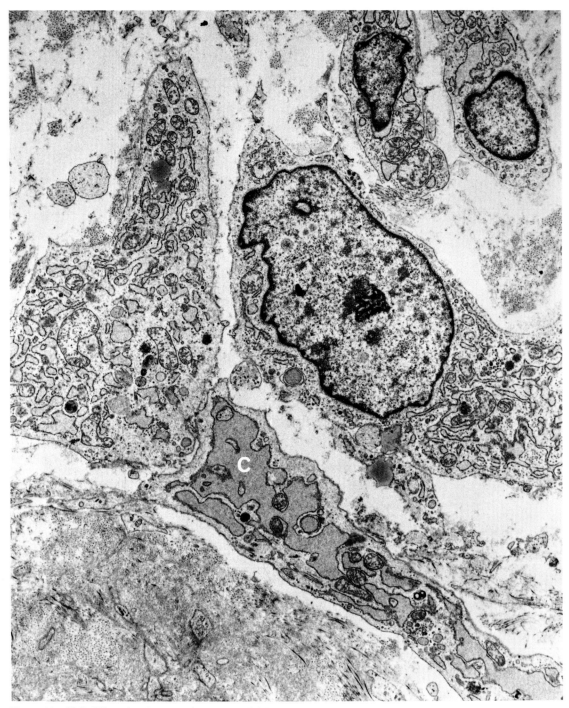

Figure 29 *Well-differentiated osteogenic sarcoma. A fair
amount of rough endoplasmic reticulum is present in the
tumour cells. In one cell the cristernae (C) of the rough
endoplasmic reticulum are grossly dilated.* ×7000 *(From
Ghadially and Mehta, 1970)*

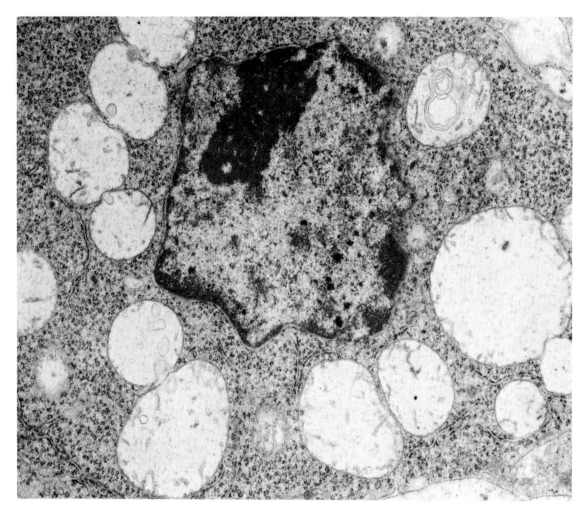

Figure 30   *Seminoma. Numerous mitoses seen by light microscopy indicated a rapidly growing tumour. This is borne out at the ultrastructural level by the finding of a fair number of cells such as the one depicted here, which show an enlarged marginated nucleolus and innumerable polyribosomes in the cytoplasm. Note also the large swollen mitochondria.* ×23 000

A well-developed rough endoplasmic reticulum may be looked upon as an expression of cell differentiation and functional activity, for immature or undifferentiated cells such as stem cells, blast cells, embryonic cells and cells in culture have, as a rule, a poor complement of rough endoplasmic reticulum as compared with their normal, mature, functioning (secretory) counterparts. Such immature cells, particularly fast-growing populations of cells, generally have an abundance of free polyribosomes in the cytoplasm. This presumably reflects the active synthesis of endogenous proteins needed for cell growth and division. The above-mentioned concepts also apply to tumours, where an inverse relationship has often been noted between the amount of rough endoplasmic reticulum present and the growth rate and malignancy of the tumour (Oberling and Bernhard, 1961; Bernhard, 1969).

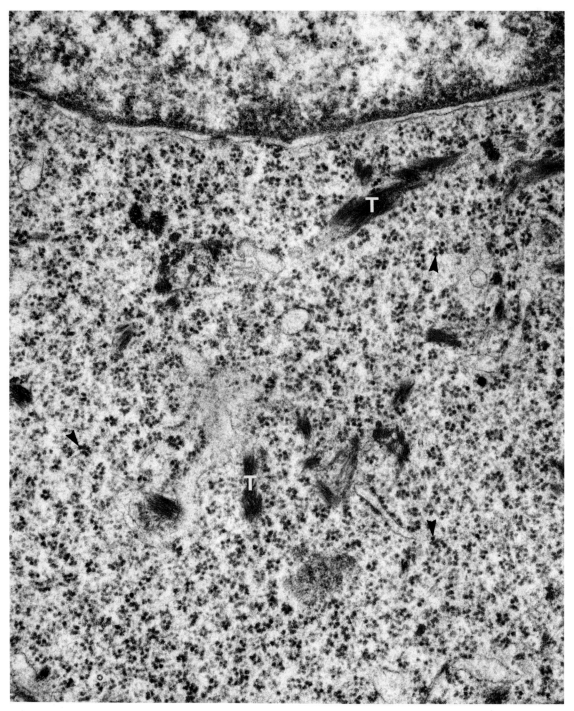

Figure 31   *Light microscopically this was a poorly differen-tiated squamous cell carcinoma of the lip (same case as Figure 13). Electron microscopically the presence of characteristic desmosomes and tonofibrils (T) confirms the diagnosis of squamous cell carcinoma. Numerous mitoses seen with the light microscope and the abundant poly-ribosomes (arrowheads) with the electron microscope indicate a fast-growing lesion. ×61 000*

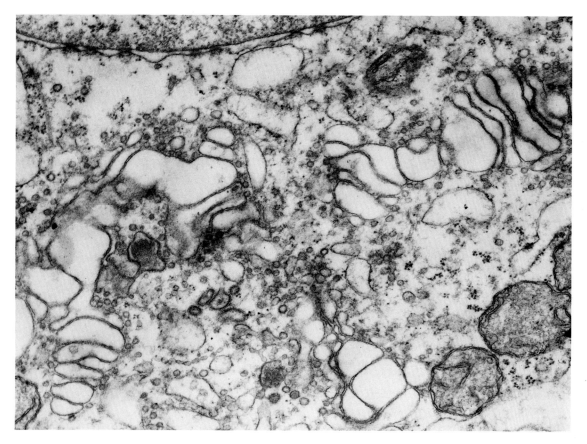

Figure 32   *An example of hypertrophy and dilatation of the Golgi complex found in a singularly well differentiated hepatocellular carcinoma. Fixed in osmium (phosphate buffer), stained with lead citrate. ×35 000 (From Ghadially and Parry, 1966)*

Perhaps the most frequently studied model illustrating the above-mentioned concept is the rat hepatoma (Dalton, 1964; Hruban, Swift and Slesers, 1965; Ma and Webber, 1966; Flaks, 1968). Here the cells of very well-differentiated slow-growing examples of this tumour have been found to contain a well-developed rough endoplasmic reticulum resembling that found in normal hepatocytes, but in highly anaplastic fast-growing variants only an occasional vesicle of rough endoplasmic reticulum is seen and the cytoplasm contains little besides some mitochondria and innumerable polyribosomes. In extreme examples of this kind there is little difficulty in drawing meaningful positive correlations between ultrastructural signs of poor differentiation and growth rate or malignancy, but when intermediate

examples of tumours with moderate degrees of such changes and differences in growth rates are compared, exceptions or apparent exceptions to our concepts are soon found. Such differences may be real or may be due to the small sample examined with the electron microscope not being truly representative of the whole tumour mass.*

As stated earlier, the comments made regarding the rough endoplasmic reticulum relate mainly to tumours arising from cells fairly well endowed with rough endoplasmic reticulum to begin with. However, the remarks about the polyribosomes lying free in the cytoplasm are generally applicable to all tumours (*Figures 30* and *31*). If numerous polyribosomes are

*This perennial difficulty must be constantly kept in mind when one evaluates tumour biopsies.

seen, it is an indication of rapid growth. This change goes hand in hand with hypertrophy and margination of the nucleolus and correlates well with the number of mitoses seen by light microscopy. It is worth noting that solitary ribosomes lying free in the cytoplasm have a converse connotation — namely a suppressed or deranged messenger RNA production and protein synthesis. (For examples and discussion see Ghadially, 1975.)

Golgi complex

This organelle is best developed in secretory cells; it has numerous functions (see Ghadially, 1975), but the best-known ones are modifying, condensing and packaging materials to form secretory granules. Thus, the Golgi complex, like the rough endoplasmic reticulum may be regarded as an indicator of cellular differentiation and functional activity. In keeping with this is the oft-made observation that immature cells or undifferentiated cells (e.g. stem cells or blast cells) have a poorly developed Golgi complex as compared with their normal mature counterparts. Similarly, fast-growing cells such as cells in tissue culture and anaplastic tumour cells, where the accent is on growth and multiplication rather than on differentiation and function, also tend to have a poorly developed Golgi complex.

Light microscopic studies on tumours (Ludford, 1929, 1952; Severinghaus, 1937; Dalton and Edwards, 1942; Bothe *et al.*, 1950) have shown many variations in size and distribution of the Golgi complex but none that can be considered specific for the neoplastic state. Electron microscopic studies have done little besides confirm and clarify these findings (Haguenau and Bernhard, 1955; Haguenau and Lacour, 1955; Howatson and Ham, 1955, 1957; Selby, Biesele and Grey, 1956; Dalton and Felix, 1957; Epstein, 1957a, b; Suzuki, 1957; Dalton, 1959, 1961; Oberling and Bernhard, 1961; Bernhard, 1969).

From a review of the literature and personal observations on tumours of man and experimental animals, the following tentative conclusions are drawn: (1) in fast-growing anaplastic tumours the Golgi complex is almost invariably poorly developed or difficult to identify; (2) there is a rough correlation between the degree of differentiation and the size of the Golgi complex in a given tumour type, the less differentiated tumours having poorer Golgi complexes; (3) relatively well-differentiated malignant tumours and benign tumours usually have a well-developed Golgi complex if the parent tissue of

origin is also well endowed in this respect; and (4) marked hypertrophy, dilatation and distortion of the Golgi complex are, at times, found in some tumours.

We (Ghadially and Parry, 1966) have seen hypertrophy, dilatation and distortion of Golgi complexes in a human hepatoma (*Figure 32*) and such changes have also been reported by other workers in some examples of: (1) mouse and rat hepatomas (Dalton and Edwards, 1942; Bothe *et al.*, 1950; Dalton, 1961, 1964); (2) Rous sarcoma (Bernhard, 1969); and (3) experimentally produced pituitary adenomas (Severinghaus, 1937). It must, however, be stressed that, as a general rule, tumours are poorly endowed with Golgi complexes as compared with their cell of origin.

Lysosomes

Little is known about the occurrence of primary lysosomes in tumours, since acid phosphatase reaction would be needed to confidently identify them. A few electron-dense bodies acceptable as secondary lysosomes are seen in most tumours. Sometimes they seem to be totally absent, as in the case of a hepatoma we studied (Ghadially and Parry, 1966), while in granular cell myoblastoma the cytoplasm is loaded with lysosomes (Chapter 9). Phagocytic activity is also generally diminished or lost in malignant histiocytes *vis-à-vis* their normal counterparts.

References

ARCOS, J. C., MATHISON, J. B., TISON, M. J. and MOULEDOUX, A. M. (1969). Effect of feeding amino azo dyes on mitochondrial swelling and contraction. Kinetic evidence for deletion of membrane regulatory sites. *Cancer Res.*, 29, 1288

BERNHARD, W. (1969). Ultrastructure of the cancer cell. In: *Handbook of Molecular Cytology*, ed. A. Lima-De-Faria. Amsterdam: North-Holland

BERNHARD, W. and GRANBOULAN, N. (1963). The fine structure of the cancer cell nucleus. *Expl. Cell Res.* Suppl., 9, 19

BOTHE, A. E., DALTON, A. J., HASTINGS, W. S. and ZILLESEN, F. O. (1950). Study of Golgi material and mitochondria in malignant and benign prostatic tissue. *J. Natn. Cancer Inst.*, 11, 239

BOUTEILLE, M. (1972). Ultrastructural localization of proteins and nucleoproteins in the interphase nucleus. *Karclinska Symposium on Research Methods in Endocrinology, 5th Symposium, May 29—31. Gene Transcription in Reproductive Tissue*

CASPERSSON, T. O. (1950). *Cell Growth and Cell Function. A Cytochemical Study.* New York: Norton

CASPERSSON, T. O. and SANTESSON, L. (1942). Studies on protein metabolism in the cells of epithelial tumours. *Acta Radiol.* Suppl., 46, 1

CASPERSSON, T. O. and SCHULTZ, J. (1940). Ribonucleic acids in both nucleus and cytoplasm and the function of the nucleolus. *Proc. Natn. Acad. Sci. U.S.A.,* 26, 507

COOPER, N. C. (1956). Early cytological changes produced by carcinogenesis. *Bull. N. Y. Med. Soc.,* 32, 79

COWDRY, E. V. and PALETTA, F. X. (1941). Changes in cellular nuclear and nucleolar sizes during methylcholanthrene epidermal carcinogenesis. *J. Natn. Cancer Inst.,* 1, 745

DALTON, A. J. (1959). Organization in benign and malignant cells. *Lab. Invest.,* 8, 510

DALTON, A. J. (1961). Golgi apparatus and secretion granules. In: *The Cell,* ed. J. Brachet and A. E. Mirsky. New York: Academic Press

DALTON, A. J. (1964). An electron microscopical study of a series of chemically induced hepatomas. In *Cellular Control Mechanisms and Cancer,* ed. P. Emmelot and O. Muhlbock. New York: American Elsevier

DALTON, A. J. and EDWARDS, J. E. (1942). Mitochondria and Golgi apparatus of induced and spontaneous hepatomas in mouse. *J. Natn. Cancer Inst.,* 2, 565

DALTON, A. J. and FELIX, M. D. (1957). Electron microscopy of mitochondria and the Golgi complex. *Symposia Soc. Expl Biol.,* 10, 148

DASKAL, I., MERSKI, J. A., HUGHES, B. B. and BUSCH, H. (1975). The effects of cycloheximide on the ultrastructure of rat liver cells. *Expl Cell Res.,* 93, 395

DEVLIN, T. M. and PRUSS, M. P. (1962). Oxidative phosphorylation and ATPase activity of mitochondria from rat hepatomas. *Proc. Am. Assoc. Cancer Res.,* 3, 315

EMMELOT, P., BOS, C. J., BROMBACHER, P. J. and HAMPE, J. F. (1959). Studies on isolated tumour mitochondria; biochemical properties of mitochondria from hepatomas with special reference to a transplanted rat hepatoma of the solid type. *Br. J. Cancer,* 13, 348

EPSTEIN, M. A. (1957a). The fine structure of the cells in mouse sarcoma 37 ascitic fluids. *J. Biophys. Biochem. Cytol.,* 3, 567

EPSTEIN, M. A. (1957b). The fine structural organization of Rous tumour cells. *J. Biophys. Biochem. Cytol.,* 3, 851

FAWCETT, D. W. (1966). On the occurrence of a fibrous lamina on the inner aspect of the nuclear envelope in certain cells of vertebrates. *Am. J. Anat.,* 119, 129

FAWCETT, D. W. (1967). *An Atlas of Fine Structure. The Cell, its Organelles and Inclusions.* Philadelphia: Saunders

FIALA, S. and FIALA, A. E. (1967). Structural and metabolic distinction between Morris hepatoma 5123A and normal rat liver. *Int. J. Cancer,* 2, 344

FLAKS, B. (1968). Formation of membrane-glycogen arrays in rat hepatoma cells. *J. Cell Biol.,* 36, 410

GHADIALLY, F. N. (1958). A comparative morphological study of the kerato-acanthoma of man and similar experimentally produced lesions in the rabbit. *J. Path. Bact.,* 75, 441

GHADIALLY, F. N. (1961). The role of hair follicle in origin and evolution of some cutaneous neoplasms of man and experimental animals. *Cancer,* 14, 801

GHADIALLY, F. N. (1971). Keratoacanthoma. In *Dermatology in General Medicine,* ed. T. B. Fitzpatrick and D. P. Johnson. New York: McGraw-Hill

GHADIALLY, F. N. (1975). *Ultrastructural Pathology of the Cell.* London: Butterworths

GHADIALLY, F. N., BARTON, B. W. and KERRIDGE, D. F. (1963). The etiology of keratoacanthoma. *Cancer,* 16, 603

GHADIALLY, F. N., BHATNAGER, R. and FULLER, J. A. (1972). Waxing and waning of nuclear fibrous lamina. *Archs Path.,* 94, 303

GHADIALLY, F. N., FULLER, J. A., KIRKALDY-WILLIS, W. H. (1971). Ultrastructure of full thickness defects in articular cartilage. *Archs Path.,* 92, 356

GHADIALLY, F. N. and LALONDE, J. M. A. (1979). Single-membrane-bound pseudoinclusions in the nucleus. *J. Submicrosc. Cytol.,* 11, 413

GHADIALLY, F. N., ORYSCHAK, A. F. and MITCHELL, D. M. (1974). Nuclear fibrous lamina in pathological human synovial membrane. *Virchows Arch. Abt. B. Zellpath.* 15, 223

GHADIALLY, F. N. and PARRY, E. W. (1966). Ultrastructure of a human hepatocellular carcinoma and surrounding non-neoplastic liver. *Cancer,* 19, 1989

GRANBOULAN, N. and BERNHARD, W. (1961). Cytochimie ultrastructurale. Exploration des structures nucleaires par digestion enzymatique. *C. R. Séanc. Soc. Biol.,* 155, 1767

HAGUENAU, F. and BERNHARD, W. (1955). L'appareil de Golgi dans les cellules normales et cancereuses de vertèbres. *Archs Anat. Microsc. Morph. Exp.,* 44, 27

HAGUENAU, F. and LACOUR, F. (1955). Cytologie electronique de tumeurs hypophysaires experimentals; leur appareil de Golgi. In: *Symposium on the Fine Structure of Cells* (Symposium held at the 8th Congress of Cell Biology, Leiden 1954). New York: Interscience

HEINE, U., SEVERAK, L., KONDRATIC, J. and BONAR, R. A. (1971). The behaviour of HeLa-S$_3$ cells under the influence of supranormal temperatures. *J. Ultrastruct. Res.,* 34, 375

HOWATSON, A. F. and HAM, A. W. (1955). Electron microscope study of sections of two rat liver tumours. *Cancer Res.,* 15, 62

HOWATSON, A. F. and HAM, A. W. (1957). The fine structure of cells. *Can. J. Biochem. Physiol.,* 35, 549

HRUBAN, Z., SWIFT, H. and SLESERS, A. (1965). Effect of Triparanol and diethanolamine on the fine structure of hepatocytes and pancreatic acinar cells. *Lab. Invest.,* 14, 1652

JEZEQUEL, A. M. and MARINOZZI, V. (1963). A propos de certains composants granulaires du moyau reveles par la fixation aux aldehydes. *J. Microsc.,* 2, 34 (abstract)

KIELLEY, R. K. (1952). Oxidative phosphorylation by mitochondria of transplantable mouse hepatoma and mouse liver. *Cancer Res.,* 12, 124

LEHNINGER, A. L. (1960). Energy transformation in the cell. Reprinted from *Scientific American,* No. 69 (May 1960). San Francisco: Freeman

LEHNINGER, A. L. (1961). How cells transform energy. Reprinted from *Scientific American.* No. 91 (September 1961). San Francisco: Freeman

LEHNINGER, A. L. (1965). *The Mitochondrion. Molecular Basis of Structure and Function.* New York, Amsterdam: Benjamin

LUDFORD, R. J. (1929). Vital staining of normal and malignant cells: staining of malignant tumours with trypan blue. *Proc. R. Soc.,* **B104**, 493

LUDFORD, R. J. (1952). Pathological aspects of cytology. In: *Cytology and Cell Physiology,* ed. G. Bourne, 2nd edn, pp. 373–418. London: Oxford University Press

MA, M. H. and WEBBER, A. J. (1966). Fine structure of liver tumours induced in the rat by 3-methyl-4-dimethylaminoazobenzene. *Cancer Res.,* **26**, 935

MacCARTY, W. C. (1937). Further observations on the macronucleolus of cancer. *Am. J. Cancer,* **31**, 104

MONTELLA, G. (1954). Lo studio del nucleo cellulare nei tumori. *Tumori,* **40**, 232

MURAD, T. M. and SCARPELLI, D. G. (1967). The ultrastructure of medullary and scirrhous mammary duct carcinoma. *Am. J. Path.,* **50**, 335

NORTON, W. N., DASKAL, I., SAVAGE, H. E., SEIBERT, R. A., BUSCH, H. and LANE, M. (1977). Effects of Galactoflavin-induced riboflavin deficiency upon rat hepatic cell ultrastructure. *Virchows Arch. B. Cell Path.,* **23**, 353

NOVIKOFF, A. B. (1961). Mitochondria (chondriosomes). In: *The Cell,* Vol. 2, ed. J. Brachet and A. E. Mirsky, p. 299. London: Academic Press

OBERLING, Ch. and BERNHARD, W. (1961). The morphology of the cancer cells. In: *The Cell,* Vol. 5, ed. J. Brachet and A. E. Mirsky, p. 405. New York: Academic Press

ORYSCHAK, A. F., GHADIALLY, F. N. and BHATNAGER, R. (1974). Nuclear fibrous lamina in the chondrocytes of articular cartilage. *J. Anat.,* **118**, 511

ORYSCHAK, A. F., MITCHELL, D. M. and GHADIALLY, F. N. (1976). Nuclear fibrous lamina in the rheumatoid synovium. *Archs Path.,* **100**, 218

PATRIZI, G. and POGER, M. (1967). The ultrastructure of the nuclear periphery. The Zonula Nucleum Limitans. *J. Ultrastruct. Res.,* **17**, 127

PEDERSEN, P. L., GREENAWALT, J. W., CHAN, T. L. and MORRIS, H. P. (1970). A comparison of some ultrastructural and biochemical properties of mitochrondria from Morris hepatomas 9618A, 7800 and 3924A. *Cancer Res.,* **30**, 2620

PERRY, R. P. (1964). Role of the nucleolus in ribonucleic acid metabolism and other cellular processes. *Natn. Cancer Inst. Monogr.,* **14**, 73

PERRY, R. P. (1966). On ribosome biogenesis. *Natn. Cancer Inst. Monogr.,* **23**, 527

PERRY, R. P. (1969). Nucleoli: the cellular sites of ribosome production. In: *Handbook of Molecular Cytology,* ed. A. Lima-De-Faria. Amsterdam: North-Holland

PIANESE, G. (1896). Beitrag zur Histologie und Aetiologie des Carcinoms. Histologische und Experimentalle Untersuchungen. Aus dem Italieneschen ubersetzt von R. Teuscher. I-II Histologische Untersuchungen. *Zieglers Beitr.,* **142**, Suppl. 1, 1

RACKER, E. (1968). The membrane of the mitochondrion. Reprinted from *Scientific American* **218k**, 32

REDDY, J. K. and SVOBODA, D. J. (1968). The relationship of nucleolar segregation to ribonucleic acid synthesis following the administration of selected hepatocarcinogens. *Lab. Invest.,* **19**, 132

REJTHAR, A. and BLUMAJER, J. (1974). Difference in density of nuclear pores in normal and malignant fibroblasts of Syrian hamsters. *Neoplasma,* **21**, 479

ROUILLER, Ch. (1960). Physiological and pathological changes in mitochondrial morphology. *Int. Rev. Cytol.,* **9**, 227

RUSSELL, W. (1890). An address on a characteristic organism of cancer. *Br. Med. J.,* **2**, 1356

SELBY, C. C., BIESELE, J. J. and GREY, C. E. (1956). Electron microscope studies of ascites tumor cells. *Ann. N. Y. Acad. Sci.,* **63**, 748

SEVERINGHAUS, A. E. (1937). Cellular changes in the anterior hypophysis with special reference to its secretory activities. *Physiol. Rev.,* **17**, 556

SIEKEVITZ, P. (1957). Powerhouse of the cell. Reprinted from *Scientific American,* No. 36 (July 1957). San Francisco: Freeman

SORDAHL, L. A., BLAILOCK, Z. R., LIEBELT, A. G. KRAFT, G. H. and SCHWARTZ, A. (1969). Some ultrastructural and biochemical characteristics of tumor mitochondria isolated in albumin-containing media. *Cancer Res.,* **29**, 2002

STOWELL, R. E. (1949). Alterations in nucleic acids during hepatoma formation in rats fed *p*-dimethylaminoazobenzene. *Cancer,* **2**, 121

SUZUKI, T. (1957). Electron microscopic cyto-histopathology. III. Electron microscopic studies on spontaneous mammary carcinoma of mice. *Gann,* **48**, 39

ŠVEJDA, J., VRBA, M. and BLUMAJER, J. (1975). A freeze-etch study of the occurrence of nuclear pores in normal and tumor cells. *Neoplasma,* **22**, 385

SWIFT, H. (1959). Studies on nucleolar function. In *Symposium on Molecular Biology,* ed. R. E. Zirkle. Chicago: University of Chicago Press

SWIFT, H. (1963). Cytochemical studies on nuclear fine structure. *Expl Cell Res.* Suppl., **9**, 54

WARBERG, O. (1956). The metabolism of tumors (English translation). *Science, N. Y.,* **123**, 309

WARBERG, O. (1962). Uber die Fakultative Anaerobiose de Krebszellen und ihre Amuedung auf die Chemotherapie. In: *On Cancer and Hormones. Essays in Experimental Biology,* pp. 29-34, Chicago: University of Chicago Press

WATSON, M. L. (1962). Observations on a granule associated with chromatin in the nuclei of cells of rat and mouse. *J. Cell Biol.,* **13**, 162

Part 3

Ultrastructural analysis of diagnostic problems

5
Is it a carcinoma or a sarcoma? (A study of cell junctions in normal and neoplastic tissues[*])

A problem in diagnostic histopathology is the differentiation of anaplastic carcinoma from sarcoma. In such cases one resorts to reticulin staining to see whether tumour cells are arranged in groups within a reticulin framework (as expected in a carcinoma) or whether reticulin fibres can be demonstrated between individual cells (as seen in some sarcomas). As is well known, the results of such staining can at times be difficult to interpret or equivocal. Further, in the case of lymphosarcoma one cannot even theoretically expect to find reticulin fibres between individual cells and the cells can be very closely packed indeed (see *Figure 137* in Chapter 12 and *Figures 142, 145* and *146* in Chapter 13).

Ultrastructural investigation of the situation is in a sense an extension or a substitute for reticulin staining, for with the electron microscope one can clearly visualize what lies between the cells (i.e. tumour matrix and basal lamina or external lamina†), how closely the cells lie together and whether they are linked by junctions or not.

Basal lamina and external lamina

The tumour matrix and features of the basal and external lamina are best dealt with when individual

---

*At times certain ultrastructural features can unequivocally establish the histogenesis of a tumour. For example, if characteristic secretory granules or other structures were found, we would know what particular variety of tumour it is (e.g. APUDoma, acinic cell carcinoma, melanoma, etc.). Such features, although they indirectly resolve or render redundant the question 'is it a carcinoma or sarcoma?', do not concern us here (these matters are dealt with in later chapters). Here we address ourselves to the fundamental or common differences which distinguish carcinomas from sarcomas as two major tumour groups, and this means a study of cell junctions and cell relationships.

†The basal lamina and the external lamina are part of the cell coat (glycocalyx). It is a moot point as to whether one considers them a component of the matrix or a part of the cell membrane and, hence, the cell itself.

---

tumours are considered in later chapters. However, a few general remarks about the latter are worth making here. Electron microscopy shows a polysaccharide-rich layer at the base of various epithelia; this is called the 'basal lamina'. (It usually shows two components — the lamina lucida and the lamina densa.) The basement membrane as seen by the light microscope comprises the basal lamina and underlying collagen fibrils.

In epithelial neoplasms groups of closely packed cells may be found separated from the stroma by a basal lamina. This may be quite thin, interrupted or almost absent; or, on the other hand, it can be quite prominent and/or reduplicated (see Chapter 3, *Figures 8* and *9*). As is well known, cells of mesenchymal tissues and their tumours tend to lie independently with a matrix between them. Electron microscopy shows that some mesenchymal cells have a polysaccharide-rich coat or layer around them (called the 'external lamina'), while others do not. This is a point of diagnostic value. For example, one can distinguish fibroblastic tumours from tumours of Schwann cells by the fact that in the latter instance quite a prominent external lamina is usually present. Thus, a study of the basal and external lamina is of value in distinguishing not only carcinomas from sarcomas, but also different types of sarcomas.

Cell junctions

The accurate evaluation of cell junctions is an important factor in deciding whether a tumour is a carcinoma or a sarcoma. The theory behind this is that since cell junctions, such as desmosomes and tight junctions, are characteristic of epithelia, it follows that demonstration of such junctions in an anaplastic tumour should be diagnostic of carcinoma, while the absence of junctions would argue strongly in the favour of a sarcoma.

By and large this is correct, but the situation is somewhat complicated because: (1) there is a marked reduction in the number of junctions in malignant tumours as compared with the normal tissue of origin; (2) morphological changes occur in junctions — the desmosomes lose some of their characteristic features, while tight junctions tend to open up (leaky junctions); (3) desmosome-like junctions are at times seen between normal mesenchymal cells and in certain pathological states affecting such cells; (4) quite a few tumours (including some sarcomas) besides carcinomas have been found to contain desmosome-like structures.

Thus, more than a passing knowledge about the morphology and distribution of cell junctions is essential for proper evaluation of the significance of cell junctions in tumours. Hence, such matters will be dealt with now. (For a more detailed account see Ghadially, 1975.)

Cell junctions in epithelial tissues

The existence of cell junctions has long been known to light microscopists. Perhaps the best-known example of this is the so-called 'intercellular bridge' found in the epidermis. Such bridges present as fine processes or fibrils traversing a clear space between adjacent cells, and it is this which gives the prickly appearance to prickle cells. The belief that these bridges represent tonofilaments crossing over from the cytoplasm of one cell into the next one, or that the cytoplasm of neighbouring cells is continuous at such sites, is not borne out by electron microscopy. It would appear that this phenomenon is largely a shrinkage artefact, the bridges being no more than plaques or zones of firm attachment (in the past referred to as 'granules of Ranvier' or 'nodes of Bizzozero', now understood to be desmosomes: *Figure 33*) which have become rotated and drawn out as the cells shrink away from each other during fixation and dehydration.

Another example of junctions seen at light microscopy is the terminal bar demonstrable by classic histological methods near the surface of various epithelia, particularly the small intestine. In ultrathin sections the terminal bar is seen to be a junction complex, comprising three morphologically distinct types of junctions. Starting from the lumen of the gut, one finds a tight junction followed by an intermediate junction and some desmosomes (*Figures 34 and 35*). Similar junction complexes have been

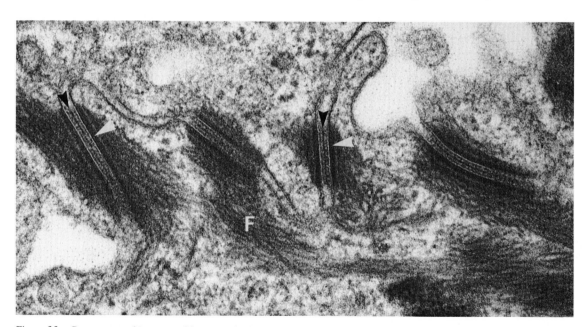

Figure 33   *Desmosomes from normal human skin. Note dense plaques (white arrowheads), tonofibrils (F) and the dense line, called the 'intermediate line' (black arrowheads) which bisects the material in the intercellular gap. ×96 000 (From Ghadially, 1975)*

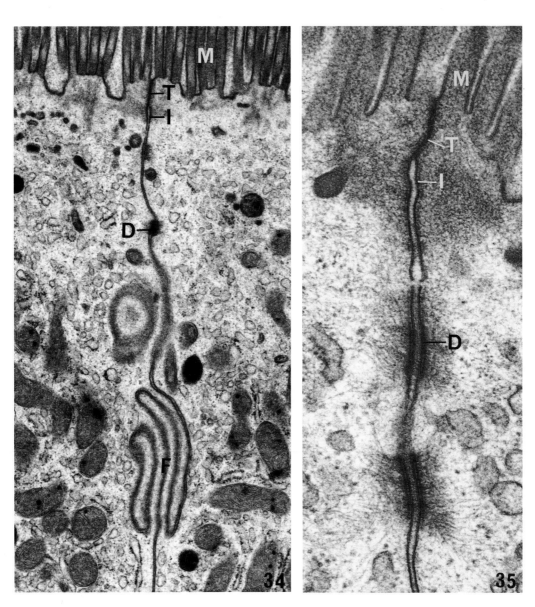

Figure 34 and 35   *The terminal bar of the junction complex between adjacent intestinal epithelial cells of man is illustrated here. The tight junction (T) is seen near the lumen of the gut lined by microvilli (M). It presents as a dense line both in the low-power (Figure 34) and in the high-power (Figure 35) views shown. The fusion of the outer leaflets of the plasma membrane characteristic of this type of junction is not revealed in these electron micrographs. Below the tight junction lies an intermediate junction (I)* *and desmosomes (D). The desmosomes show dense plaques and filaments on their cytoplasmic surface. Less well oriented filamentous material is seen adjacent to the intermediate junction and some cytoplasmic 'fuzz' is also seen near the tight junction. In the desmosomes and intermediate junction the intercellular gap is widened. The complex interdigitating folds (F) which are also thought to help to hold cells together are seen in Figure 34. ×21 000; ×67 000 (From Ghadially, 1975)*

described in various epithelia (Farquhar and Palade, 1963, 1965). However, the constant feature here is the tight junction which seals the intercellular space from the external environment (e.g. contents of gut, duct, acinus, etc.). The arrangement, number and type of the junctions which follow are quite variable.

The tight junctions of the junction complex of epithelia are characterized by punctate and linear fusion of the outer leaflets of the cell membrane of adjacent cells. A zone of increased density (cytoplasmic fuzz) is seen adjacent to true tight junctions, and their overall width is less than the combined width of the two membranes forming the junction.

Unfortunately details of structure as described above are rarely demonstrable in routinely prepared tissues, but they can be visualized in tissues stained *en bloc* with uranium. In routine sections the tight junction appears as a dense line between cells, but so may gap junctions (where the intercellular gap is about 2 nm wide) and labile appositions, which are thought to be either transient associations of the cell membrane or an artefact of tissue preparation.* One further possibility is that such a dense line mimicking a tight junction and the cytoplasmic fuzz may in fact be little more than an overlap of two adjacent cell membranes within the section thickness.†

Desmosomes are fundamentally different from tight junctions in that the width of the intercellular gap is either unaltered or widened but not narrowed as in the tight junction. The morphology and size of desmosomes are quite variable, but they are readily identified by the presence of a dense plaque and filaments on their cytoplasmic faces. The widened intercellular space often contains a dense material and a dense line (called the 'intermediate line') which suggests a modification of the cell coat at this site. Desmosomes are button-like structures which bind cells together; hence, the desmosome is at times referred to as a 'macula adherens'.

*Differences between tight junctions, gap junctions and labile appositions can be unequivocally resolved only by the use of tracers such as lanthanum hydroxide which permeate the intercellular space and allow one to determine the degree and extent of obliteration of the intercellular space achieved in a junction. Nevertheless, in routine preparations as used in diagnostic electron microscopy one has little choice but to use the term 'tight junction' in a loose fashion when adjacent cell membranes appear to be 'fused', producing a dense line. This point must be kept in mind when one reads this chapter and, indeed, when one evaluates published reports on the ultrastructure of tumours.
†This problem can often be resolved by using a tilting stage.

Cell junctions in non-haemopoietic mesenchymal tissues

One might begin by reflecting that an obvious minimum requirement for the production of cell junctions would be close apposition of cell surfaces and, hence, one would not even expect to find junctions in such tissues. In keeping with this is the observation that in fibrous tissue, synovial tissue or cartilage, where the cells are usually separated by a fair amount of matrix, junctions are, as a rule, not seen.

However, examples may be quoted where cell junctions do develop in such tissues, and this is usually seen in situations where cellular proliferation (not necessarily neoplastic) has brought such cells close together. Thus, tight junctions or close junctions (gap said to be 2—10 nm wide) have been noted between embryonic connective tissue cells (Trelstad, Revel and Hay, 1966; Trelstad, Hay and Revel, 1967), and 'close association regions', where the cell membranes of adjacent cells were in intimate contact, have been described in adult guinea-pig fibroblasts proliferating in cell culture (Devis and James, 1964). Sites of attachment resembling intermediate junctions have been demonstrated between a variety of embryonic connective tissue cells (Ross and Greenlee, 1966).

Desmosome-like junctions (and also rare tight junctions) have been seen between the normal synovial intimal cells of some species where these cells are closely packed (for details see Ghadially, 1975, 1978), but in the normal synovial intima of man, where the cells are loosely packed with a fair amount of matrix between them, no junctions occur. However, in the hyperplastic synovial membrane of traumatic arthritis, rheumatoid arthritis and villonodular synovitis the closely packed synovial cells do develop desmosome-like junctions (Grimley and Sokoloff, 1966; Ghadially and Roy, 1969). It is thought (Ghadially, Lalonde and Dick, 1978) that in some instances these desmosome-like structures are engendered by fibrin trapped between the synovial intimal cells (*Figure 36*).

The chondrocytes of articular cartilage usually lie apart separated from one another by abundant matrix. Even between chondrocyte pairs there is a fair amount of intervening matrix. However, occasionally such cells may lie very close together and in such instances desmosome-like junctions develop between them (Palfrey and Davis, 1966, and personal observations). Similarly, on very rare occasions a junction may form between cell processes of fibroblasts or between a fibroblast and a cell process from

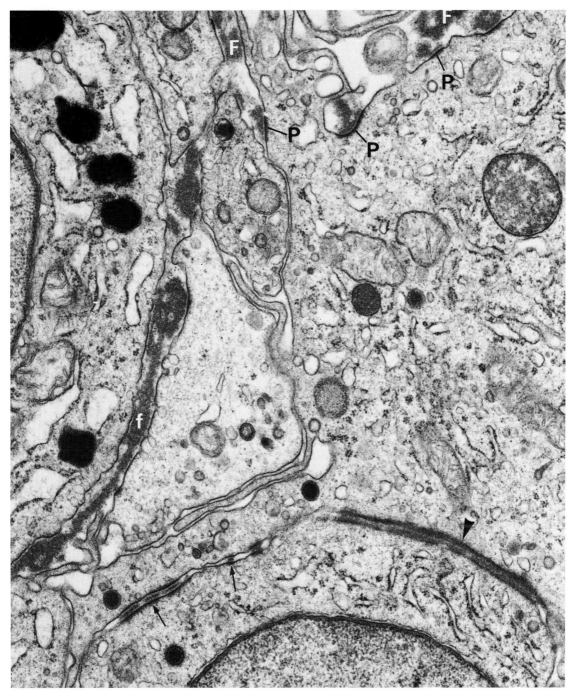

Figure 36 *Synovial membrane from a case of villonodular synovitis. A mass of fibrin (F) is seen among the synovial cells situated near the joint space. In some places dense plaques (P) have formed where the fibrin abuts the synovial membrane. A band of fibrin (f) is seen between the more deeply placed synovial cells and at an even deeper level desmosome-like structures (arrows) have formed where the intercellular space contains material acceptable as fibrin.*

Also seen is a rather long junction-like formation (arrowhead) where the plane of section is such that the contents of the intercellular space are not clearly revealed. Note the absence of converging filaments as seen in true desmosomes (e.g. in Figures 33 and 38). Compare details of intercellular gap shown here with that depicted in these true desmosomes. ×27 000 (From Ghadially, Lalonde and Dick, 1978)

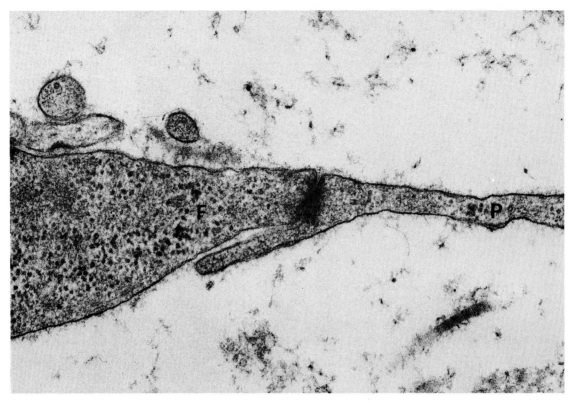

Figure 37 *Fibroadenoma of breast. A desmosome-like junction is seen between a fibroblast (F) and the cell process (P) of another fibroblast. ×40 000*

a neighbouring fibroblast. This is seen in both normal and neoplastic tissue (*Figure 37*).

In endothelia tight junctions occur,* but in most instances† they do not form continuous bands around the cells, as shown by the fact that they can be circumvented by tracers such as lanthanum or horseradish peroxidase. In mesothelia of man tight junctions and desmosome and desmosome-like junctions are present.

Cell junctions in haemopoietic tissues (including lymphoreticular tissue)

Whether junctions occur in haemopoietic tissues and their neoplasms is a matter of much dispute and uncertainty. Since this is a point of diagnostic im-

*In some species desmosomes are also found but not in man.
†An exception being capillaries in the brain.

portance in distinguishing leukaemias and lymphomas from other classes of neoplasms, it is worth looking at this controversy in some detail.

Let us begin by noting that it is difficult to understand why some workers can find junctions in these tissues but others do not. For example, junctions were not found in: (1) guinea-pig and rat bone marrow by Pease (1956); (2) human and rat spleen by Weiss (1957); (3) bone marrow of guinea-pigs by Zamboni and Pease (1961); and (4) bone marrow of albino rats by Weiss (1961). On the other hand, junctions were found in the bone marrow of: (1) rabbits, rats and guinea-pigs by Watanabe (1966); (2) rats by Weiss (1965), Ito (1965) and Ferguson, Hayes and Webber (1972); and (3) guinea-pigs by deBruyn, Michelson and Thomas (1971). It is difficult to be too precise about the type of junction or the cell type between which junctions are alleged to occur, because of differences in interpretation and nomenclature. However, it would appear that the controversy revolves mainly around tight junctions between reticulum cells or reticulo-endothelial cells.* The fact that some authors can find 'tight junctions', while others cannot, leads one to suspect that these junctions may be a preparative artefact — that is to say, they are probably labile appositions† rather than true tight junctions.

*An exception to this is the report by Veerman and van Ewijk (1975), who illustrate structures that could be tight junctions between what they call an 'interdigitating cell' and a lymphocyte.
†Labile or simple appositions of the cell membrane are thought to be either transient association of the cell membrane or an artefact producing a pentalaminar structure. Their incidence varies with preparative techniques, and such structures, comprising apposed rather than fused membranes, do not impede the passage of tracers. They lack the zone of increased cytoplasmic density (cytoplasmic fuzz) seen adjacent to true tight junctions and their overall width is not less than the combined width of the two membranes forming the junction, as is the case with true tight junctions (for references and review see Ghadially, 1975).

Desmosomes or desmosome-like structures have on rare occasions been demonstrated between dendritic reticulum cells in the germinal centres of the lymph nodes. For example: Kojima and Imai (1973) present a convincing illustration of desmosome-like structures between reticulum cells in the lymph node, while Lennert and Niedorf (1969) show a desmosome or desmosome-like structure between reticulum cells in a lymph node from a case of follicular lymphoma. The same desmosome-like structure is illustrated in Mori and Lennert (1969) and in Lennert (1973), attesting perhaps to the rarity of occurrence of desmosome or desmosome-like structures in this site. A desmosome-like structure found in a histiocytic lymphoma with sclerosis (arising from a nodular lymphoma) is illustrated by Katayama et al. (1977), but this was between the stromal cells producing the collagenous stroma.

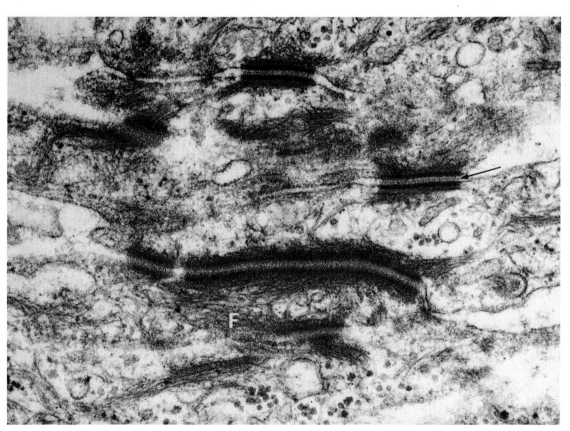

Figure 38   *Desmosomes in an epithelial thymoma. Note filaments (F) converging on plaques and the intermediate line (arrow) which is visualized when the plane of sectioning is favourable.* ×65 000 (Ghadially and Yong, unpublished electron micrograph)

In an excellent paper on nodular lymphoma Levine and Dorfman (1975) show indubitable desmosomes with dense plaques, filaments and an intermediate line in the normal human tonsil. However, in a tissue such as this the possibility of squamous epithelial cells trapped in lymphoid tissue has to be kept in mind. Carr *et al.* (1977) present an electron micrograph (their *Figure 1.6*) with a legend which reads: 'Electron micrograph of macrophage from sarcoid granuloma showing numerous lysosomes, interdigitating cytoplasmic processes and desmosomes.' No desmosome is seen in this illustration but some interesting leniar densities are present along the cell membrane of this macrophage. However, the poor quality of tissue preservation and/or preparation precludes speculations about their nature.

One may conclude by pointing out that in a majority of reports there is no mention of desmosomes or desmosome-like structures in haemopoietic tissues, nor have we (Skinnider and Ghadially, unpublished observations) seen such structures in hundreds of cases that we have studied. However, I think one has to concede that on rare occasions desmosome-like structures do occur between reticulum cells but perhaps not between various other cell types in the lymphoreticular and other haemopoietic tissues, except, of course, the reticular epithelial cell of the thymus. Here, as one would expect (because of their epithelial nature), indubitable desmosomes perfect in every detail are found and the same is also true for epithelial thymomas, where classic desmosomes with dense plaques, filaments and intermediate line are seen (*Figure 38*) (Ghadially and Illman, 1965; Levine, 1973); Bloodworth *et al.*, 1975; Llombart-Bosch, 1975).

Cell junctions in neoplasia

Desmosome and desmosome-like structures

What one might call the 'perfect' desmosome, 'classic' desmosome or 'well-differentiated' desmosome shows the following features: (1) a widened or 'unwidened' but not narrowed intercellular gap filled by dense material, which shows a line or a pattern of lines; (2) dense plaques on the cytoplasmic faces; and (3) filaments from the cytoplasm converging

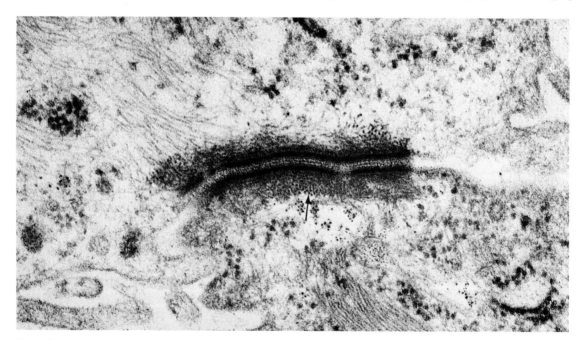

Figure 39 *Mesothelioma. Same case as Figure 5. A well-differentiated desmosome. The plane of sectioning is such that most of the filaments (arrows) converging on the desmosome are cut transversely. An intermediate line may just be discerned in the intercellular gap.* ×77 000

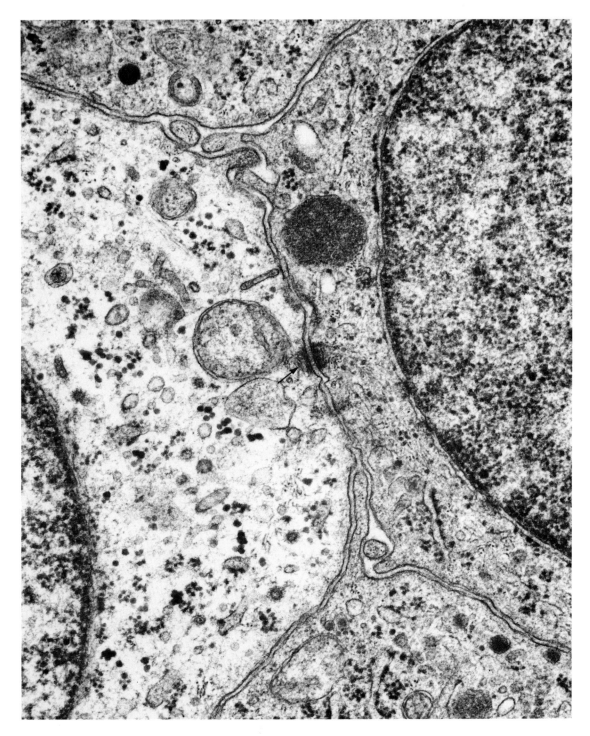

Figure 40 *Carcinoma of breast. An attenuated desmosome (arrow) with converging filaments, but without an intermediate line is seen here.* ×23 000

upon* the plaques (*Figures 33* and *38*). In human material the presence of such desmosomes virtually guarantees that one is looking at an epithelial tissue or its neoplasm. Exceptions to this are extremely rare. An example of this is illustrated in *Figure 39*, where we see a well-differentiated desmosome with an intermediate line found in a mesothelioma.

Conversely, it may be stated that even in indubitable carcinoma one does not always find 'perfect' desmosomes; indeed attenuated or altered desmosomes are quite common (*Figure 40*), this being particularly so in anaplastic carcinoma. In such desmosomes details in the intercellular gap are lacking but the filaments converging upon the plaques are still present, or *vice versa*. Such desmosomes, if frequent enough, can also be reasonably confidently accepted as suggestive of carcinoma.

In the desmosome-like junction the intercellular gap is unchanged or narrowed and the characteristic details are not visualized in the material that fills the gap. The cytoplasmic dense plaques or densities acceptable as plaques are present, but filaments converging upon the plaque are often not detectable, although some cytoplasmic fuzz may be seen. These are the so-called 'desmosomes' or 'desmosome-like' structures which one at times finds in mesenchymal tissues and a wide variety of tumours (*Figures 41* and *42*), including some sarcomas.† These desmosome-like structures are of little diagnostic value but they constitute a potential hazard in that they may erroneously lead one to believe that the tumour is a carcinoma. However, the presence of such structures does help to exclude lymphoma and leukaemia.

Quantitive changes in desmosomes

There is usually a marked reduction in the number of desmosomes in malignant tumours (i.e. carcinomas) as compared with the parent tissue of origin, this being particularly so in anaplastic tumours. In some benign tumours, however, there may be an increase in the number of junctions. For example: (1) Chapman, Drusin and Todd (1963) report an increase in the number of desmosomes in human

warts; (2) Fisher, McCoy and Wechsler (1972) found that desmosomes were plentiful in keratoacanthomas; and (3) according to Takaki, Masutani and Kawada (1971), desmosomes are increased in numbers in keratoacanthomas. Such differences may be of some diagnostic value, for keratoacanthoma is at times mistaken for squamous carcinoma (Ghadially, 1971).

Intracytoplasmic desmosomes and desmosome-like structures

Intracytoplasmic desmosomes may occur when cells connected by desmosomes fuse to produce multinucleate giant cells. After fusion the intervening cell membranes suffer fragmentation and dissolution but the less vulnerable desmosomes tend to persist awhile.

Intracytoplasmic desmosomes may also be found in tumours (*Figure 43*). While the occurrence of a characteristic desmosome in an intracellular situation is a strong indicator of epithelial origin, it is not an indicator of malignancy. For example, intracytoplasmic desmosomes have been seen in the cells of human keratoacanthoma (Bülow and Klingmüller, 1971; Takaki, Masutani and Kawada, 1971; Fisher, McCoy and Wechsler, 1972). Intracytoplasmic desmosomes have also been seen in dyskeratotic cells undergoing mitosis in Bowen's disease (Seiji and Mizuno, 1969), and it has been suggested that such dyskeratotic cells may lose contact with neighbouring epidermal cells during mitosis and incorporate the desmosomes into their cytoplasm.

Little is known about intracytoplasmic desmosome-like structures (*Figure 44*), but one may speculate either that they derive by incorporation of desmosome-like structures into the cytoplasm or that they are a stage in the dissolution of 'typical' desmosomes, after they have been internalized.

Tight junctions and terminal bars

There is a reduction in the number of tight junctions (and gap junctions) in neoplasia and there is a tendency for such junctions to 'open up' or become 'leaky'. The elegant studies of Martinez-Palomo (1970) have demonstrated this by using lanthanum as a tracer to delineate clearly the intercellular space. In routinely prepared tumour tissue (adenomas and adenocarcinomas) also, one often finds appearances which suggest that tight junctions have become 'leaky' (*Figures 45* and *46*), but proof of this can only be provided by tracer techniques.

Modified terminal bars (comprising tight junctions

---

*Some people speak about 'tonofilaments attached to desmosomes', but this is not strictly correct, for most of the filaments seem to loop through the plaques of the desmosome (Kelly, 1966). Hence, alternative terms such as 'radiating from' or 'converging upon', seem preferable (see, for example, Fawcett, 1967).

†Such structures have also been found in 3-methylcholanthrene-induced mouse sarcoma (Clarke, 1970).

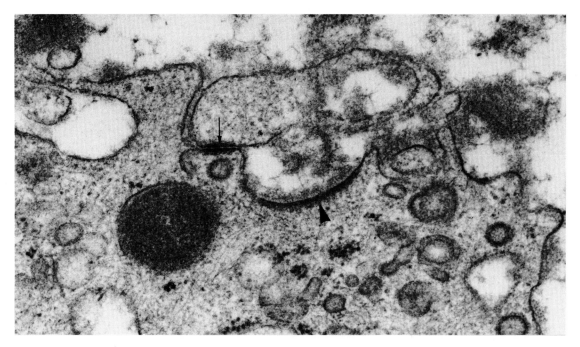

Figure 41　*A desmosome-like structure (arrow) in an atrial myxoma. Note the absence of converging filaments and an intermediate line in the intercellular gap. A dense plaque (arrowhead) is seen on the cytoplasmic face of the cell membrane. ×60 000*

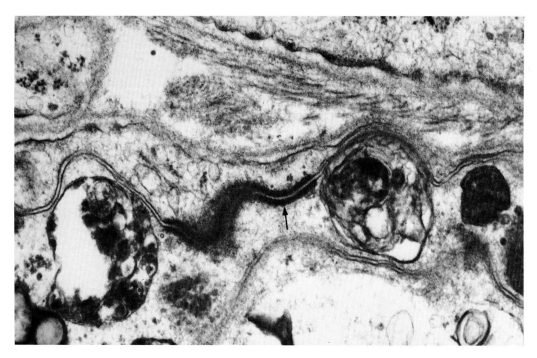

Figure 42　*A desmosome-like structure in a Schwannoma (arrow). ×46 000*

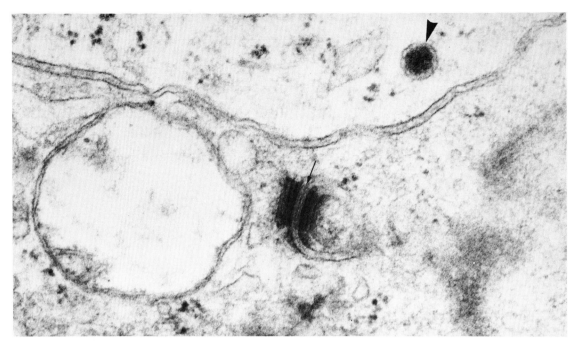

Figure 43　*An intracytoplasmic desmosome found in a secondary deposit of an APUDoma (anaplastic carcinoid of the oesophagus) in a lymph node. The intermediate line is just discernible (arrow). Note also the APUD granule (arrowhead). ×31 000*

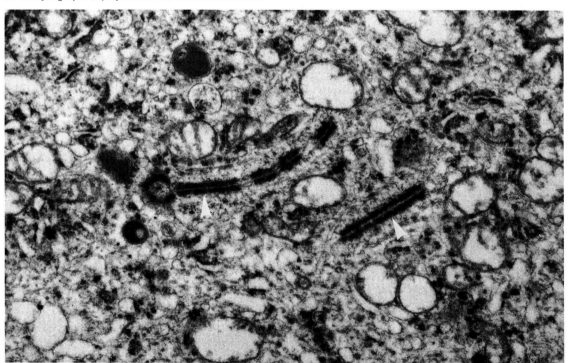

Figure 44　*Intracytoplasmic desmosome-like structures found in a phaeochromocytoma (arrowheads). ×68 000*

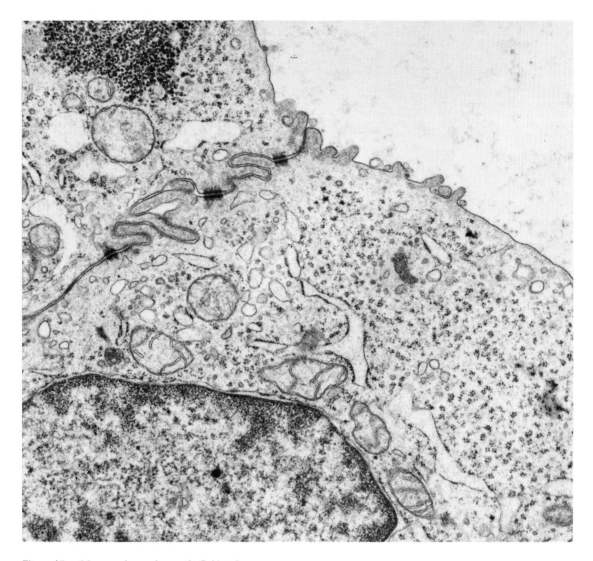

Figure 45 *Adenocarcinoma in ascetic fluid; primary probably in stomach or colon. Two tumour cells are seen, linked by a terminal bar and interdigitations of adjacent cell membranes. Note short microvilli, numerous polyribosomes and sparse rough endoplasmic reticulum.* ×25 000

or altered tight junctions followed by desmosomes, attenuated desmosomes or desmosome-like structures) and also interdigitations of adjacent cell membranes together comprise highly characteristic features which frequently assist in the diagnosis of adenocarcinoma. However, the occurrence of cellular locking by interdigitations and tight junctions is not 'diagnostic of adenocarcinoma', as stated by Gyorkey

et al. (1975) for such features (i.e. tight junctions or terminal bars) have been seen in: (1) adenoma and adenocarcinoma; (2) some APUDomas (personal observations); (3) transitional cell papilloma and carcinoma (*Figure 47*) (Tannenbaum, Tannenbaum and Carter, 1978); (4) synovial sarcoma (Gabbiani *et al.*, 1971; Klein and Huth, 1974; Kubo, 1974; Dische, Darby and Howard, 1978) and mesothelioma

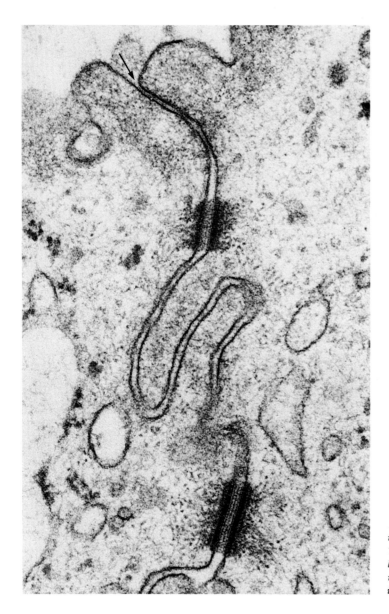

Figure 46 *Adenocarcinoma. High-power view of terminal bar shown in Figure 45. The tight junction (arrow) is probably leaky. Note the well-formed desmosomes with converging filaments and good detail in the intercellular gap.* ×49 000

(*Figure 48*) (Mackay, Bennington and Skoglund 1971).*

Consider now the interdigitations of the plasma membrane seen usually near the terminal bars.

*Mackay, Bennington and Skoglund (1971) correctly identify these structures as 'terminal bars', but in some other studies, although the illustrations show structures acceptable as tight junctions or terminal bars, the authors speak only about desmosomes (e.g. *Figures 4* and *5* in Nistal, Contreras and Paniagua, 1978, and *Figure 4* in Legrand and Pariente, 1974).

Theoretically one might expect that this kind of specialization might persist in benign tumours, become altered in not too aggressive versions of a tumour, and disappear in anaplastic highly malignant examples. There is some validity in such contentions and this does seem to be so in some groups of related tumours varying only in degrees of differentiation and malignancy.

However as a broad overall generalization this is not acceptable because even in normal tissues the degree and extent of such interdigitations vary

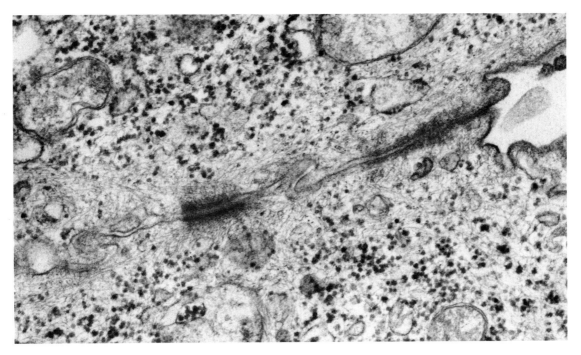

Figure 47   *Transitional cell carcinoma of urinary bladder.*
The tumour cells are linked by a terminal bar comprising a
tight junction and a desmosome. ×50 000

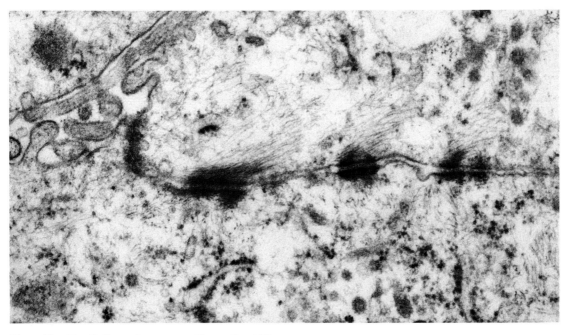

Figure 48   *Mesothelioma. Same case as Figures 5 and 39.*
Note terminal bar comprising a structure acceptable as a
tight junction followed by desmosomes or desmosome-like
structures. ×53 000

from tissue to tissue and certainly some quite benign tumours (e.g. fibroadenoma of the breast) may not show interdigitations between the tumour cells.

Absence of cell junctions

We noted earlier that cell junctions are very rarely encountered in haemopoietic tissues and then only between dendritic reticulum cells. It is therefore not surprising that in lymphomas and leukaemias, cell junctions are not seen even though the cells are very closely packed together. Our own experience (Skinnider and Ghadially, unpublished observations) and that of many others (e.g. Gyorkey *et al.*, 1975) support this view. Needless to say, this is a point of great diagnostic value, for if junctions of any kind are present, this would argue against the diagnosis of a lymphoma or leukaemia. However, it would be a mistake to imagine that the absence of junctions is automatically diagnostic of lymphoma or leukaemia, for even the ubiquitous desmosome-like junction are not present in every sarcoma and one can, theoretically at least, envisage a carcinoma so undifferentiated that it produces no cell junctions.

References

BLOODWORTH, J. M. B. Jr., HIRATSUKA, H., HICKEY, R. C. and WU, J. (1975). Ultrastructure of human thymus, thymic tumours and myasthenia gravis. *Path. Ann.* 10, 329

BÜLOW, M. V. and KLINGMÜLLER, G. (1971). Elektronenmikroskopische untersuchungen des Keratoakanthoms. Vorkommen intracytoplasmatischer Desmosomen. *Arch. Derm. Forsch.*, 241, 292

CARR, I., HANCOCK, B. W., HENRY, L. and MILFORD WARD, A. (1977). *Lymphoreticular Disease*. Oxford: Blackwell Scientific

CHAPMAN, G. B., DRUSIN, L. M. and TODD, J. E. (1963). fine structure of the human wart. *Am. J. Path.*, 42, 619

CLARKE, M. A. (1970). Specialized intercellular junctions in tumor cells. An electron microscope study of mouse sarcoma cells. *Anat. Rec.*, 166, 199

DEBRUYN, P. P. H., MICHELSON, S. and THOMAS, T. B. (1971). The migration of blood cells of the bone marrow through the sinusoidal wall. *J. Morph.*, 133, 417

DEVIS, R. and JAMES, D. W. (1964). Close association between adult guinea pig fibroblasts in tissue culture, studied with the electron microscope. *J. Anat.*, 98, 63

DISCHE, F. E., DARBY, A. J. and HOWARD, E. R. (1978). Malignant synovioma: Electron microscopical findings in three patients and review of the literature. *J. Path.*, 124, 149

FARQUHAR, M. G. and PALADE, G. E. (1963). Junctional complexes in various epithelia. *J. Cell. Biol.*, 17, 375

FARQUHAR, M. G. and PALADE, G. E. (1965). Cell junctions in amphibian skin. *J. Cell. Biol.*, 26, 263

FAWCETT, D. W. (1967). *An Atlas of Fine Structure. The Cell, its Organelles and Inclusions.* Philadelphia: Saunders

FERGUSON, R. J., HAYES, E. R. and WEBBER, R. H. (1972). The nature of the reticulum cell of the bone marrow of the rat: An electron microscopic study of the effects of methotrexate. *Acta Anat.*, 83, 556

FISHER, E. R., McCOY, M. M., II and WECHSLER, H. L. (1972). Analysis of histopathologic and electron microscopic determinants of keratoacanthoma and squamous cell carcinoma. *Cancer*, 29, 1387

GABBIANI, G., KAYE, G. I., LATTES, R. and MAJNO, G. (1971). Synovial sarcoma. *Cancer*, 28, 1031

GHADIALLY, F. N. (1971). Keratoacanothoma. In: *Dermatology in General Medicine*, ed. T. B. Fitzpatrick, pp. 425–436. New York: McGraw-Hill

GHADIALLY, F. N. (1975). *Ultrastructural Pathology of the Cell.* London: Butterworths

GHADIALLY, F. N. (1978). Fine structure of joints. In: *The Joints and Synovial Fluid,* ed. L. Sokoloff. New York: Academic Press

GHADIALLY, F. N. and ILLMAN, O. (1965). Naturally occurring thymomas in the European hamster. *J. Path. Bact.*, 90, 465

GHADIALLY, F. N., LALONDE, J.-M. A. and DICK, C. E. (1978). A mechanism of formation of desmosome-like structures between synovial cells. *Experientia*, 34, 1212

GHADIALLY, F. N. and ROY, S. (1969). *Ultrastructure of Synovial Joints in Health and Disease.* London: Butterworths

GRIMLEY, P. M. and SOKOLOFF, L. (1966). Synovial giant cells in rheumatoid arthritis. *Am. J. Path.*, 49, 931

GYORKEY, F., MIN, K.-W., KRISKO, I. and GYORKEY, P. (1975). The usefulness of electron microscopy in the diagnosis of human tumors. *Hum. Path.*, 6, 421

ITO, U. (1965). Electron microscopic study on benzene intoxicated rat bone marrow with special reference to its reticuloendothelial structure. *Bull. Tokyo Med. Dent. Univ.*, 12, 1

KATAYAMA, I., CECCACCI, L., VALU, A. G. and HORNE, E. O. (1977). Histiocytic lymphoma with sclerosis arising from a nodular lymphoma with a special stromal reaction. *Cancer*, 40, 2203

KELLY, D. E. (1966). Fine structure of desmosomes, hemidesmosomes and adepidermal globular layer in developing newt epidermis. *J. Cell Biol.*, 28, 51

KLEIN, W. and HUTH, F. (1974). The ultrastructure of malignant synovioma. *Beitr. Path. Anat.*, 153, 194

KOJIMA, M. and IMAI, Y. (1973). Genesis and function of germinal center. *Gann Monogr. Cancer Res.*, 15, 1

KUBO, T. (1974). A note on fine structure of synovial sarcoma. *Acta path. Jap.*, 24, 163

LEGRAND, M. and PARIENTE, R. (1974). Étude au microscope électronique de 18 mésothéliomes pleuraux. *Pathologie-Biologie*, 22, 409

LENNERT, K. (1973). Follicular lymphoma. A tumor of the germinal centers. *Gann Monogr. Cancer Res.*, 15, 217

LENNERT K. and NIEDORF, H. R. (1969). Nachweis von desmosomal verknupften Reticulumzellen im follikulären Lymphom (Brill Symmers). *Virchows Arch. Abt. B. Zellpath.*, 4, 148

LEVINE, G. D. (1973). Primary thymic seminoma – a neoplasm ultrastructurally similar to testicular seminoma and distinct from epithelial thymoma. *Cancer*, 31, 729

LEVINE, G. D. and DORFMAN, R. F. (1975). Nodular lymphoma: An ultrastructural study of its relationship to germinal centers and a correlation of light and electron microscopic findings. *Cancer*, **35**, 148

LLOMBART-BOSCH, A. (1975). Epithelio-reticular cell thymoma with lymphocytic 'Emperipolesis'. An ultra-structural study. *Cancer*, **36**, 1794

MACKAY, B., BENNINGTON, J. L. and SKOGLUND, R. W. (1971). The adenomatoid tumour: Fine structural evidence for a mesothelial origin. *Cancer*, **27**, 109

MARTINEZ-PALOMO, A. (1970). Ultrastructural modifications of intercellular junctions in some epithelial tumours. *Lab. Invest.*, **22**, 605

MORI, Y. and LENNERT, K. (1969). *Electron Microscopic Atlas of Lymph Node Cytology and Pathology*. Berlin: Springer

NISTAL, M., CONTRERAS, F. and PANIAGUA, R. (1978). Adenomatoid tumour of the epididymis: histochemical and ultrastructural study of 2 cases. *Br. J. Urol.*, **50**, 121

PALFREY, A. J. and DAVIS, D. V. (1966). The fine structure of chondrocytes. *J. Anat.*, **100**, 213

PEASE, D. C. (1956). An electron microscopic study of red bone marrow. *Blood*, **11**, 501

ROSS, R. and GREENLEE, T. K. (1966). Electron microscopy: attachment sites between connective tissue cells. *Science, N. Y.*, **153**, 997

SEIJI, M. and MIZUNO, F. (1969). Electron microscopic study of Bowen's disease. *Archs Derm.*, **99**, 3

TAKAKI, Y., MASUTANI, M. and KAWADA, A. (1971). Electron microscopic study of keratoacanthoma. *Arch. Derm., Stockholm*, **51**, 21

TANNENBAUM, M., TANNENBAUM, S. and CARTER, H. W. (1978). SEM, BEI and TEM ultrastructural charac-teristic of normal, preneoplastic and neoplastic human transitional epithelia. In *Scanning Electron Microscopy*, **11**, p. 949. Ed. O. Johari and R. P. Becker. Chicago: IIT Research Institute

TRELSTAD, R. L., HAY, E. D. and REVEL, J. P. (1967). Cell contact during early morphogenesis in the chick embryo. *Devl Biol.*, **16**, 78

TRELSTAD, R. L., REVEL, J. P. and HAY, E. D. (1966). Tight junctions between cells in the early chick embryo as visualized with the electron microscope. *J. Cell. Biol.*, **31**, C6

VEERMAN, A. J. P. and van EWIJK, W. (1975). White pulp compartments in the spleen of rats and mice: A light and electron microscopic study of lymphoid and non-lymphoid celltypes in T- and B-areas. *Cell Tiss. Res.*, **156**, 417

WATANABE, Y. (1966). An electron microscopic study of the reticuloendothelial system in the bone marrow. *Tohoku J. Expl Med.*, **89**, 167

WEISS, L. (1957). A study of the structure of splenic sinuses in man and in albino rat with the light microscope and the electron microscope. *J. Biophys. Biochem. Cytol.*, **3**, 599

WEISS, L. (1961). An electron microscopic study of the vascular sinuses of the bone marrow of the rabbit. *Bull. Johns Hopkins Hosp.*, **108**, 171

WEISS, L. (1965). The structure of bone marrow. Functional relationships of vascular and hematopoietic compartments in experimental hemolytic anemia. An electron microscopic study. *J. Morph.*, **117**, 467

ZAMBONI, L. and PEASE, D. C. (1961). The vascular bed of red bone marrow. *J. Ultrastruct. Res.*, **5**, 65

6

Is it a squamous cell carcinoma or an adenocarcinoma?

The two main possibilities which cross one's mind when examining a poorly differentiated carcinoma are embodied in the question asked in this chapter; the answer to which becomes quite important when one examines a metastatic tumour, for it helps narrow down the search for the primary. The adenocarcinoma which one first thinks about is the common mucinous adenocarcinoma and it is the distinction between this and the squamous cell carcinoma which forms the subject of this chapter.*

At the light microscopic level one seeks for secretory granules (with special staining reactions such as PAS if needed) and suggestions of alveolar and tubular differentiation to support the diagnosis of 'poorly differentiated adenocarcinoma' or indications of keratinization and the so-called 'intercellular bridges' to support the diagnosis of 'poorly differentiated squamous cell carcinoma'. If the tumour is so poorly differentiated that light microscopy fails to establish the diagnosis, one can with much profit continue the search for such clues of differentiation by electron microscopy, because: (1) secretory granules too few and/or too small to detect with the light microscope may be revealed by the electron microscope; (2) alveoli with a small lumen formed by cells linked together by terminal bars might be undetectable by light microscopy but they are easily revealed by electron microscopy; and (3) in the case of squamous cell carcinoma, even though light microscopy may not show the so-called 'intercellular bridges', one might find their equivalent in desmosomes and tonofilaments converging upon them† with an electron microscope.

*Adenomas and adenocarcinomas which produce other secretory products (e.g. APUDomas, acinic cell carcinoma and alveolar cell carcinoma) are dealt with in subsequent chapters.
†It is customary to speak about 'tonofilaments attached to desmosomes' but this is not strictly correct, for most of the filaments seem to loop through the plaques of the desmosomes (Kelly, 1966). Hence, alternative terms such as 'converging upon' or 'radiating from' seem preferable (see, for example, Fawcett, 1967).

Types of granules in adenocarcinoma and squamous cell carcinoma

Even in quite poorly differentiated adenocarcinoma one can with diligent search find a few granules acceptable as mucous granules and this can be of diagnostic value.ƒ However, there are two problems one has to contend with: (1) the marked pleomorphism of mucous granules; and (2) the alterations in morphology engendered by the neoplastic state.

Mucous granules are so pleomorphic that it would take innumerable illustrations to show all the forms and sizes that these granules can assume.** Fortunately, in a cystadenoma of the ovary I studied, the cells contained a virtually complete repertoire of granule types (*Figures 49* and *50*). This is a convenient way of showing varieties and developmental stages of mucous granules, but it must be stressed that in normal tissues one finds only one or two versions of the granule in a cell, the commonest being the large lucent granules shown in *Figures 49* and *50*.

In adenocarcinoma also, one may find one or two varieties of granules. Thus, for example, in the adenocarcinoma of the lung illustrated in *Figures 51* and *52* (diagnosed as a poorly differentiated squamous carcinoma by light microscopy) it will be noted that both small electron-dense granules and larger medium-density granules are present. In some poorly differentiated adenocarcinomas it becomes quite difficult to unequivocally identify mucous granules. Here one finds lucent vacuoles containing small amounts of flocculent or particulate material which presumably represents a much diluted or altered mucus produced by the tumour (*Figure 10*). Finally, even such vacuoles are lost and the diagnosis of adenocarcinoma has to rest on other findings.

ƒThis usually but not invariably establishes the diagnosis of mucinous adenocarcinoma, for mucous granules can be found in other tumours, such as some APUDomas.
**A point that sometimes distinguishes mucous granules from many others is their tendency to fuse together.

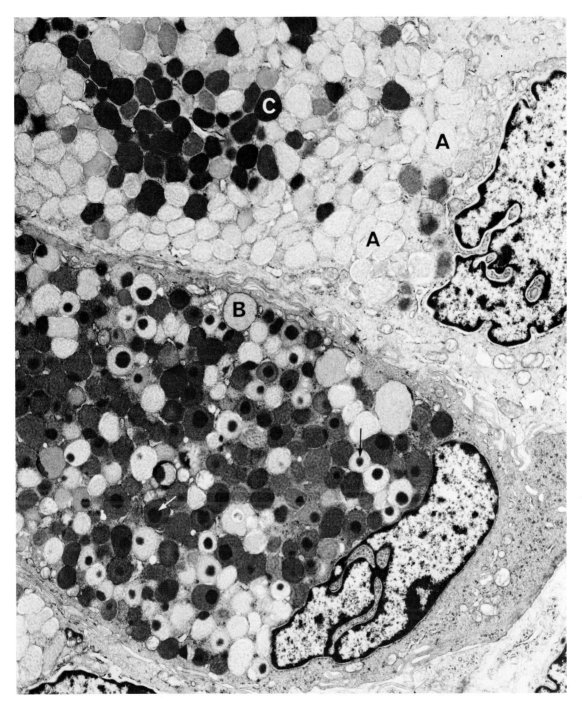

Figure 49   *Mucous cystadenoma of ovary, showing mucous granules of varying morphology. Note large pale granules with a reticular (A) or very fine particulate content (B) (difficult to discern at this low magnification), dense granules (C) and an assortment of 'bull's-eye' granules (arrows) with a central or eccentric core set in a light or dense matrix. ×13 000*

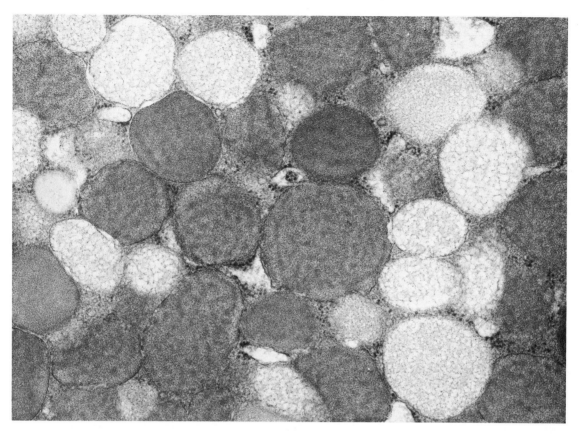

Figure 50 *Mucous cystadenoma of ovary. Same case as Figure 49. This high-power view of mucous granules is presented to show the characteristic reticular pattern and other patterns seen in mucous granules.* ×44 000

An interesting sequence of changes in the morphology of mucous granules has been demonstrated in the colonic mucosa during transformation from the normal to the adenomatous and, finally, to the cancerous state (Mughal and Filipe, 1978). In the normal mucosa the mucous granules are large and lucent and the contents have a faintly reticulated appearance, but as the neoplastic change progresses, bull's-eye granules and dense granules begin to appear. However, it must be stressed that such changes are not specific for the neoplastic state.

In passing, it is worth noting that some of these dense granules seen in mucus-secreting cells and their carcinomas bear some resemblance to the electron-dense zymogen granules found in acinic cells (see Chapter 17), and the 'bull's-eye' type of granule is also at times seen in acinic cells. However,

I am not aware of an instance where an error in diagnosis has occurred on this account, but some thought should be given to this matter before arriving at a diagnosis.

Large irregular electron-dense granules called 'keratohyaline granules' are found in the keratinocytes of the superficial zones of the normal epidermis. I have not seen such granules in the neoplastic keratinocytes of squamous cell or basal cell carcinomas, but I have seen them in keratinocytes from adjacent or overlying epidermis (*Figure 53*). However this may be because most of the squamous cell carcinomas that I have studied have been quite poorly differentiated tumours.

Most published reports on squamous cell carcinomas make no statement about keratohyaline granules. Chen and Harwick (1977) state that they have seen them but provide no illustration to support this, while Vérin *et al.* (1973) comment about their absence in squamous cell carcinomas and Sato and Seiji (1973) report that keratohyaline granules are absent in the dyskaryotic cells of Bowen's disease and leukoplakia. The problem is compounded by the fact that some workers imagine that tonofilaments or tonofibrils are the same as or similar to keratin (see, for example, *Figure 1.8* and accompanying legend in Carr *et al.*, 1977, where indubitable tonofibrils shown in the illustration are described as 'aggregates of microfibrils resembling keratin'). This is not correct, for tonofilaments are not rich in sulphur as is keratin and such filaments occur even in non-keratinizing epithelia. However, keratohyaline (contains proline and amino acids rich in sulphhydryl groups) is deposited as an electron-dense substance in and around tonofibrils which probably serve as a scaffolding for its deposition (Rhodin, 1974; Weiss and Greep, 1977). Attention should be drawn to yet another structure, the membrane-coating granule. Here, again, we do not know whether such granules occur in squamous cell carcinomas. The only comment on this point is by Chen and Harwick (1977), who state that '...membrane coating granules were not observed'.

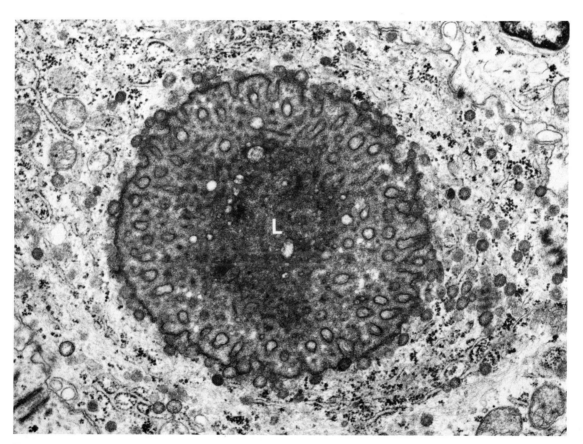

Figure 51 *Poorly differentiated adenocarcinoma of lung that was diagnosed as a squamous cell carcinoma by light microscopy. Note intracytoplasmic lumen (L) into which are discharging numerous quite small, dense mucous granules.* ×24 000

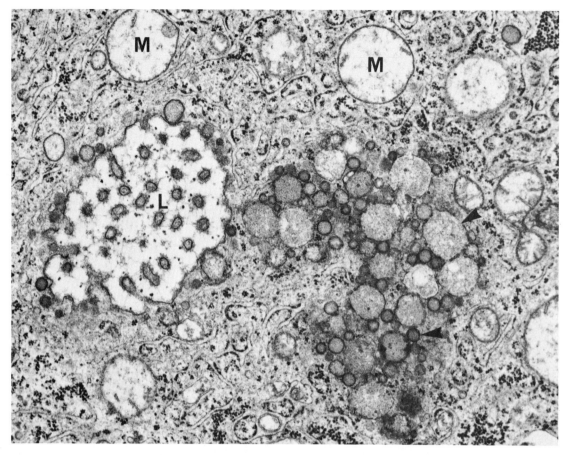

Figure 52 *Poorly differentiated adenocarcinoma of lung. Same case as Figure 51. Note intracellular lumen (L), small and large mucous granules (arrowheads) and swollen mitochondria (M).* ×25 000

Intercellular canaliculi, lumina or spaces

At the light microscopical level the tubular and alveolar pattern of cell arrangement bounding a lumen or canaliculus is a feature of well-differentiated adenocarcinoma but these features cannot be unequivocally identified in a poorly differentiated tumour. Electron microscopy reveals that even in such tumours this pattern of differentiation is still present but the intercellular lumina are too small and/or distorted and/or ill-defined to be appreciated by the light microscope. Unequivocal identification of such lumina (*Figure 54*) bounded by the apices of surrounding cells (the borders of which are connected by tight junctions or terminal bars) is quite easy by electron microscopy. Sparse or numerous microvilli arising from the cell apices are seen within the lumina, which also often contain

secretory products. This feature (i.e. lumina bounded by cells linked by tight junctions) helps to distinguish adenocarcinoma from squamous cell carcinoma, but one should remember that such lamina and modified terminal bars also occur in transitional cell carcinoma, mesothelioma and synovial sarcoma (for details and references see Chapter 5).

Intercellular lumina bounded by cells united by terminal bars do not occur in squamous cell carcinoma, but intercellular spaces occupied by long slender microvilli may be found. Such intercellular spaces (*Figures 55* and *56*) are seen in squamous cell carcinoma, basal cell carcinoma and, to a much lesser extent, also in the normal epidermis. As already mentioned (p. 52), in the case of the normal epidermis this is a shrinkage artefact and it is this which creates the clear spaces across which the so-called 'intercellular bridges' span.

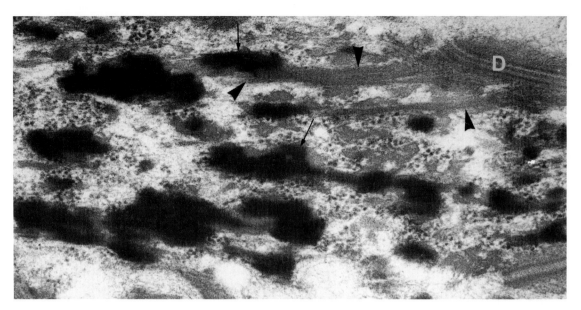

Figure 53 *Keratinocyte from the superficial zone of the epidermis (overlying a basal cell carcinoma) showing a desmosome (D) and keratohyaline granules (arrows),* *formed by the deposition of electron-dense keratohyaline in and around altered tonofibrils (arrowheads) where the filamentous substructure is no longer evident. ×58 000*

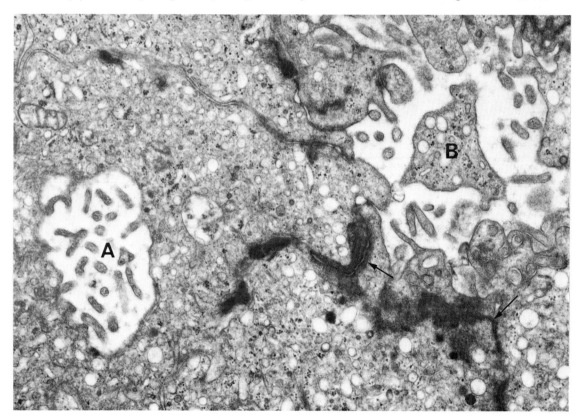

Figure 54 *Poorly differentiated mucinous cystadeno-carcinoma of the ovary showing intracytoplasmic lumen (A) with associated microvilli and an intercellular lumen* *containing a cell projection or fragment (B) and microvilli. Note the modified terminal bars (arrows) linking adjacent cells. ×22 000*

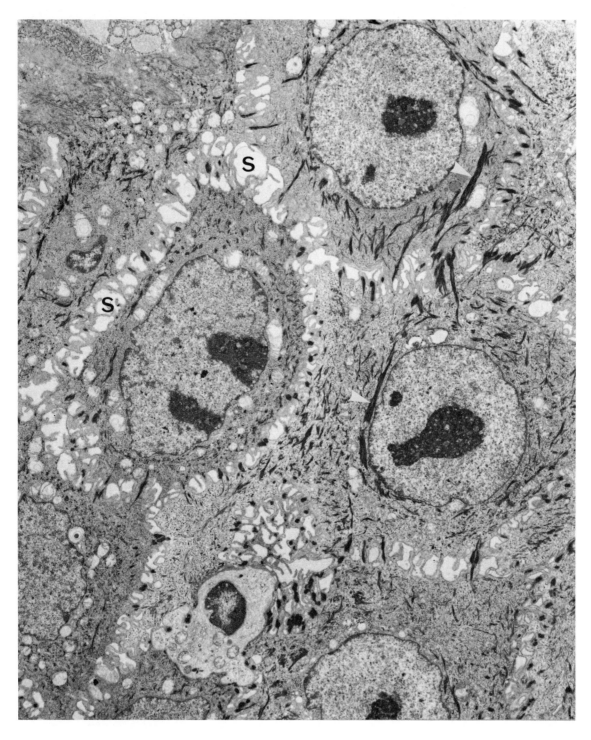

Figure 55   *Squamous cell carcinoma of the lip, showing
intercellular spaces (S), tonofibrils (arrowheads) and
enlarged and marginated nucleoli.* × 7000

74

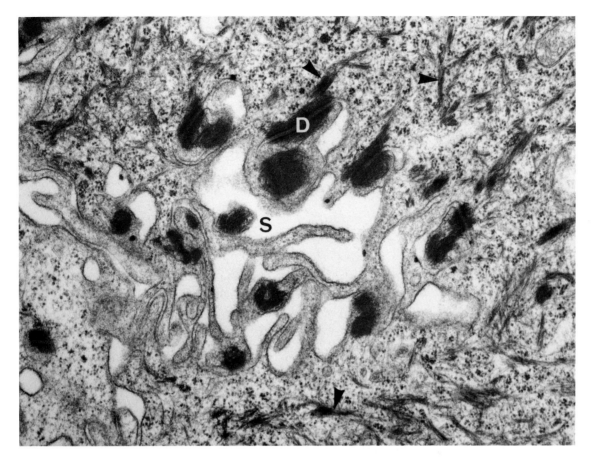

Figure 56 *Squamous cell carcinoma. Same case as Figure 55. Note intercellular spaces (S), desmosomes (D), tonofibrils (arrowheads) and polyribosomes in the cytoplasmic matrix.* ×36 000

In the case of neoplasms of keratinocytes such spaces tend to be larger. This, too, is largely but perhaps not entirely a shrinkage artefact, the larger size being accounted for by a sparsity of desmosomes and/or poor adhesion between tumour cells. The distinguishing features between these spaces and the ones seen in adenocarcinoma are: (1) absence of tight junctions, and (2) absence of secretory material.

Intracellular or intracytoplasmic lumina

In sectioned material these structures appear as vacuoles or cystic spaces bounded by a single membrane bearing a few or numerous microvilli (*Figures 51, 52* and *54*). These structures* probably derive by invaginations of the plasma membrane or by expansion and fusion of Golgi stacks and vacuoles (Harris *et al.*, 1978). From routine sections it is difficult to say whether communication with the extracellular space is present or not. Intracellular lumina are of frequent occurrence in adenocarcinomas from various sites (especially breast carcinomas); rare examples may be found in adenomas

*In passing, one might note that the well-known signet ring cells seen in some adenocarcinomas may contain a collection of mucous granules or a large intracellular lumen containing mucus.

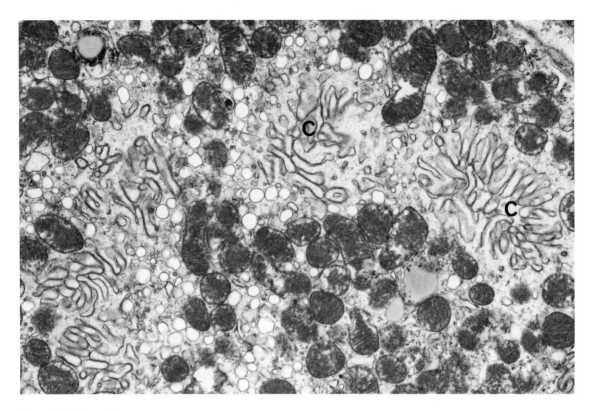

Figure 57 *Normal human gastric parietal cell. An extensive and elaborate intracellular canalicular system (C) lined by numerous microvilli is a striking but normal feature of this cell type.* ×16 000

and also at times in normal secretory cells (*Figure 57*). Such structures have not been found in squamous cell carcinoma.

Filaments

A few filaments may be seen radiating from the desmosomes of an adenocarcinoma and a few intracytoplasmic filaments may also be present. Squamous cell carcinoma is characterized by the presence of tonofilaments, which can usually be distinguished from other intracytoplasmic filaments by the fact that they are usually more electron-dense and have a marked tendency to aggregate and form fibrils. Tonofilaments or tonofibrils may be seen converging upon desmosomes or apparently lying free in the cytoplasmic matrix (*Figure 55*). Tonofibrils are more

frequently encountered and better developed in well-differentiated squamous cell carcinoma. However, even in quite poorly differentiated versions of this tumour, such as those found in the nasopharynx, it is possible to find a few characteristic tonofibrils and desmosomes (Michaels and Hyams, 1977). Hence, this is a point of diagnostic value.

Interdigitations of the cell membrane

This topic has already been discussed earlier (Chapter 5). The only additional point worth making is that such interdigitations are of no value in distinguishing adenocarcinoma from squamous cell carcinoma. Some squamous epithelia (e.g. oral) have quite extensive and elaborate interdigitations, and, as stated earlier, interdigitations are seen between secretory cells also.

References

CARR, I., HANCOCK, B. W., HENRY, L. and WARD, M. A. (1977). *Lymphoreticular Disease*. Oxford: Blackwell Scientific

CHEN. S.-Y. and HARWICK, R. D. (1977). Ultrastructure of oral squamous-cell carcinoma. *Oral Surg., Oral Med., Oral Path.*, **44**, 744

FAWCETT, D. W. (1967). *An Atlas of Fine Structure. The Cell, its Organelles and Inclusions*. Philadelphia: Saunders

HARRIS, M., VASUDEV, K. S., ANFIELD, C. and WELLS, S. (1978). Mucin-producing carcinomas of the breast: ultrastructural observations. *Histopathology*, **2**, 177

KELLY, D. E. (1966). Fine structure of desmosomes, hemidesmosomes and an adepidermal globular layer in developing newt epidermis. *J. Cell Biol.*, **28**, 51

MICHAELS, L. and HYAMS, V. J. (1977). Undifferentiated carcinoma of the nasopharynx: a light and electron microscopical study. *Clin. Otolar.*, **2**, 105

MUGHAL, S. and FILIPE, M. I. (1978). Ultrastructural study of the normal mucosa—adenoma—cancer sequence in the development of familial polyposis coli. *J. Natn. Cancer Inst.*, **60**, 753

RHODIN, J. A. G. (1974). *Histology: A text and atlas.* London, Toronto and New York: Oxford University Press

SATO, A. and SEIJI, M. (1973). Electron microscopic observations of malignant dyskeratosis in leukoplakia and Bowen's disease. *Acta Dermat., Stockholm,* Suppl. 73, p. 101

VÉRIN, Ph., GENDRE, Ph., REBOUL, J., AZALOUX, H. and BASSOULET, J. (1973). Étude en microscopie électronique des épithéliomas basocellulaires et spinocellulaires de la peau des paupières et de la face. *Archs Ophthal., Paris,* **33**, 183

WEISS, L. and GREEP, R. O. (1977). *Histology.* New York: McGraw-Hill

7
Is it a melanoma?

Malignant melanoma figures prominently in the differential diagnosis of an anaplastic tumour. However, the diagnosis of a markedly hypomelanotic or frankly amelanotic melanoma is difficult, because in such instances the melanin granules tend to be too few and/or too small and/or too poorly melanized to be identifiable by the light microscope. Since false positive reactions are common with both the Fontana–Masson stain and the DOPA reaction (Rodriguez and McGavran, 1969), and since both pigmented and non-pigmented melanomas can be tyrosinase-negative (Mackay *et al.*, 1971), the diagnosis of melanoma may be missed and the tumour falsely diagnosed as some other tumour.

The converse situation where a pigmented lesion not containing melanin is misdiagnosed as a melanoma is rare but not unknown. An example where a 'black adenoma' of the adrenal was misdiagnosed as metastatic melanoma on frozen section is reported by Tannenbaum (1973). Electron microscopy revealed that the pigment granules were lysosomes (residual bodies) containing lipofuscin and not melanin granules or melanosomes. More frequently, however, it is an amelanotic melanoma that is mistaken for some other tumour.

It has repeatedly been shown (e.g. Gyorkey *et al.*, 1975; Bonikos, Bensch and Kempson, 1976; Dambrain, Cordier and Noel, 1977) that when all else has failed, the diagnosis of malignant melanoma can be established by electron microscopy. Briefly, this rests on demonstrating organelles of a characteristic morphology called 'melanosomes' in the tumour cells. Although this is usually quite simple, there are pitfalls, so caution is needed.

A melanoma is a tumour of melanocytes. This has been shown to be so for not only human melanomas, but also melanomas of all vertebrates (Gordon, 1948; Ghadially and Gordon, 1957). Hence, it is important to remember that what one is really trying to demonstrate is that the tumour cells are neoplastic melanocytes; demonstration of melanosomes is just one part (albeit an important part) of this exercise.

Our diagnostic difficulties stem from two facts: (1) melanosomes can be found in cells other than melanocytes; and (2) the characteristic internal structure which permits identification of the melanosome may be so markedly altered in the neoplastic state that it becomes quite difficult to confidently assert that a given organelle is in fact a melanosome and not, say, for example, a lysosome. Thus, a diligent search may be required to find at least a few organelles with a morphology unequivocally acceptable as that of the melanosome.

In order to better appreciate these matters, it is worth recalling certain aspects of normal and pathological melanology.

Melanosomes

The concept that melanin synthesis occurs in a specialized organelle of the melanocyte called the melanosome was first proposed by Seiji, Fitzpatrick and Birbeck (1961). It is now clear that this organelle contains tyrosinase, an enzyme which is involved in the oxidation of the colourless amino acid tyrosine to the pigmented polymers we call melanins (eumelanins are brownish-black; plaeomelanins are yellowish-red). DOPA (3,4-dihydroxyphenylalanine) is an intermediate compound formed during the first stage of this oxidative reaction. Thus, when either DOPA or tyrosine is presented to cells containing tyrosinase, they show increased pigmentation. This is the basis of the DOPA reaction (Bloch, 1927) and the tyrosinase reaction (Fitzpatrick *et al.*, 1950); both reveal the presence of the only known enzyme involved in melanin synthesis, namely tyrosinase.

The latest classification of melanosomes (Fitzpatrick *et al.*, 1971) recognizes four stages of melanosome development. The first or earliest stage of development contains no melanin. The last stage is the fully mature melanin granule where the internal structure of the melanosome is totally masked or destroyed by melanin deposition (*Figures 58–64*). The earlier stages possess an active tyrosinase system;

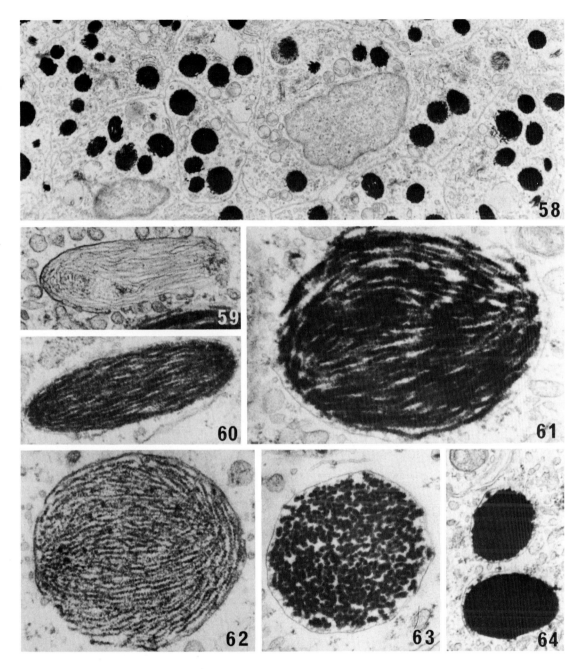

Figures 58—64   *Pigmented epithelium of the eye of a 10-week-old human fetus (From Ghadially, 1975).*
Figure 58 numerous solitary melanosomes are present in the melanocytes. ×6500. Figure 59 A Stage II melanosome showing membranous formations in its interior. ×39 000.
Figures 60—63 Stage III melanosomes. The differences in appearance seen can be related to: (1) the size and shape of the melanosome, (2) the plane of sectioning and (3) amount of melanin present. ×39 000; ×40 000; ×45 000; ×40 000. Figure 64 Stage IV melanosomes (melanin granules) are seen here. ×27 000

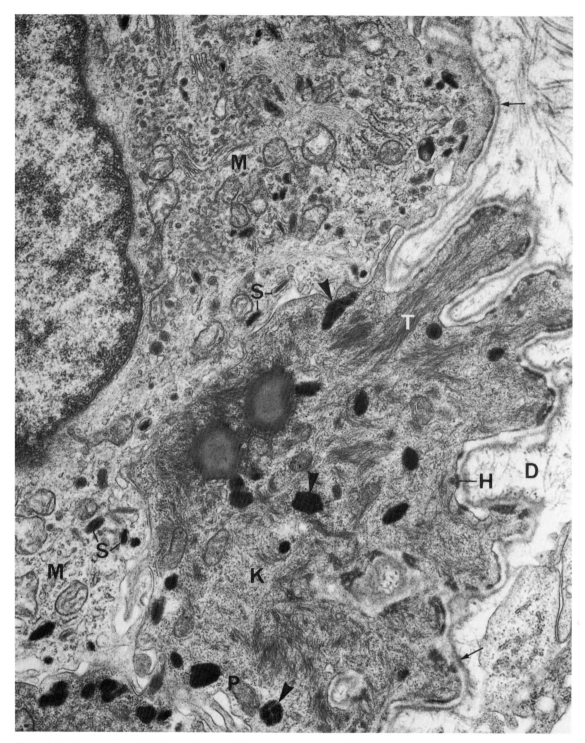

Figure 65   *Normal caucasoid skin showing a melanocyte (M) and a keratinocyte (K) separated from the dermis (D) by a basal lamina (arrows). The melanocyte has a paler appearance and contains numerous solitary melanosomes (S). The keratinocyte has a darker appearance and con-* *tains bundles of tonofilaments forming tonofibrils (T) and hemidesmosomes (H) along its basal border. Numerous compound melanosomes (arrowheads) are present in the keratinocyte. ×25 000 (From Ghadially, 1975)*

the last stage does not. It is now generally held* that tyrosinase is synthesized by the polyribosomes of the rough endoplasmic reticulum and transported via this organelle to the Golgi complex, where it is parcelled off into small vesicles (melanosome stage I†). The vesicles then enlarge and elongate to form an oval organelle (melanosome stage II, or pre-melanosome∮) in which develops a characteristic patterned membranous structure, the three-dimensional morphology of which is difficult to interpret. The internal structure has been regarded as a folded membrane, a concentric sheet or a helical tubular structure with a space of about 10 nm between each turn of the coil.** Deposition of melanin on the membranous structure heralds the next stage (melanosome stage III, or partially melanized melanosome), and the completion of this process produces a uniformly electron-dense granule without discernible internal structure (melanosome stage IV, mature melanosome or melanin granule).

Melanocytes

It is now generally accepted that the melanocyte (normal or neoplastic) is the only cell capable of producing melanosomes; a probable exception to this is the Schwann cell, but more about that later. Hence, in melanocytes one finds solitary or discrete melanosomes (*Figures 58* and *65*) in various stages of development. The other features of interest are as follows: (1) melanocytes do not form desmosomes or other types of cell junctions with one another or with adjacent cells such as keratinocytes;†† (2) the cytoplasmic matrix of the melanocyte is much lighter (less electron-dense) than that of the keratinocyte; (3) tonofilaments are absent, and intracytoplasmic filaments of other types are usually sparse or absent; and (4) the Golgi complex is fairly well developed,

*For other theories of melanosome formation see Jimbow *et al.* (1976).
†The stage I melanosome cannot be confidently identified on morphological grounds alone, but it can be demonstrated by cytochemical methods.
∮The term 'premelanosome' is unnecessary and confusing and, hence, should not be used. The organelle in which melanin synthesis occurs should obviously be called a melanosome.
**In sectioned material various appearances are seen in stages II and III melanosomes. A common appearance is that of a series of parallel or concentric zigzag or dotted lines. Another appearance seen is that of striated or banded material lying in the melanosome.
††Epidermal cells producing keratin are collectively referred to as keratinocytes. This includes basal cells and prickle cells.

particularly if active synthesis of melanosomes is occurring.

Distribution of solitary and compound melanosomes in various cell types

Melanosomes may occur as discrete solitary organelles or they may occur in groups surrounded by a single membrane. The latter arrangement is referred to as a compound melanosome or a melanosome complex. Compound melanosomes are typically seen in melanophages (e.g. dermal macrophages which have ingested melanin) and, in fact, they are heterolysosomes containing phagocytosed melanosomes (*Figure 66*). Solitary melanosomes are rarely seen in melanophages, and even rarer is the finding of a compound melanosome in a melanocyte. The latter presumably represents an autolysosome (autophagic vacuole) where a portion of cytoplasm containing a few melanosomes is sequestrated within the melanocyte.

In the keratinocytes of Caucasoids and Mongoloids compound melanosomes occur (the melanosomes suffer degradation into small electron-dense particles within these lysosomal bodies), but in the keratinocytes of Negroids and Australoids solitary melanosomes larger than in Caucasoids are found. All the melanosomes in keratinocytes, whether solitary or compound, are derived secondarily from adjacent melanocytes; they are not synthesized in the keratinocyte. Similarly, on a rare occasion one might see a melanosome or a melanosome complex in a Langerhans cell, but this, too, is derived from the melanocyte.

Compound melanosomes have been seen in Schwann cells (see, for example, illustrations in Sato *et al.*, 1977) and one can see no reason why one may not also find an occasional solitary melanosome in this cell type, but clearly these are derived from adjacent melanocytes. The idea that Schwann cells can synthesize melanosomes or that they can transform into melanocytes and produce melanosomes is attractive, for both these cell types stem from the neural crest; however, unequivocal proof of this is lacking.

This subject is reviewed by Hahn *et al.* (1976), and they claim that '. . .electron microscopy revealed various stages of development of melanosomes in neoplastic cells of Schwann, the first direct demonstration in human material that these cells are melanogenic'. Unfortunately, not a single illustration in their paper supports this contention, the appearances depicted being more in keeping with the

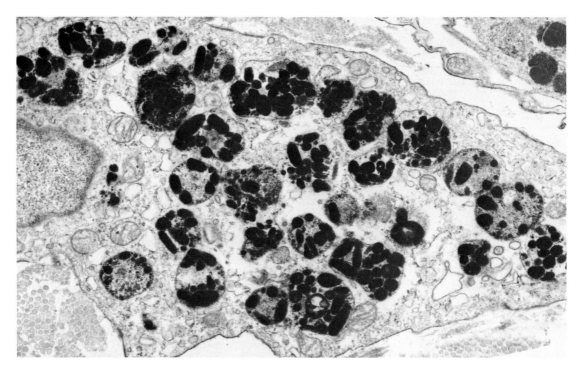

Figure 66   *Dermal macrophage (melanophage) from human skin containing compound melanosomes.* ×15 000

morphology of lysosomes. Certainly, not a single melanosome with characteristic internal structure is depicted in this paper.

To support such contentions these authors (and many others) quote the study of Nakai and Rappaport (1963), who purported to show that the intradermal blue-naevi-like melanotic lesions (they very rarely metastasize) which develop in carcinogen-painted hamster skin arise from Schwann cells. This is quite surprising, since it has repeatedly been shown by many workers that these tumours arise from the perifollicular collection of melanocytes of the small pigmented spot which occur in only a few species such as the Syrian hamster, the Chinese hamster and the Mongolian gerbil, and it is only in these animals that these intradermal melanotic lesions develop as a result of chemical carcinogenesis (Ghadially and Barker, 1960; Illman and Ghadially, 1960, 1966; Quevedo *et al*., 1961, 1968; Ghadially and Illman, 1963, 1966; Oberman and Riviere, 1966; Parish and Searle, 1966). The theory of the Schwann cell origin of these tumours is untenable because it does not explain this species difference nor does it take into account the abundant melanocytes present in this region.

Ultrastructure of melanoma and diagnostic pitfalls

In melanomas one finds two types of cells — neoplastic melanocytes and non-neoplastic melanophages. As in the normal state, the former are characterized by the presence of solitary melanosomes, the latter by compound melanosomes (*Figures 67–71*). On the basis of this difference, with the electron microscope one can quite confidently distinguish melanocytes and melanophages, and this is of diagnostic value.

For example, when lymph node deposits are evaluated in cases of melanoma, if only melanophages are found, then obviously a true neoplastic secondary deposit has not developed, but if neoplastic melanocytes are found, it has. However, it must be remembered that in the case of blue naevi secondary deposits in the regional lymph node may contain both melanophages and melanocytes, yet the tumour may not be truly malignant in the sense that it is highly unlikely to spread to distant sites and kill the patient. (For references see Silverberg *et al*., 1971.)

We have seen that both solitary and compound

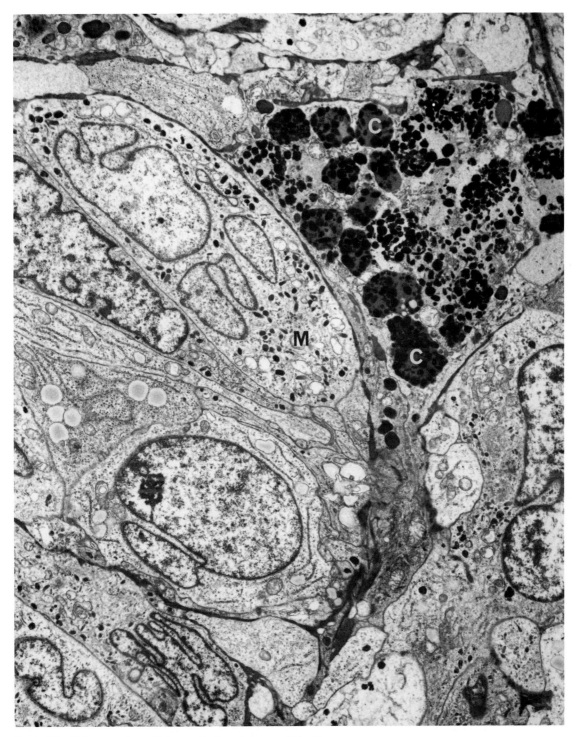

Figure 67   *Melanoma of eye. Note neoplastic melanocytes (M) with*
irregular nuclei and numerous solitary melanosomes. Compound
melanosomes (C) are present in a melanophage. ×8000

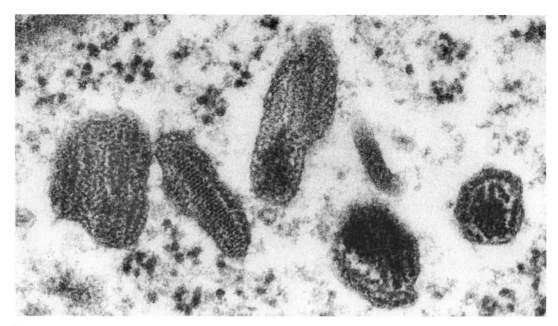

Figure 68   *High-power view of melanosomes from tumour shown in Figure 67. Note the characteristic transverse striations and zig-zag pattern.* ×*111 000*

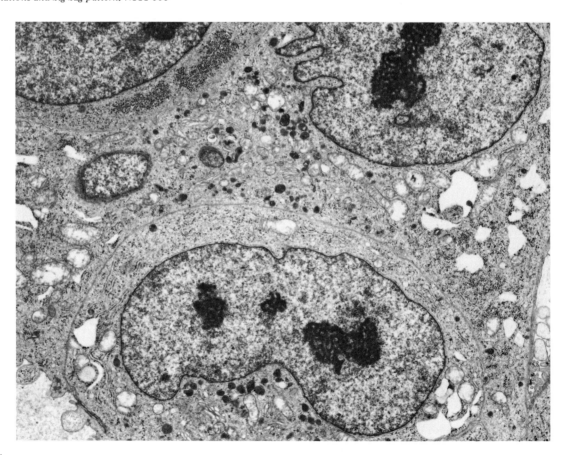

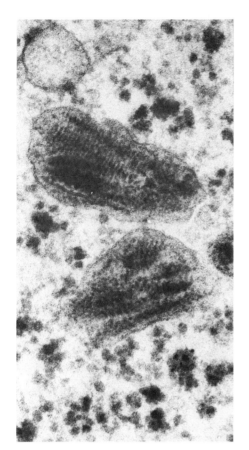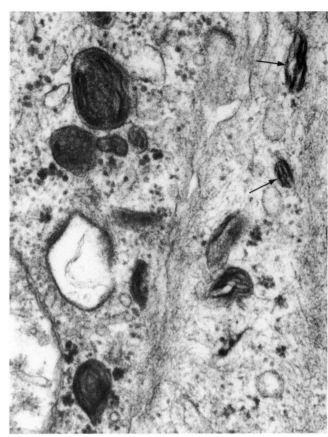

Figures 70 and 71   Malignant melanoma. High-power views
from tumour illustrated in Figure 69. The characteristic
striated pattern seen in Figure 70 (left) unequivocally establishes that these structures are melanosomes, but the patterns
seen in Figure 71 (right) can be mimicked by myelinoid
membranes seen in other situations, although some of these
(arrows) are almost certainly altered or atypical melanosomes. ×105 000; ×69 000

◀ Figure 69   (bottom, facing page) Neoplastic melanocytes
from a malignant effusion in the peritoneal cavity (primary
in the skin) showing numerous small electron-dense bodies.
At high magnification quite a few of these showed the
characteristic structure of melanosomes. The diagnosis of
amelanotic melanoma was considered that could not be
established by light microscopy. It would appear that the
difficulty in diagnosis stems from the fact that most of the
melanosomes are less than 0.25 μm in size. Other points of
interest include enlarged irregular nuclei with large multiple
nucleoli expected in a malignant tumour and the absence
of cell junctions between cells. ×8000

melanosomes may be found in keratinocytes. It is, therefore, not surprising that melanosomes may be found in some examples of squamous and basal cell carcinoma (Lightiger, Mackay and Tessmer, 1970; Bleehen, 1975; Deppe, Pullmann and Steigleder, 1976; Jauregui and Klintworth, 1976), because active melanocytes become incorporated in such tumours. However, the presence of melanosomes in these tumour cells poses no great diagnostic problem, because such tumours of keratinocytes contain tonofilaments and desmosomes, while melanomas do not show these features.

Consider now the problem of morphological alterations in melanosomes engendered by the neo-plastic state. Clearly, the demonstration of oval or cigar-shaped electron-dense bodies within tumour cells is not good enough to base a diagnosis of melanoma on, for these could be lysosomes. For unequivocal identification of a melanosome one should demonstrate the characteristic internal structure. For example, the transversely banded pattern seen in the single membrane bound organ-elles depicted in *Figures 68* and *70* clearly identifies them as melanosomes. Some of the laminated structures shown in *Figure 71* could be altered melanosomes but caution is needed, for myelino-somes (i.e. lysosomes containing myelinoid membranes) have a similar appearance and small whorls of myelinoid membranes can so easily be created as an artefact of glutaraldehyde fixation (Chapter 1).

Finally, it may be worth pointing out that certain profiles of the rod-shaped tubular body (which is the specific organelle of vascular endo-thelia) bear some superficial resemblance to melanosomes, for it can be quite electron-dense and show a striated appearance (*Figure 72*). I have seen this organelle mistakenly identified as: (1) melanosomes injected into the endothelial cells by melanocytes; (2) lysosomal granules extruded into endothelial cells from macrophages; and (3) an organism of probable aetiological significance in rheumatoid arthritis (Highton, Caughey and Rayns; 1966). This, of course, is not a serious or even a

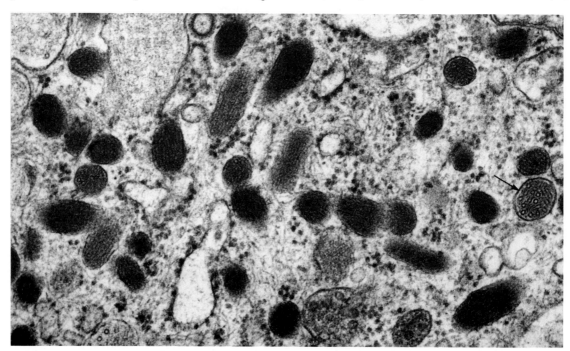

Figure 72 *Rod-shaped tubulated bodies in a capillary endothelial cell. Note their density and the longitudinally striated appearance produced by microtubules in their interior. A transversely sectioned (arrow) rod-shaped tubulated body shows the microtubules more distinctly.* ×66 000

genuine problem in the diagnosis of melanoma, but it is worth remembering that this organelle can present many and varied appearances (see Ghadially, 1975) which can be confusing, particularly if the plane of section is such that the vessel bearing these cells is not easily recognized.

References

BLEEHEN, S. S. (1975). Pigmented basal cell epithelioma, *Br. J. Derm.,* **93**, 361

BLOCH, B. (1927). Das Pigment. *Jadassohns Handb. Haut-Greschl. Krankh.,* **1**, 434

BONIKOS, D. S., BENSCH, K. G. and KEMPSON, R. L. (1976). The contribution of electron microscopy to the differential diagnosis of tumours. *Beitr. Path. Anat.,* **158**, 417

DAMBRAIN, R., CORDIER, A and NOEL, H. (1977). Ultrastructure du mélanome malin achromique de la gencive. Intérét en diagnostic différentiel. *Rev. Stomatol.,* **78**, 519

DEPPE, R., PULLMANN, H. and STEIGLEDER, G. K. (1976). Dopa-positive cells and melanin in basal cell epithelioma (BCE). *Archs Derm. Res.,* **256**, 79

FITZPATRICK, T. B., BECKER, S. W. Jr., LERNER, A. B. and MONTGOMERY, H. (1950). Tyrosinase in human skin: demonstration of its presence and its role in human melanin formation. *Science, N.Y.,* **112**, 223

FITZPATRICK, T. B., QUEVEDO, W. C. Jr., SZABO, G. and SEIJI, M. (1971). Biology of the melanin pigmentary system. In: *Dermatology in General Medicine,* ed. T. B. Fitzpatrick, K. A. Arndt, W. H. Clarke, A. Z. Eisen, E. J. Van Scott and J. H. Vaughan, p. 117. New York: McGraw-Hill

GHADIALLY, F. N. (1975). *Ultrastructural Pathology of the Cell.* London: Butterworths

GHADIALLY, F. N. and BARKER, J. F. (1960). The histogenesis of experimentally induced melanotic tumours in the Syrian hamster (*Cricetus auratus*). *J. Path. Bact.,* **79**, 263

GHADIALLY, F. N. and GORDON, M. (1957). A localized melanoma in a hybrid fish *Lebistex* X *Molliensia. Cancer Res.,* **17**, 597

GHADIALLY, F. N. and ILLMAN, O. (1963). The histogenesis of experimentally produced melanotic tumours in the Chinese hamster (*Cricetulus criseus*). *Br. J. Cancer,* **17**, 727

GHADIALLY, F. N. and ILLMAN, O. (1966). Small pigmented spots in hamsters. In: *Structure and Control of the Melanocyte,* ed. G. Della Porta and O. Muhlbock, pp. 259–268. Berlin: Springer

GORDON, M. (1948). Effects of five primary genes on the site of melanomas in fishes and the influence of two color genes on their pigmentation. In: *The Biology of Melanomas,* ed. R. W. Miner and M. Gordon. *Spec. Pubs N.Y. Acad. Sci.,* **4**, 216

GYORKEY, F., MIN, K.-W., KRISKO, I. and GYORKEY, P. (1975). The usefulness of electron microscopy in the diagnosis of human tumors. *Hum. Path.,* **6**, 421

HAHN, J. F., NETSKY, M. G., BUTLER, A. B. and SPERBER, E. E. (1976). Pigmented ganglioneuroblastoma: relation of melanin and lipofuscin to schwannomas and other tumours of neural crest origin. *J. Neuropath.,* **35**, 393

HIGHTON, T. C., CAUGHEY, D. E. and RAYNS, D. G. (1966). A new inclusion body in rheumatoid synovia. *Ann. Rheum Dis.,* **25**, 149

ILLMAN, O. and GHADIALLY, F. N. (1960). Coat colour and experimental melanotic tumour production in the hamster. *Br. J. Cancer,* **14**, 483

ILLMAN, O. and GHADIALLY, F. N. (1966). Effect of oestrogen on the small pigmented spots in hamsters. *Nature, Lond.* **211**, 1303

JAUREGUI, H. O. and KLINTWORTH, G. K. (1976). Pigmented squamous cell carcinoma of cornea and conjunctiva. *Cancer,* **38**, 778

JIMBOW, K., QUEVEDO, W. C. Jr., FITZPATRICK, T. B. and SZABO, G. (1976). Some aspects of melanin biology: 1950-1975. *J. Invest. Derm.,* **67**, 72

LICHTIGER, B., MACKAY, B. and TESSMER, C. F. (1970). Spindle-cell variant of squamous carcinoma. *Cancer,* **26**, 1311

MACKAY, B., LICHTIGER, B., TESSMER, C. F. and CHANG, J. P. (1971). The pathologic diagnosis of metastatic malignant melanoma. *Cancer Bull.,* **23**, 30

NAKAI, T. and RAPPAPORT, H. (1963). A study of the histogenesis of experimental melanotic tumours resembling cellular blue nevi. The evidence in support of their neurogenic origin. *Am. J. Path.,* **43**, 175

OBERMAN, B. and RIVIERE, M. R. (1966). Experimental melanoma in hamsters. In: *Structure and Control of the Melanocyte,* ed. G. Della Porta and O. Muhlbock, pp. 268–272. Berlin: Springer

PARISH, D. J. and SEARLE, C. E. (1966). The carcinogenicity of beta-propiolactone and 4-nitroquinoline N-Oxide for the skin of the golden hamster. *Br. J. Cancer,* **20**, 206

QUEVEDO, W. C. Jr., BIENIEKI, T. C., FAUSTO, N. and MAGALINI, S. I. (1968). Induction of pigmentary changes in the skin of the mongolian gerbil by chemical carcinogens. *Experientia,* **24**, 585

QUEVEDO, W. C. Jr., CAIRNS, J. M., SMITH, J. A., BOCK, F. G. and BURNS, R. J. (1961). Induction of melanotic tumours in the white (partial albino) Syrian hamster. *Nature, Lond.,* **189**, 936

RODRIGUEZ, H. A. and McGAVRAN, M. H. (1969). A modified DOPA reaction for the diagnostic and investigation of pigment cells. *Am. J. Clin. Path.,* **52**, 219

SATO, S., OGIHARA, Y., HIRAGA, K., NISHIJIMA, A. and HIDANO, A. (1977). Fine structure of unmyelinated nerves in neonatal skin. *J. Cutaneous Path.,* **4**, 1

SEIJI, M., FITZPATRICK, T. B. and BIRBECK, M. S. C. (1961). The melanosome: a distinctive subcellular particle of mammalian melanocytes and the site of melanogenesis. *J. Invest. Derm.,* **36**, 243

SILVERBERG, G. D., KADIN, M. E., DORFMAN, R. F., HANBERY, J. W. and PROLO, D. J. (1971). Invasion of the brain by a cellular blue nevus of the scalp. *Cancer,* **27**, 349

TANNENBAUM, M. (1973). Ultrastructural pathology of the adrenal cortex. *Path. Ann.,* **8**, 109

8
Is it an APUDoma?
What type of APUDoma is it?

Before answering these questions it is essential to recall some points regarding the classification and nomenclature of APUD cells (amine precursor uptake and decarboxylation) and their tumours. It is at present believed that there are about 24 types of APUD cells (Dobbins, 1978) and that this endocrine cell system is derived from the neural crest (Pearse, 1974). In the past these cells were referred to (depending on site and staining reactions) by various terms, such as 'argentaffin cells', 'argyrophile cells', 'chromaffin cells' and 'kultschitzky cells'. The tumours from these cells* include carcinoids, islet cell tumours, pituitary adenomas, parathyroid adenomas,† medullary thyroid carcinoma, paragangliomas and phaeochromocytomas, but now one tries to classify them under various terms with a functional connotation, such as 'gastrinoma', 'glucagonoma', 'insulinoma' and 'calcitoninoma' (C cell tumour).

Although the term 'APUDoma' is useful, for it brings together a confusing collection of diverse neoplasms into a comprehensible group, it does not appear practical to pursue the classification of these tumours on the basis of hormone produced too far, for in many instances more than one hormone is produced or stored by a tumour.

Is it an APUDoma?

A forte of the electron microscopist is his ability to confidently diagnose an APUDoma when histological and histochemical tests have failed to establish the diagnosis, probably because of paucity of

secretory granules in the tumour. APUDomas have been discovered by electron microscopy when one was not even suspected on the basis of clinical and histopathological findings. Further, our concepts regarding the histogenesis of some tumours have been altered by the APUD concept and electron microscopy. For example, we now know that the medullary carcinoma of the thyroid is a calcitonin producing APUDoma of C cell origin and that the oat cell carcinoma of the lung is an APUDoma, with a behaviour and prognosis probably different from that of other anaplastic carcinomas of the lung (more about this later). Such feats are possible because APUD cells and their tumours contain granules which are readily identifiable on the basis of their size and ultrastructural morphology.

Such APUD granules include: (1) small, round, uniformly electron-dense granules 100—250 nm in diameter; (2) larger uniformly electron-dense granules measuring 200—400 nm in diameter (3) uniformly electron-dense granules which are pleomorphic (pear-shaped, dumb-bell shaped and egg-shaped); (4) dense core granules, which, as their name implies, have a dense core, but the periphery is lucent or of medium density;* and (5) electron-lucent granules containing an electron-dense crystalline core (beta cells of pancreas only).

Although one can often at a glance diagnose an APUDoma with the electron microscope, there are some pitfalls which one must guard against. As we have seen, APUD granules are, by and large, electron-dense structures bound by a single membrane and as such there is a real danger of mistaking lysosomes for APUD granules, or vice versa. Here the saving grace is that APUD granules show only small variations in size and morphology, whereas lysosomes tend to be pleomorphic, in size and content. If sufficient numbers are present in the specimen, there

---

*The melanocyte is also considered to be a member of the APUD system, but melanomas are best considered separately (Chapter 7).
†The parathyroid chief cell has granules ultrastructurally characteristic of APUD cells and produces a peptide hormone but some authors are reluctant to accept these cells as part of APUD system, because of their cytochemical properties. However, other investigators have recommended their inclusion in the APUD system (e.g. Weichert, 1970).

---

*The dense core granule is sometimes looked upon as a dense granule lying in an ill-fitting membrane or a loose-fitting vesicle or membrane.

is usually no difficulty in deciding what one is looking at, but when only rare 'dense granules' are present, the distinction between lysosome and APUD granule becomes difficult or impossible.

Small osmiophilic lipid droplets may at times cause problems, but these are not as a rule bound by a membrane and to the experienced eye at least the texture is quite different. Further, lipid droplets vary quite a bit in size, which contrasts with the rather restricted size range of APUD granules.

Apart from the secretory granules discussed above, there are no other ultrastructural features in APUDomas which are of diagnostic import. These tumours usually contain a modest amount of rough endoplasmic reticulum and Golgi complex. Although endocrine cells do not pour out their secretion in a system of ducts, one does occasionally find inter-cellular lumina with accompanying tight junctions and desmosomes and also intracytoplasmic lumina.* In this respect the APUDomas resemble other adenomas and adenocarcinomas (see Chapter 6).

APUD cells are widely distributed and one finds occasionally such cells 'accidentally included' in a variety of neoplasms,† but this presents no diagnostic problems once it is recognized that the mere presence of APUD cells does not in itself automatically establish the diagnosis of APUDoma (Lillie and Glenner, 1960). Noteworthy also is the fact that some APUD cells contain not only the characteristic secretory granules, but also mucous granules; but this, too, does not cause confusion once this fact is realized.

Finally, there is the problem of paucity and im-maturity of APUD granules. Often APUDomas associated with severe hormonal syndromes contain sparse immature-looking granules (i.e. the electron-dense granules may not be quite so electron-dense, or in the case of insulinoma the characteristic crystalline core may not be formed). Conversely, APUDomas associated with mild hormonal dis-turbance may contain numerous well-developed granules. Such differences may be explained by sup-posing that hormones are being produced (not necessarily in excessive amounts) but are not being stored in granules and that the hormones are released

continually or in an uncontrolled manner from the tumour.

Yet another possibility is that the secretory product produced by the neoplastic cells may not be structurally and functionally identical with that produced by their normal counterparts (Gould, 1977) or that a 'prohormone' (i.e. an 'immature' precursor product) is produced which is not trans-formed into the biologically active hormone.

What type of APUDoma is it?

We have seen that there are only a few morpho-logically distinct types of granules but some two dozen varieties of APUD cells, all presumably capable of producing tumours. Further, the morphology of these granules varies according to the method of fixation, the freshness of the tissue and the secretory phase or cycle of the cell. Thus, on morphological grounds alone, one can hardly hope to establish exactly which particular type of APUD cell a given tumour is derived from. Besides, as is only to be expected, the secretory granule produced by a tumour cell is hardly likely to be the exact replica of that found in the normal state. Therefore, as a rule the precise histogenesis of an APUDoma cannot be established by electron microscopy alone, but in conjunction with clinical and biochemical studies quite interesting and valuable data can be obtained. This and other points of interest will be revealed as we study some of the APUDomas. A detailed de-scription of all APUDomas is outside the scope of this small book.

Islet cells and islet cell tumours

Normal islet cells

There is much confusion regarding the number of cell types present in the normal islet and the no-menclature of these cells. Morphologically three or perhaps four cell types may be recognized. They are: (1) Alpha cell (*Figures 73* and *74*) containing dense core granules. The halo around the core is quite lucent in osmium-fixed material but of a medium density after glutaraldehyde fixation. (2) Beta cell (*Figure 73*) with its highly characteristic granules containing a crystalline core. (3) The chromophobic (C cell) cell, which lacks granules. (4) The delta cell (*Figure 75*), which has granules of variable density where the appearance ranges from light and punctate or flocculent to dense and compact.

---

*See, for example, Suzuki and Matsuyama (1971), who illustrate an intracellular lumen lined with microvilli in a beta cell tumour of the pancreas.

†For example, APUD cells form an integral element in 3.1 per cent of gastric and 2.5 per cent of intestinal carcinomas (Kubo and Watanabe, 1971).

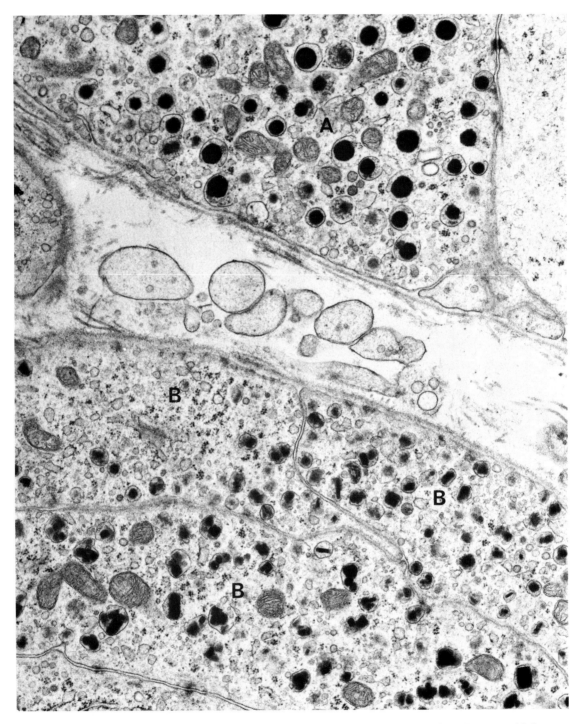

Figure 73   *Human pancreatic islet, fixed in osmium (cacodylate buffer) and stained with uranium and lead. Note alpha cell (A) containing dense core granules with a lucent halo and beta cells (B) containing granules with a crystalline core. Compare with glutaraldehyde-fixed material shown in Figure 74. ×27 000 (Ghadially and Larsen, unpublished electron micrograph)*

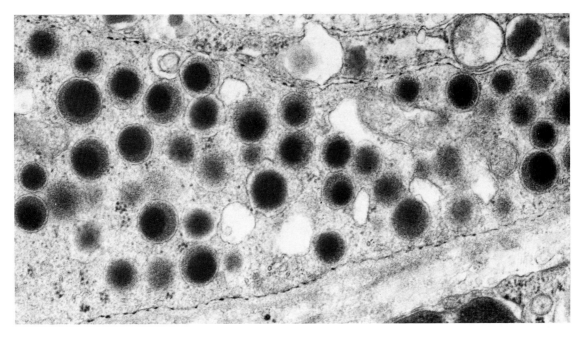

Figure 74 *Human pancreatic islet. Same case as Figure 73 but fixed in glutaraldehyde, post-fixed in osmium and stained with uranium and lead. The halo of the alpha cell granules shown here is of medium density and not lucent as seen in Figure 73. This is because some proteinaceous material leaches out during osmium fixation, as explained in Chapter 1. ×45 000*

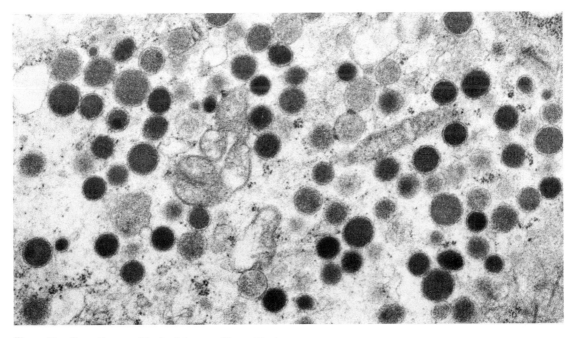

Figure 75 *From the same block of tissue as Figure 74. A delta cell showing granules of varying densities. ×36 000*

In the past most workers regarded chromophobic cells and delta cells as a stage of the development or secretory cycle of the alpha cell; therefore, all non-beta granulated (i.e. without crystalline core) cells were designated alpha cells (Greider and Elliott, 1964; Like, 1967; Toker, 1967; Waisman, 1969). This situation began to change with the advent of immunofluorescence techniques and the term 'A$_1$ cells' (probably the same as D cells) was given to cells which presumably produced gastrin and 'A$_2$ cells' (probably the same as A cells) to cells which presumably produce glucagon (for references see Grieder, Bencosme and Lechago, 1970). Other authors, however, have contended that the converse is correct (for references and discussion see Zeitoun and Lehy, 1970). This controversy stems from the difficulty of establishing a correlation between cells which give a positive Hellman—Hellerström reaction and their corresponding ultrastructural appearance.

There seems little point in continuing with this new classification (i.e. A$_1$ and A$_2$ cells) and arguing whether it is the A$_1$ or the A$_2$ cell which is the equivalent of the D cell. The situation is now becoming even more complex, for Capella et al. (1977) claim that up to seven types of APUD cells occur in the pancreas. According to these authors, these include '. . .glucagon A cells, insulin B cells, somatostatin D cells, pancreatic peptide F cells and 5-hydroxytryptamine E.C. cells. In addition D$_1$ cells which have been proposed as the cell type producing VIP and possible P cells of unknown function are seen.'

As may be expected, the problem becomes more acute when one is trying to classify neoplasms arising

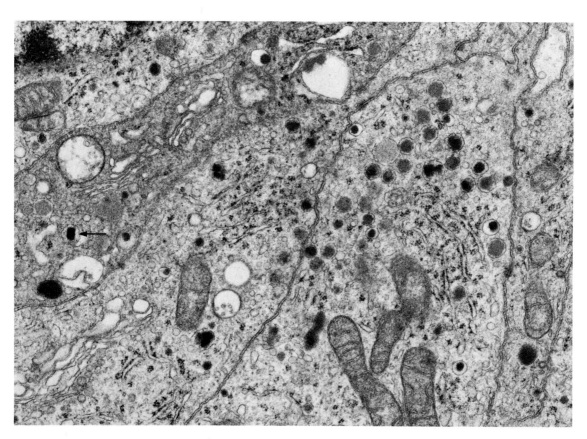

Figure 76 *Insulinoma, from a patient with marked hyper-insulinaemic hypoglycaemia. The tumour cells show pleomorphic granules of little diagnostic value save one* (arrow) *which shows the characteristic cystalline core.* ×24 000

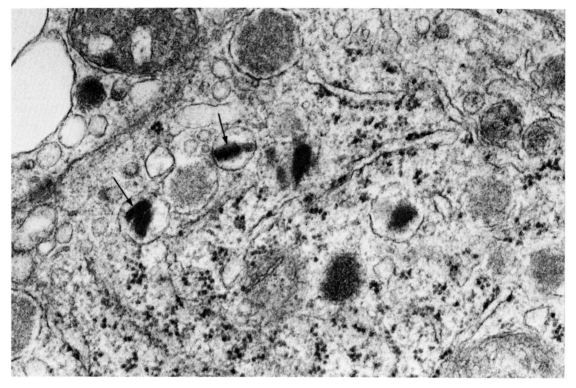

Figure 77 *Same tumour as in Figure 76, showing granules with crystalline cores (arrows).* ×59 000

from these cells, for changes in granular size and morphology are engendered by the neoplastic state. The task of sorting things out is not helped by case reports based on formalin-fixed autopsy material (e.g. Kawaoi, Okano and Uchida, 1977) and papers purporting to show granular differences in illustrations not much larger than some postage stamps (e.g. Harano *et al.*, 1975).

Insulinoma (beta cell tumour)

Innumerable studies on insulinomas have been published but there are only a few in which correlations between immunoradiological assay, histology and ultrastructure have been attempted. The outstanding paper here is by Creutzfeldt *et al.* (1973), who studied 28 human insulinomas in this fashion. They found that in 13 cases the tumour cells contained typical beta cell granules, while in another 7 cases both typical and atypical granules (i.e. granules of various morphology but lacking a crystalline core) were found. These 20 cases could be diagnosed as 'insulinoma' by electron microscopic appearances alone. In another 4 cases they found atypical granules

only, while in the remaining 4 cases the tumours were virtually agranular; here the diagnosis rested on clinical and biochemical findings.

The insulinoma illustrated in *Figures 76* and *77* comes from a patient who had a severe hyperinsulinaemic hypoglycaemia. The tumour cells showed a variety of granules, such as dense core granules, dense granules and granules whose contents were of a low density. Such granules are of no diagnostic value, for one can find occasional examples of such granules not only in beta cells, but also in a variety of other APUD cells, including alpha cells and delta cells. Careful search, however, did reveal a few granules with a crystalline core, and this establishes unequivocally the diagnosis of insulinoma.

The difficulty of finding crystalloid-containing granules in some insulinomas can be explained on the basis of what is known about the mechanics of insulin secretion and tumour biology. It is thought that when insulin is produced and secreted rapidly, it is not stored in granules, at least not long enough to crystallize. In such circumstances typical beta granules are not seen (Fawcett, Long and Jones, 1969).

The concentration of insulin or proinsulin-like compounds is lower in insulinomas than in normal islet tissue (Creutzfeldt *et al.*, 1973); the raised level of insulin in the blood probably reflects a reduced capacity of tumour cells to store insulin which is rapidly released in an uncontrolled fashion, via either the granular or the pre-granular route.

An islet cell carcinoma which produced insulin and glucagon has been reported by Boden *et al.* (1977). Immunoreactive glucagon could be extracted from all parts of the tumour but immunoreactive insulin was present in only one section of the tumour. Thus, it seems likely that there was a dual population of cells in this tumour.

Indeed, the general consensus of most students of human islet cell tumours has been that when multiple hormones are produced, each stems from a separate cell (e.g. Bordi and Bussolati, 1974). In contrast to this is the report by Amherdt *et al.* (1971) on the ultrastructure of a transplantable islet cell tumour of the hamster which contained insulin, glucagon and catecholamines. A heterogenous population of granules (70—250 nm) was seen in the tumour cells, so the authors suggest that either multi-hormone synthesis was occurring in individual cells or '. . .one or several of the hormones found in the tumours may have been synthesized elsewhere and accumulated accidentally in this particular tissue'.

Other islet cell tumours

On the basis of radioimmunoscopy and clinical data at least three* well-defined categories of functionally distinct islet cell tumours seem to occur. These are: (1) the so-called 'ulcerogenic tumour' of the Zollinger—Ellison syndrome; (2) the so-called 'diarrhoeagenic tumour' of the Verner—Morrison syndrome; and (3) the quite rare glucagonoma.

Several hormones, such as gastrin, cholecystokinin, glucagon and secretin or combinations of these, have been implicated in the production of these syndromes, but the unequivocal association between a hormone and the neoplastic proliferation of a particular cell type in the islet has not been unequivocally established in all instances. However, gastrin appears to be the principal hormone involved in the Zollinger—Ellison syndrome and the delta cell appears to be the most likely candidate for the production of this hormone (for references see review

*Excluding hypoglycaemic hyperinsulinaemia due to an insulinoma, which has already been dealt with.

94

by Greider, Rosai and McGuigan, 1974). The situation regarding the diarrhoeagenic tumour seems more complex, for quite a few hormones have been implicated in the production of the Verner—Morrison syndrome, such as secretin, gastrin and glucagon (Zollinger *et al.*, 1968; Sircus, 1969; Cleator *et al.*, 1970; Barbezat and Grossman, 1971). Greider, Rosai and McGuigan (1974) studied 34 ulcerogenic tumours and 5 diarrhoeagenic tumours; they could find no constant morphological, histochemical or ultrastructural difference between these two types of neoplasm.

A glucagonoma producing hyperglucagonaemia (patient had mild diabetes and dermatitis) is described by McGavran *et al.* (1966). They describe this as an alpha cell carcinoma but the dense granules (average diameter 200 nm) did not have a halo around them. An islet cell tumour producing ACTH glucagon and gastrin has been described by Belchetz *et al.* (1973). Two cell types were seen, one containing dense granules 120—200 nm in diameter and the other containing dense granules 330—500 nm in diameter. Neither type of granule had a halo around it. However, in a tumour thought to be a metastasizing ACTH-secreting islet cell carcinoma Rawlinson (1973) found that the cells contained granules (180—200 nm in diameter) with a central electron-dense core and a halo. Secretion of more than one hormone is a recognized feature of quite a few islet cell tumours (Law *et al.*, 1965; O'Neal *et al.* 1968).

Conclusions regarding differential diagnosis of islet cell tumours

It will be apparent from the above that the electron microscopist can confidently identify only certain cases of insulinoma when at least a few characteristic beta cell granules with a crystalline core are present. In the absence of this finding, the tumour can still be an insulinoma or a tumour producing a variety of other hormones. Hope lies, however, in the development of immunological techniques at the ultrastructural level, for by such methods one might be able to characterize the hormone content of the secretory granules in these tumours.

Carcinoid tumours

At one time it was thought that the carcinoid was a distinctive tumour of the terminal ileum and caecal appendix and that it originated from Kultschitzky

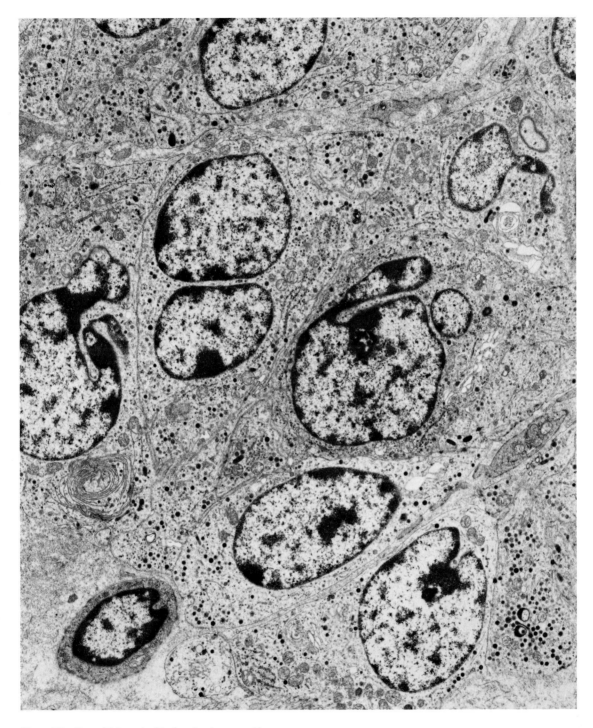

Figure 78   *Bronchial carcinoid, showing innumerable*
APUD granules. ×9000

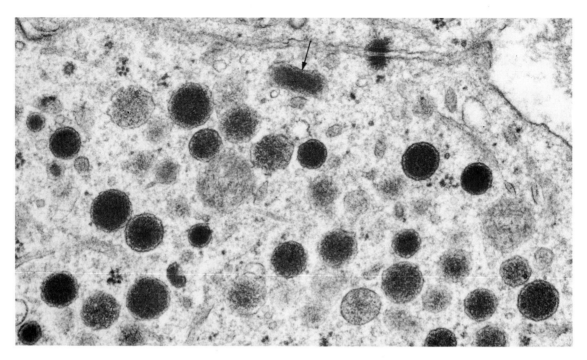

Figure 79 *Same case as Figure 78, showing APUD granules. Most of the granules are small and round; some have a barely discernible halo. There is, however, one granule which is tending towards a dumb-bell shape (arrow).* ×58 000

cells (now called 'enterochromaffin cells' or 'EC cells'). These cells are characterized by quite dense secretory granules, some of which are spherical, while others are of dumb-bell shape, oval or elongated. A very slender halo or no halo is evident.

Carcinoids are now considered to be a variety of APUDoma; some, but perhaps not all, arise from EC cells, but about such matters one cannot be too certain, for eleven varieties of APUD cells are said to occur in the gut (Dobbins, 1978) and some three varieties are said to occur in the lung (Capella *et al.*, 1978). Besides this there is the usual vexatious problem of morphological variations engendered by the neoplastic process which make it quite difficult to relate a given APUDoma to its presumed precursor cell.

However, certain broad patterns of biological behaviour and granule morphology are worth noting (Williams and Sandler, 1963; Black, 1968; Orloff, 1971; Rosai *et al.*, 1976). One can divide carcinoid tumours into three groups: (1) Fore-gut carcinoids (stomach, duodenum, thymus and bronchus) (*Figures 78* and *79*). Main product 5-HTP, may secrete histamine. Associated with peptic ulcer,

Cushing's syndrome or pluriglandular adenomatosis. Secretory granules said to be small and uniformly round (argyrophil + argentaffin−). (2) Mid-gut carcinoids (jejunum, ileum, appendix and right hemicolon). Main product serotonin. Associated with the classic malignant carcinoid syndrome. Granules said to be large and pleomorphic (argyrophil−, argentaffin+). (3) Hind-gut carcinoids (left hemicolon and rectum). No known secretory product. Almost never associated with endocrine disturbances. Granules said to be large and round by electron microscopic examination (argentaffin−, argyrophil−).

It is now clear that while a majority (95 per cent) of the carcinoid tumours occur in the gastrointestinal tract (including pancreas, gall-bladder and perhaps liver), some (5 per cent) also occur in the bronchus,* thymus, ovary, thyroid and sacrococcygeal region (teratoma) (Peskin and Kaplan, 1969; Orloff, 1971;

*We now know that some of the tumours designated as 'bronchial adenoma' are in fact carcinoid tumours and that the term 'adenoma' is a misnomer, because these tumours show low-grade malignancy. Ultrastructural study can easily distinguish these from the truly benign adenoma arising from the mucous glands (Pritchett and Key, 1978).

Johnston and Waisman, 1971; Weichert, Roth and Harkin, 1971; Tolis *et al.*, 1972; Fu *et al.*, 1974; Livnat *et al.*, 1977). Carcinoids are easily diagnosed by electron microscopy but from the morphology of the granules it is not possible to say in which organ the tumour arose.

Anaplastic carcinoid (oat cell carcinoma)

As we have already noted, the small cell undifferentiated (oat cell) carcinoma of the bronchus is now regarded as a poorly differentiated APUDoma (carcinoid) and not a tumour derived from the basal cells of the bronchial mucosa, as had been universally accepted in the past.

Although the endocrine nature of this tumour was suspected as a result of the light microscopic studies of Azzopardi (1959) and the multifarious hormonal disturbances seen in patients bearing this neoplasm, it was the demonstration (Bensch *et al.*, 1968) of APUD granules (dense core granules called

'neurosecretory granules' or 'neurosecretory-like granules' by some workers) and the demonstration (Hattori *et al.*, 1972) of substantial amounts of serotonin in extracts from the tumour which established the idea that the well-known oat cell carcinoma of the bronchus is in fact a poorly differentiated carcinoid.

Intermediate forms where it has been difficult (by light microscopy) to decide whether a given tumour is an oat cell carcinoma or a carcinoid (so-called 'atypical carcinoid') have long been known to histopathologists. This conceptual dilemma is now resolved, for we can look upon these (carcinoids, atypical carcinoids and oat cell carcinomas) as one tumour, differing only in degrees of differentiation and malignancy. The degree of differentiation can be assessed by the number of secretory granules present in a given tumour (Arrigoni, Woolner and Bernatz, 1972). Rarity of secretory granules or their absence in a majority of tumour cells deserves the designation of 'oat cell carcinoma' or 'anaplastic carcinoid'. Somewhat more granules would be seen in the so-called

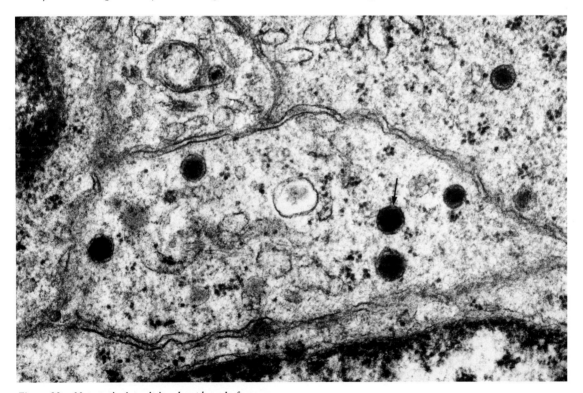

Figure 80 *Metastatic deposit in a lymph node from an anaplastic carcinoid of the oesophagus. Note the characteristic APUD granules. The granule indicated by an arrow is approximately 135 nm in diameter.* ×59 000

'atypical carcinoid', while plentiful granules in virtually all tumour cells would be designated as 'carcinoid of the lung' or 'carcinoid of the bronchus' (i.e. one variety of so-called 'bronchial adenoma').

The diagnostic problem of distinguishing oat cell carcinoma (anaplastic carcinoid) from other anaplastic pulmonary neoplasms is of growing practical importance, for this affects prognosis and therapy. This problem can be solved by electron microscopy but an adequate sample of the tumour tissue must be available for study. The finding of occasional dense core granules would establish the diagnosis of oat cell carcinoma (anaplastic carcinoid), while their total absence would favour the idea that it was an anaplastic carcinoma from some non-APUD cell line.

Rosai *et al.* (1976) have pointed out that 'oat cell carcinomas' or 'small cell carcinomas' have been described in the larynx, oesophagus, salivary glands, pancreas, gastrointestinal tract and uterine cervix, so it seems possible that some of these, too, may be anaplastic carcinoids. This is particularly likely to be so for undifferentiated tumours of various organs associated with Cushing's syndrome are known to occur.

Figure 80 shows APUD granules in a lymph node metastasis from an anaplastic carcinoid of the oesophagus. On the basis of light microscopy various diagnoses such as anaplastic carcinoma, anaplastic sarcoma and melanoma were offered. Ultrastructural study of the lesion in the lymph node revealed the presence of dense core granules. About one in three or four cells had one or two granules in the cytoplasm but in a few instances as many as five such granules were present and this is shown in *Figure 80*.

Phaeochromocytoma

There is quite a close morphological and histochemical resemblance between a phaeochromocytoma (*Figures 81* and *82*) and the adrenal medulla. Two principal types of secretory granule-containing (catecholamine granules or chromaffin granules) cells

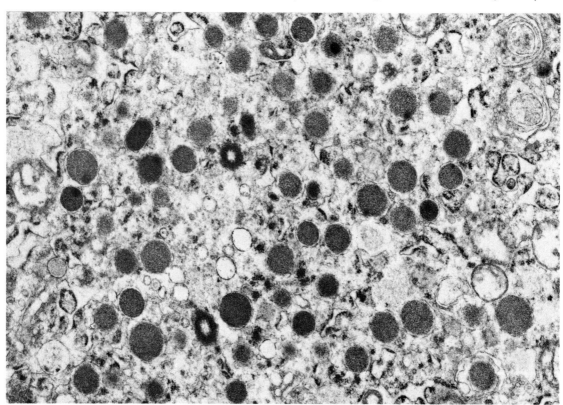

Figure 81   *Phaeochromocytoma. Cell containing epinephrine granules.* ×*24 000 (Ghadially and Larsen, unpublished electron micrograph)*

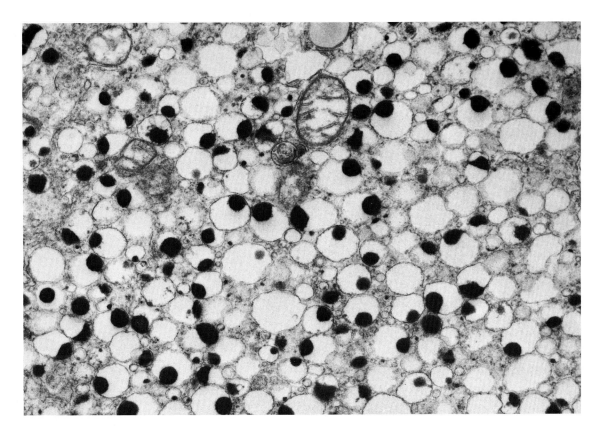

Figure 82 *Phaeochromocytoma. Same case as Figure 81.*
Cell containing norepinephrine granules. × 24 000 (Ghadially
and Larsen, unpublished electron micrograph)

are found in the normal adrenal medulla, and phaeochromocytoma (Misugi, Misugi and Newton, 1968; Tannenbaum, 1970; DeLellis *et al.*, 1973). With the electron microscope these granules present as: (1) Quite large round or elongated medium-density granules with a particulate substructure. (A very thin halo is usually discernible. This granule is thought to contain epinephrine.). (2) A small electron-dense granule lying in a vacuole. One might regard this as a variety of dense core granule with an unusually large halo; often the electron-dense granule is eccentrically placed or abuts the enveloping membrane. These granules are thought to contain norepinephrine.

The normal adrenal medulla contains more epinephrine than norepinephrine but phaeochromocytomas usually contain more norepinephrine than epinephrine (Wurtman, 1965; Tannenbaum, Spiro and Lattimer, 1966), and this correlates well with the population of the two cell types seen with the

electron microscope. This is evidenced by the work of Tannenbaum (1970), who studied 14 phaeochromocytomas. In five cases of norepinephrine-containing phaeochromocytomas, cells containing granules with large holes were found, but in two cases of 'biochemically pure' epinephrine-containing phaeochromocytomas oval or elongated granules about 270 nm long were seen. This is about 100 nm larger than the corresponding epinephrine granules in the normal adrenal medulla. Tannenbaum (1970) designated seven cases as 'mixed' type of phaeochromocytoma, for they contained both types of cells. Biochemical analysis of tumour homogenates correlated well with morphological findings. Thus, one might be able to guess what hormone is being produced by looking at ultrathin sections of a phaeochromocytoma, the main limiting factor being the smallness of the sample examined with the electron microscope.

APUDamyloid

Amyloid (called 'APUDamyloid' to distinguish it from immunamyloid) is found in the stroma of some but not all APUDomas. The incidence of APUD-amyloid in calcitoninoma is said to be virtually 100 per cent (Hazard, Hawk and Crile, 1959; Albores-Saavedra *et al.*, 1964; Williams, Brown and Doniach, 1966; Gonzales-Licea, Hartmann and Yardley, 1968; Müller, 1969; Steiner, 1969; Pearse, Ewen and Polak, 1972; Meyer, Hutton and Kenny, 1973). This has led some to imagine that if amyloid is present in the stroma of an APUDoma, this is diagnostic of calcitoninoma.

This is incorrect for amyloid has been documented to occur (albeit less frequently) in some: (1) phaeochromocytomas (Paloyan *et al.*, 1970); (2) carotid body tumours (Capella and Solcia, 1971); (3) bronchial carcinoids (Štěrba, 1968); (4) 'islet cell tumours' (Porta, Yerry and Scott, 1962); (5) insulinomas (Steiner, 1969; Pearse, Ewen and Polak, 1972; Le Charpentier *et al.*, 1974; Teisa and Kaye, 1978); (6) gastrinomas (Pearse *et al.*, 1972); and (7) pituitary adenomas (Bilbao *et al.*, 1975; Schober and Nelson, 1975).

APUD amyloid, like immunamyloid, gives dichromic staining with Congo red and is metachromatic with methyl violet. The ultrastructural morphology of the amyloid fibrils appears similar for both types of amyloid. However, there are quite a few chemical differences, the main one being the absence from APUDamyloid of tryptophan and tyrosin (Pearse *et al.*, 1972). Immunofluorescence tests for specific hormones in APUDamyloid are negative, and Pearse *et al.* (1972) have hypothesized that '...non-hormone polypeptide products of the endocrine tumour cells which are, in some cases, non-functional sequences derived from prohormones, constitute the polypeptides of the apudamyloid fibril'.

References

ALBORES-SAAVEDRA, J., ROSE, G. G., IBANEZ, M. L., RUSSELL, W. O., GREY, C. E. and DMOCHOWSKI, L. (1964). The amyloid in solid carcinoma of the thyroid gland — staining characteristics, tissue culture and electron microscopic observations. *Lab. Invest.*, **13**, 77

AMHERDT, M., ORCI, L., TRACK, N. S., LAMBERT, A. E., KANAZAWA, Y. and STAUFFACHER, W. (1971). An ultrastructural study of the islet cell tumour of the golden hamster. *Horm. Metab. Res.*, **3**, 252

ARRIGONI, M. G., WOOLNER, I. B. and BERNATZ, P. E. (1972). Atypical carcinoid tumours of the lung. *J. Thorac. Cardiovasc. Surg.*, **64**, 413

AZZOPARDI, J. G. (1959). Oat cell carcinoma of the bronchus. *J. Path. Bact.*, **78**, 513

BARBEZAT, G. O. and GROSSMAN, M. I. (1971). Cholera-like diarrhoea induced by glucagon plus gastrin. *Lancet*, **i**, 1025

BELCHETZ, P. E., BROWN, C. L., MAKIN, H. L. J., TRAFFORD, D. J. H., STUART MASON, A., BLOOM, S. R. and RATCLIFFE, J. G. (1973). ACTH, glucagon and gastrin production by a pancreatic islet cell carcinoma and its treatment. *Clin. Endocr.* **2**, 307

BENSCH, K. G., CORRIN, B., PARIENTE, R. and SPENCER, H. (1968). Oat-cell carcinoma of the lung, its origin and relationship to bronchial carcinoid. *Cancer*, **22**, 1163

BILBAO, J. M., HORVATH, E., HUDSON, A. R. and KOVACS, K. (1975). Pituitary adenoma producing amyloid-like substance. *Archs Path.*, **99**, 411

BLACK, W. C. (1968). Enterochromaffin cell types and corresponding carcinoid tumours. *Lab. Invest.* **19**, 473

BODEN, G., OWEN, O. E., REZVANI, I., ELFENBEIN, B. I. and QUICKEL, K. E. (1977). An islet cell carcinoma containing glucagon and insulin. Chronic glucagon excess and glucose homeostasis. *Diabetes*, **26**, 120

BORDI, C. and BUSSOLATI, G. (1974). Immunofluorescence, histochemical and ultrastructural studies for the detection of multiple endocrine polypeptide tumours of the pancreas. *Virchows Arch. B. Zellpath.*, **17**, 13

CAPELLA, C., HAGE, E., SOLCIA, E. and USELLINI, L. (1978). Ultrastructural similarity of endocrine-like cells of the human lung and some related cells of the gut. *Cell Tiss. Res.*, **186**, 25

CAPELLA, C. and SOLCIA, E. (1971). Optical and electron microscopical study of cytoplasmic granules in human carotid body, carotid body tumours and jugular tumours. *Virchows Arch. B. Cell Path.*, **7**, 37

CAPELLA, C., SOLCIA, E., FRIGERIO, B., BUFFA, R., USELLINI, L. and FONTANA, P. (1977). The endocrine cells of the pancreas and related tumours. *Virchows Arch. A, Path. Anat. Histol.*, **373**, 327

CLEATOR, I. G. M., THOMSON, C. G., SIRCUS, W. and COOMBES, M. (1970). Bio-assay evidence of abnormal secretin-like and gastrin-like activity in tumour and blood in cases of 'choleraic diarrhoea'. *Gut*, **11**, 206

CREUTZFELDT, W., ARNOLD, R., CREUTZFELDT, C., DEUTICKE, U., FRERICHS, H. and TRACK, N. S. (1973). Biochemical and morphological investigations of 30 human insulinomas. *Diabetologia*, **9**, 217

DeLELLIS, R. A., MERK, F. B., DECKERS, P., WARREN, S. and BALOGH, K. (1973). Ultrastructure and in vitro growth characteristics of a transplantable rat pheochromocytoma. *Cancer*, **32**, 227

DOBBINS, W. O. (1978). Diagnostic pathology of the intestine and colon. In: *Diagnostic Electron Microscopy*, Vol. 1, ed. B. F. Trump and R. T. Jones, pp. 253–339. New York: Wiley

FAWCETT, D. W., LONG, J. A. and JONES, A. L. (1969). The ultrastructure of endocrine glands. *Rec. Progr. Horm. Res.*, **25**, 318

FU, Y-S., McWILLIAMS, N. B., STRATFORD, T. P. and KAY, S. (1974). Bronchial carcinoid with choroidal metastasis in an adolescent. *Cancer, 33*, 707

GONZALEZ-LICEA, A., HARTMANN, W. H. and YARDLEY, J. H. (1968). Medullary carcinoma in the thyroid. Ultrastructural evidence of its origin from the parafollicular cell and its possible relation to carcinoid tumors. *Am. J. Clin Path., 49*, 512

GOULD, V. E. (1977). Neuroendocrinomas and neuro-endocrine carcinomas. *Path. Ann., 12*(Pt 2), 33

GREIDER, M. H., BENCOSME, S. A. and LECHAGO, J. (1970). The human pancreatic islet-cells and their tumors I. The normal pancreatic islets. *Lab. Invest., 22*, 344

GREIDER, M. H. and ELLIOTT, D. W. (1964). Electron microscopy of human pancreatic tumors of islet cell origin. *Am. J. Path., 44*, 663

GREIDER, M. H., ROSAI, J. and McGUIGAN, J. E. (1974). The human pancreatic islet cells and their tumors. II. Ulcerogenic and Diarrheagenic tumors. *Cancer, 33*, 1423

HARANO, Y., KOHAMA, M., ARAKI, N., SAKAMOTO, A., HOSHI, M., SHICHIRI, M., SHIMA, K., OKAMURA, J. and SHIGETA, Y. (1975). Qualitative abnormality of insulin secretion in a case with insulinoma. *Endocr. Jap., 22*, 175

HATTORI, S., MATSUDA, M., TATEISHI, R., NISHIHARA, H. and HORAI, T. (1972). Oat-cell carcinoma of the lung; clinical and morphological studies in relation to its histogenesis. *Cancer, 30*, 1014

HAZARD, J. B., HAWK, W. A. and CRILE, G. Jr. (1959). Medullary (solid) carcinoma of the thyroid. A clinico-pathologic entity. *J. Clin. Endocr., 37*, 205

JOHNSTON, W. H. and WAISMAN, J. (1971). Carcinoid tumor of the vermiform appendix with Cushing's syndrome. *Cancer, 27*, 681

KAWAOI, A., OKANO, T. and UCHIDA, T. (1977). Immunohistological study of the ACTH producing islet cell carcinoma of the pancreas. *Acta Path. Jap., 27*, 265

KUBO, T. and WATANABE, H. (1971). Neoplastic argentaffin cells in gastric and intestinal carcinomas. *Cancer, 27*, 447

LAW, D. H., LIDDLE, G. W., SCOTT, H. W. Jr. and TAUBER, S. D. (1965). Ectopic production of multiple hormones (ACTH, MSH and gastrin) by a single malignant tumor. *New Engl. J. Med., 273*, 292

LE CHARPENTIER, Y., LOUVEL, A., de SAINT-MAUR, P. P., DAUDET-MONSAC, M., LÉGER, L. and ABELANET, R. (1974). Étude ultrastructurale d'un insolome à stroma amyloide. *Virchows Arch Path. Anat., 362*, 169

LIKE, A. A. (1967). The ultrastructure of the secretory cells of the islets of Langerhans in man. *Lab. Invest., 16*, 937

LILLIE, R. D. and GLENNER, G. G. (1960). Histological reaction in carcinoid tumors of the human gastrointestinal tract. *Am. J. Path., 36*, 623

LIVNAT, E. J., SCOMMEGNA, A., RECANT, W. and JAO, W. (1977). Ultrastructural observations of the so-called strumal carcinoid of the ovary. *Archs Path. Lab. Med., 101*, 585

McGAVRAN, M. H., UNGER, R. H., RECANT, L., POLK, H. C., KILO, C. and LEVIN, M. E. (1966). A glucagon-secreting alpha cell carcinoma of the pancreas. *New Engl. J. Med., 274*, 1408

MEYER, J. S., HUTTON, W. E. and KENNY, A. D. (1973). Medullary carcinoma of thyroid gland: Subcellular distribution of calcitonin and relationship between granules and amyloid. *Cancer, 31*, 433

MISUGI, K., MISUGI, N. and NEWTON, W. A. (1968). Fine structural study of neuroblastoma, ganglioneuroblastoma and pheochromocytoma. *Archs Path., 86*, 160

MÜLLER, M. (1969). Etude clinique et anatomo-pathologique de 31 carcinomes medullaries a stroma amyloide de la thyroide. *Schweiz. Med. Wschr., 99*, 433

O'NEAL, L. W., KIPNIS, D. M., LUSE, S. A., LACY, P. E. and JARETT, L. (1968). Secretion of various endocrine substances by ACTH-secreting tumors — gastrin, melanotropin, norepinephrine, serotonin, parahormone, vasopressin, glucagon. *Cancer, 21*, 1219

ORLOFF, M. J. (1971). Carcinoid tumors of the rectum. *Cancer, 28*, 175

PALOYAN, E., SCANU, A., STRAUSS, F. H., PICKLEMAN, J. R. and PALOYAN, D. (1970). Familial pheochromocytoma, medullary thyroid carcinoma and parathyroid adenomas. *J. Am Med. Assoc., 214*, 1443

PEARSE, A. G. E. (1974). The APUD cell concept and its implications in pathology. *Path. Ann., 9*, 27

PEARSE, A. G. E., EWEN, S. W. B. and POLAK, J. M. (1972). The genesis of apudamyloid in endocrine polypeptide tumours: histochemical distinction from immunamyloid. *Virchows Arch. Abt. B. Zellpath., 10*, 93

PESKIN, G. W. and KAPLAN, E. L. (1969). The surgery of carcinoid tumors. *Surg. Clins. N. Am., 49*, 137

PORTA, A. E., YERRY, R. and SCOTT, R. F. (1962). Amyloidosis of functioning islet cell adenomas of the pancreas. *Am. J. Path., 41*, 623

PRITCHETT, P. S. and KEY, B. M. (1978). Mucous gland adenoma of the bronchus. Ultrastructural and histochemical studies. *Am J. Med. Sci., 15*, 43

RAWLINSON, D. G. (1973). Electron microscopy of an ACTH-secreting islet cell carcinoma. *Cancer, 31*, 1015

ROSAI, J., LEVINE, G., WEBER, W. R. and HIGA, E. (1976). Carcinoid tumors and oat cell carcinomas of the thymus. *Path. Ann., 11*, 201

SCHOBER, R. and NELSON, D. (1975). Fine structure and origin of amyloid deposits in pituitary adenoma. *Archs Path., 99*, 403

SIRCUS, W. (1969). Peptide secreting tumours with special reference to the pancreas. *Gut, 10*, 506

STEINER, H. (1969). Endokrin aktive Tumoren mit Amyloidstroma. Eine morphologische Untersuchung von Insulinomen und einem Calcitonin produzierenden Tumor. *Virchows Arch. Path. Anat., 348*, 170

ŠTĚRBA, J. (1968). Metastasierendes Bronchialkarzinoid mit Amyloid im Stroma. *Zbl. Allg. Path. 111*, 555

SUZUKI, H. and MATSUYAMA, M. (1971). Ultrastructure of functioning Beta cell tumors of pancreatic islets. *Cancer, 28*, 1302

TANNENBAUM, M. (1970). Ultrastructural pathology of adrenal medullary tumors. *Path. Ann., 5*, 145

TANNENBAUM, M., SPIRO, D. and LATTIMER, J. K. (1966). Norepinephrine and epinephrine secreting tumors of the adrenal medulla. An electron microscopic and biochemical study. *Am. J. Path.*, **48**, 48

TEISA, A. and KAYE, G. I. (1978). Amyloid formation in insulinoma. *Archs Path. Lab. Med.*, **102**, 227

TOKER, C. (1967). Some observations on the ultrastructure of a malignant islet cell tumor associated with duodenal ulceration and severe diarrhea. *J. Ultrastruct. Res.*, **19**, 522

TOLIS, G. A., FRY, W. A., HEAD, L. and SHIELDS, T. W. (1972). Bronchial adenomas. *Surg. Gynecol. Obstet.*, **134**, 605

WAISMAN, J. (1969). Alpha cell granules in a pancreatic neoplasm. *Archs Path.*, **88**, 672

WEICHERT, R. F. III (1970). The neural ectodermal origin of the peptide-secreting endocrine glands: a unifying concept for the etiology of multiple endocrine adenomatosis and the inappropriate secretion of peptide hormones by non-endocrine tumors. *Am. J. Med.*, **49**, 232

WEICHERT, R. F. III, ROTH, L. M. and HARKIN, J. C. (1971). Carcinoid islet cell tumors of the duodenum and associated multiple carcinoid tumors of the ileum (An electron microscopic study). *Cancer,* **27**, 164

WILLIAMS, E. D., BROWN, C. L. and DONIACH, I. (1966). Pathological and clinical findings in a series of 67 cases of medullary carcinoma of the thyroid. *J. Clin. Path.*, **19**, 103

WILLIAMS, E. D. and SANDLER, M. (1963). The classification of carcinoid tumors. *Lancet,* i, 238

WURTMAN, R. J. (1965). Catecholamines. *New Engl. J. Med.*, **273**, 637

ZEITOUN, P. and LEHY, T. (1970). Utilization of paraffin-embedded material for electron microscopy. *Lab. Invest.*, **23**, 52

ZOLLINGER, R. M., TOMPKINS, R. K., AMERSON, J. R., ENDAHL, G. L., KRAFT, A. R. and MOORE, F. T. (1968). Identification of the diarrheoagenic hormone associated with non-beta islet cell tumors of the pancreas. *Ann. Surg.*, **168**, 502

9
Differential diagnosis of eosinophilic granular cell tumours

Correlations between light and electron microscopic appearances are singularly satisfying and worthwhile. There is the joy of seeing familiar structures in a new light and thereby resolving old mysteries; and this kind of exercise bridges the gap between the images seen with the light and the electron microscope. It is amazing how much more one can see with the light microscope after one has comprehended the significance of a phenomenon with the electron microscope. Hence, it seems worthwhile to digress a little and talk about the tinctorial and textural properties of the cytoplasm before we see why some tumour cells have an eosinophilic granular cytoplasm.

Tinctorial and textural properties of the cytoplasm

Cytoplasmic basophilia and pyroninophilia is an indicator of the presence of RNA and, hence, ribosomes. It does not matter whether these are ribosomes or polyribosomes and whether they are attached to membranes (i.e. rough endoplasmic reticulum) or lying free in the cytoplasmic matrix. Thus, for example, the diffuse basophilia of the cytoplasm of the plasma cell stems from the extensive system of rough endoplasmic reticulum which this cell possesses. The juxtanuclear zone where the Golgi complex is situated appears as a clear area (hof of the light microscopist), because no ribosomes are present in this region. The Nissl body in the neuron presents as a basophilic body, because of the focal collection of rough endoplasmic reticulum and polyribosomes lying free in the cytoplasm.

The cytoplasmic matrix itself is tinctorially neutral or only faintly eosinophilic (this depends on hydration). Diffuse or focal eosinophilia can be produced by the presence of various structures in the matrix. Thus, the diffuse eosinophilia of the muscle cell is due to the fact that this cell is packed with myofilaments. The eosinophilia of the Mallory body found in the hepatocytes of alcoholics is due to a focal collection of quite a different type of filament. Hypertrophy of the smooth endoplasmic reticulum in the hepatocytes may be diffuse or focal. In the former instance the cytoplasm shows diffuse eosinophilia; in the latter instance eosinophilic foci are seen.

Indeed, all membranous structures contribute to the eosinophilia (acidophilia) of the cytoplasm,* so it is not surprising to find that an increase in the mitochondrial population presents as fine and coarse eosinophilic granules in the cytoplasm, the latter probably reflecting the presence of unusually large mitochondria. Lysosomes, too, are usually eosinophilic (this depends to some extent on their contents), so an abundance of lysosomes will also produce an eosinophilic granular cytoplasm.

Large eosinophilic granular cells occurring in normal and neoplastic tissues have long been the subject of interest and speculation among histologists and pathologists. By and large they can be divided into two main groups:† (1) those where the granularity is due to the abundance of mitochondria (oncocytes and oncocytomas); and (2) those where the granularity is due to an abundance of lysosomes.†

Oncocytes and oncocytomas

The term 'oncocyte' was coined by Hamperl (1950) to describe the large eosinophilic (acidophilic) cells

*The basophilia of the rough endoplasmic reticulum is due to ribosomes and not the membranous component.
†Cytoplasmic granularity in tumours may be due to various other reasons, such as: (1) microcrystals and a fair number of mitochondria in alveolar soft part sarcoma (Chapter 21); (2) abundant smooth endoplasmic reticulum occurring focally or clumped due to preparative procedures in tumours of steroid-secreting cells (Chapter 16); and (3) abundant secretory granules. An example of the latter is the so-called 'pulmonary oncocytoma' described by Black (1969) where electron microscopy showed that the cytoplasmic granularity was due to the presence of numerous 'secretory vesicles'. The term 'oncocytoma' should not be used to describe such tumours.

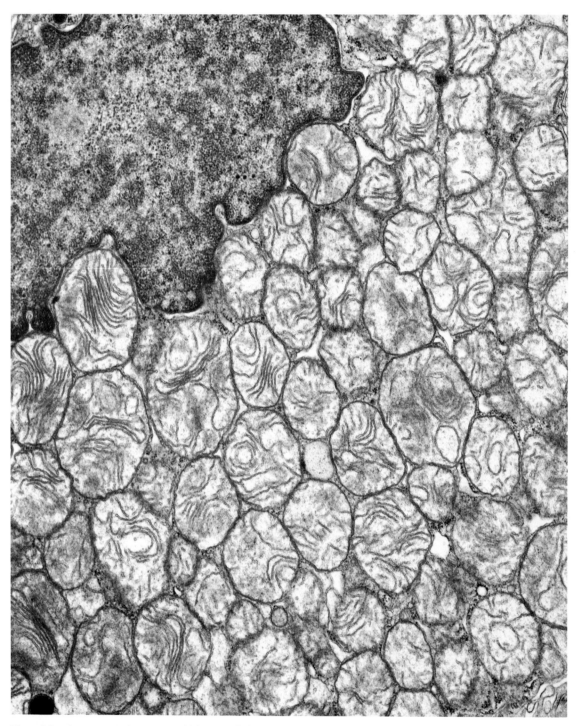

Figure 83   *An oncocyte from a bronchial mucosal gland
of man, showing cytoplasm packed with mitochondria.
Note absence of intramatrical dense granules.* ×24 000
(From Ghadially, 1975)

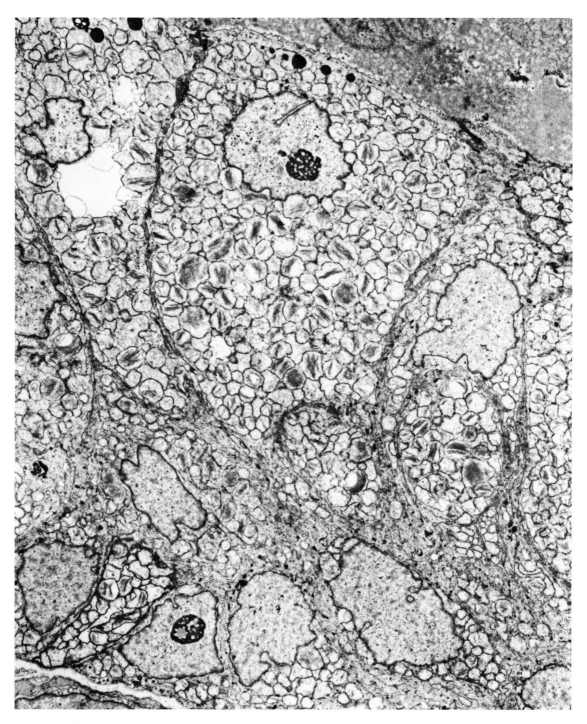

Figure 84   *Warthin's tumour (adenolymphoma of parotid gland). The cytoplasm is packed with mitochondria containing innumerable stacked cristae.* ×3700 *(From Tandler, 1966b)*

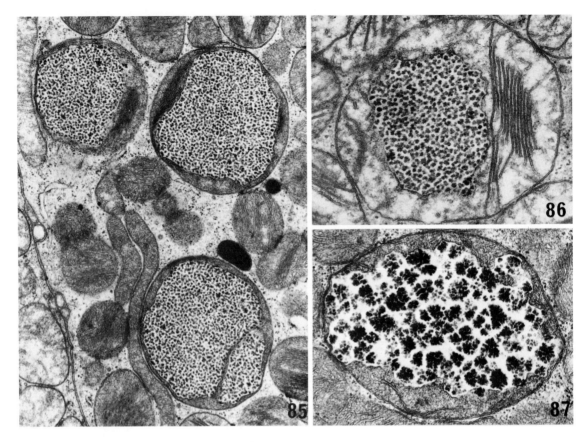

Figures 85, 86 and 87   *Glycogen-containing mitochondria from an oncocytoma of the parotid gland. Glycogen deposits in the intracristal space, not in the matrix. The electron-lucent area in which the glycogen lies is derived from an expansion of the intracristal space.* ×16 500; ×37 000; ×32 000 *(From Tandler, Hutter and Erlandson, 1970)*

of Hurthle tumours of the thyroid gland. He suggested that this was a special class of cell and that tumours of these cells should be called oncocytomas.

It is now known that these acidophilic (oxyphil) cells (*Figure 83*) with a granular cytoplasm are found in a variety of normal and pathological tissues (e.g. normal salivary gland, parathyroid gland, pancreas, liver, Graves' disease and Hashimoto's thyroiditis) and that they arise from normal epithelial cells that have already reached histological maturity. For example, in salivary glands transition from normal epithelial cells to oncocytes has been demonstrated by Tandler (1966a), and there is ultrastructural evidence that Hurthle cells derive from the thyroid epithelium (Feldman, Horvath and Kovacs, 1972).

Ultrastructurally oncocytes and cells of oncocytomas are characterized by a cytoplasm packed with innumerable mitochondria which lack intramitochondrial dense granules (*Figures 84–90*). In some instances such mitochondria may contain glycogen or lipid inclusions (*Figures 85–87* and *Figure 89*).

Tumours deserving to be called oncocytomas include: (1) Warthin's tumour (adenolymphoma of parotid gland) (Tandler and Shipkey, 1964; McGavran, 1965; Tandler, 1966b; Hübner *et al.*, 1971; Allegra, 1971; Sun, White and Thompson, 1976); (2) oxyphil cell adenoma of the major salivary glands (Tandler, Hutter and Erlandson, 1970; Kay and Still, 1973; Sun, White and Thompson, 1975); (3) oxyphil cell adenomas of parathyroid gland

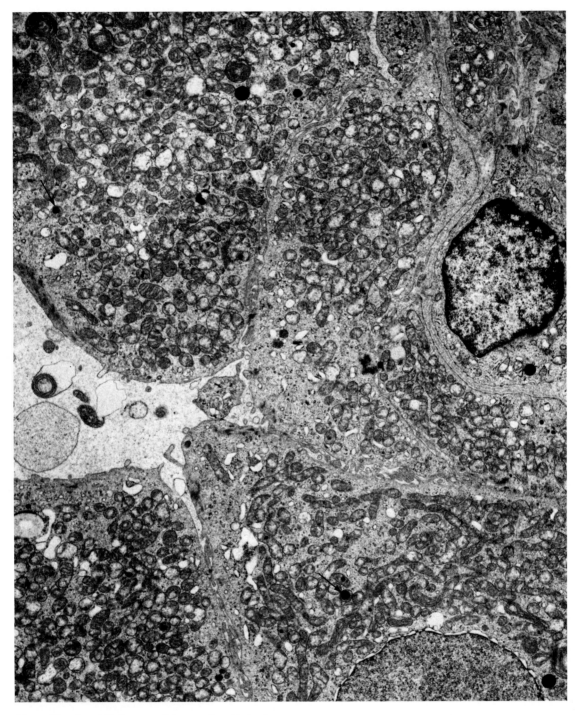

Figure 88   *Oxyphil adenoma of the parathyroid gland.*
The tumour cells are packed with innumerable mitochondria;
some of them contain lipidic inclusions (arrows). ×10 000

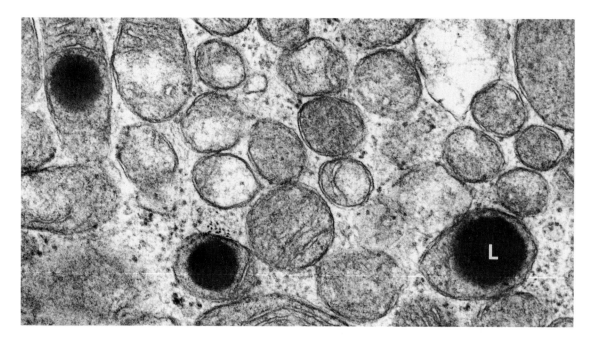

Figure 89 *Oxyphil adenoma of the parathyroid gland.*
Same case as Figure 88, showing electron-dense lipid drop-
lets (L) in three mitochondria. Note absence of matrical
dense granules. ×58 000

(Marshall, Roberts and Turner, 1967; Heinmann, Hansson and Nilsson, 1971; Arnold *et al.*, 1974; McGregor *et al.*, 1978); (4) oncocytic adenoma of pituitary gland (Kovacs and Horvath, 1973; Landolt and Oswald, 1973; Kovacs, Horvath and Bilbao, 1974; Scanarini and Mingrino, 1974; Bauserman *et al.*, 1978; Roy, 1978); (5) Hurthle tumours of the thyroid (Tonietti, Baschieri and Salabe, 1967; Michel-Bechet, Valenta and Athouel-Haon, 1971; Feldman, Horvath and Kovacs, 1972; Valenta *et al.*, 1974); and (6) bronchial oncocytoma (Fechner and Bentinck, 1973). In most of these cases virtually every tumour cell is an oncocyte loaded with mitochondria.

However, oncocytic transformation of lesser degree has been found in some examples of other neoplasms also, such as: (1) renal adenocarcinoma (Keyhani, 1969); (2) renal clear cell carcinoma Seljelid and Ericsson, 1965); and (3) fibroadenoma of the breast (Archer and Omar, 1969).

One may well ask what energy requirement so remarkable a collection of mitochondria is supposed to meet in the oncocyte. Conflicting results have

been obtained by histochemical studies and studies on isolated mitochondria. Some studies suggest that there is a high level of oxidative activity, while others have found that the mitochondria are deficient in various ways and have a low level of succinoxidase activity. Tandler, Hutter and Erlandson (1970) give an excellent critique on this subject and conclude that these mitochondria are biochemically defective and that this is an example of compensatory hyperplasia occurring at the organelle level; on the other hand, Feldman, Horvath and Kovacs (1972) discuss the possibility that the increase in mitochondrial mass may be due to a prolonged life-span or a diminished rate of elimination of mitochondria in these cells.

The idea of organelle atrophy, hypertrophy or hyperplasia is not too difficult to accept, but it takes a lot more imagination to accept a concept of organelle neoplasia. Yet such a theory has been proposed by Sun, White and Thompson (1975) regarding oncocytomas. These authors state: 'Such a tumour can represent an intracellular "neoplasm" of mitochondria proliferating at the expense of the cell's own economy.' Be that as it may, ultrastructural

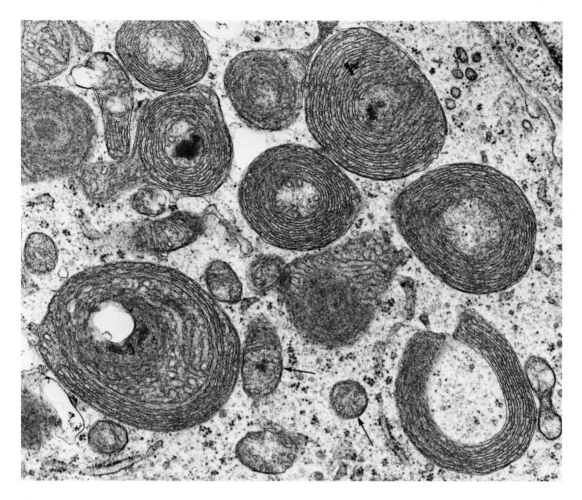

Figure 90 *Oxyphil adenoma of the parathyroid gland. Same case as Figures 88 and 89. Giant mitochondria (presumably cup-shaped) and normal-sized mitochondria (arrows) are present.* ×36 000

studies have clearly defined a group of tumours which can be confidently identified by their unique mitochondrial population.

Finally, attention should be drawn to another tumour, the hibernoma, which on ultrastructural grounds would qualify as an oncocytoma, for the cells of this tumour contain abundant mitochondria (Levine, 1972; Seemayer *et al.*, 1975). Intramatrical dense granules are not evident in the illustrations of hibernoma, but, then, they are also rare in the mitochondria of brown adipose tissue. It is difficult to say whether the mitochondria in hibernoma are biochemically defective or not. In normal brown adipose tissue the exceedingly numerous mitochondria are

related to the high energy requirements for the degradation of fat to yield the heat necessary to raise the body temperature during arousal from hibernation in hibernating animals (Smallely and Dryer, 1963; Smith and Hock, 1963) and for non-shivering thermogenesis in human neonates and other non-hibernating animals (Aherne and Hull, 1966).

Granular cell myoblastoma

These tumours are characterized by cells which contain large numbers of lysosomes in their cytoplasm (*Figures 91* and *92*). The nature and origin of these cells and the lysosomes they contain still remains an

109

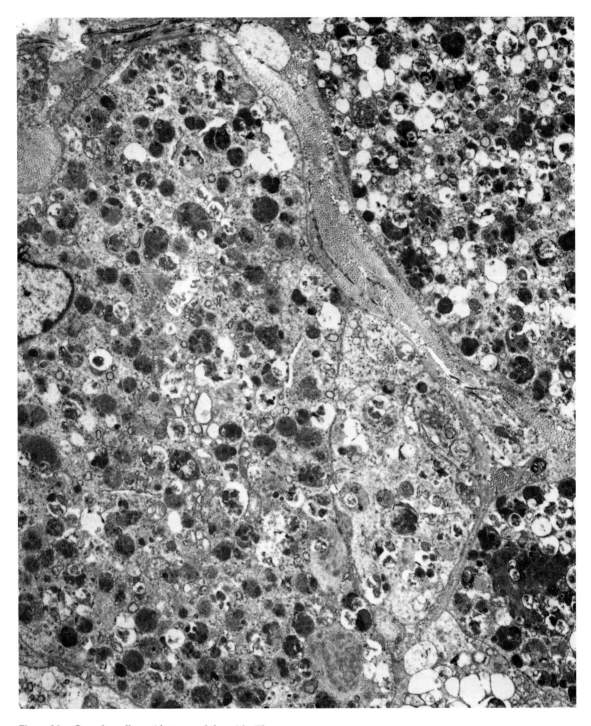

Figure 91 *Granular cell myoblastoma of the orbit. The cytoplasm of the tumour cells is packed with innumerable lysosomes.* ×9000 *(From a block of tissue supplied by Dr A. H. Cameron)*

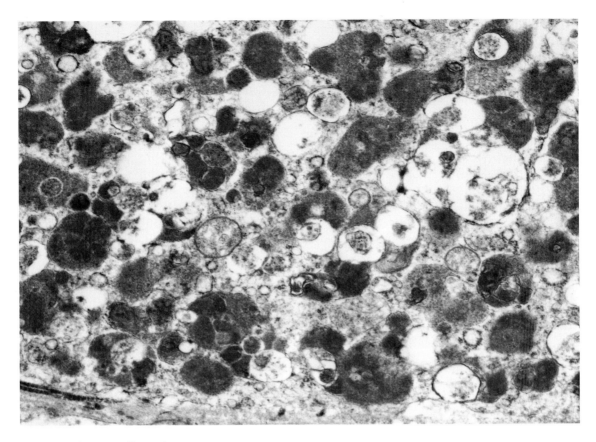

Figure 92   *Granular cell myoblastoma. Same case as*
Figure 91. High-power view of lysosomes. ×24 000 (From
a block of tissue supplied by Dr A. H. Cameron)

enigma. Various previous suggestions regarding the histogenesis of this lesion include: (1) a neoplastic or non-neoplastic derivation from adult or embryonic muscle tissue (Abrikossoff, 1926; Klemperer, 1934; Gray and Gruenfeld, 1937; (2) a non-neoplastic accumulation of histiocytic cells (Leroux and Delarue, 1939); (3) a granuloma probably due to parasitic infestation (Gullino, 1946); (4) a histiocytic storage phenomenon (Lauche, 1944); (5) a lipoid thesaurus: stored material probably myelin (Azzopardi, 1956); (6) neural origin (Fust and Custer, 1949; Bangle, 1952); (7) a degeneration of perineural and/or endoneural fibroblasts (Pearse, 1950); (8) derivation from Schwann cells or an undifferentiated mesenchymal precursor of Schwann cells (for references see Sobel and Marquet, 1974).

The neoplastic nature of these lesions is attested by the rare but well documented occurrence of malignant versions of this tumour (for references see Cadotte, 1974) and the transplantable granular cell tumour of the uterine cervix of the oestrogen-treated mouse (Dunn and Green, 1963, 1965).

Numerous ultrastructural studies on granular cell myoblastoma have been published (Fisher and Wechsler, 1962; Sobel et al., 1971; Sobel, Marquet and Schwartz, 1973; Garancis, Komorowski and Kuzma, 1970; Aparicio and Lumsden, 1969; Moscovic and Azar, 1967). The most widely accepted view is that granular cell myoblastoma is related to a schwannoma or that it is a variety of schwannoma. There are quite a few ultrastructural similarities between schwannomas and granular cell myoblastomas. For example: (1) a few or not so few lysosomes (probably containing altered myelin) are seen in schwannomas but many more occur in granular cell myoblastomas; (2) a prominent external lamina or basal lamina is a feature of schwannomas and granular cell myoblastomas, respectively; (3) Luse bodies (long-spacing collagen) are of frequent occurrence in the stroma of schwannomas and they have also been seen at times in granular cell myoblastoma* and (4) angulate bodies have been found in both granular cell myoblastomas and schwannomas. These are single membrane bound bodies containing filaments, microtubules and lipid droplets. My impression is that this is a variety of lysosome similar to that which we have described in the skin of patients with

*However, it should be noted that long-spacing collagen has been seen in a wide variety of pathological states.

rheumatoid arthritis after chrysotherapy (Ghadially et al., 1978).

There seem little reason to doubt that the single membrane bound bodies with heterogenous electron-dense contents seen in granular cell myoblastoma are in fact lysosomes. Lysosomal enzymes such as acid phosphatase and esterase have been demonstrated in the granular cells at the light microscopic level (Fisher and Wechsler, 1962; Sobel, 1969), but I have not found a report where this has been demonstrated at the ultrastructural level. Nevertheless there seems little reason to doubt that these single membrane bound bodies with heterogenous electron-dense contents are in fact lysosomes, but what function such

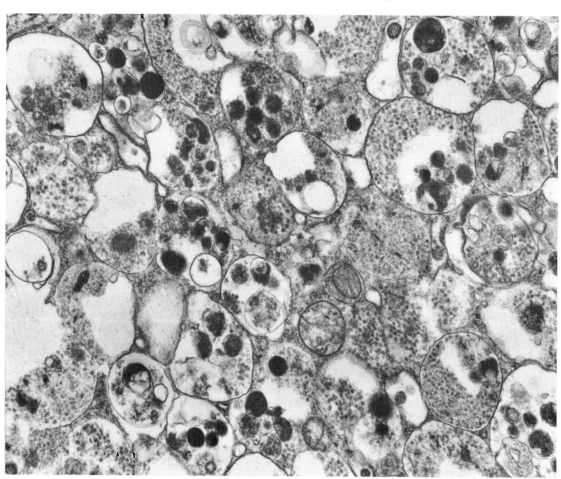

Figure 93 *Granular cell ameloblastoma. An area of cytoplasm from a tumour cell showing numerous lysosomes containing innumerable electron-dense particles, granules and small vesicles. ×16 000 (From Tandler and Rossi, 1977)*

112

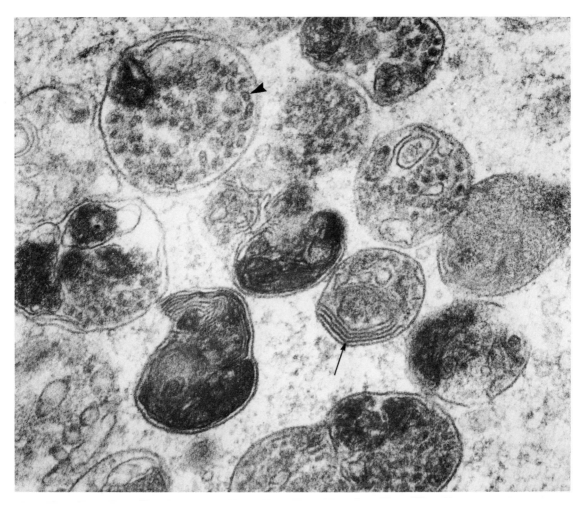

Figure 94 *Granular cell ameloblastoma. Same case as Figure 93. Lysosomes in this tumour cell contain membranous material (arrows) and numerous vesicles (arrowhead) ×59 000 (Tandler, unpublished electron micrograph)*

an increase of lysosomes serves in the granular cell is unknown. We do not even know whether they are autolysosomes or heterolysosomes (see below).

Some other granular cell tumours

Other tumours where granular cells containing numerous lysosomes occur include: (1) granular cell ameloblastoma* (Navarrete and Smith, 1971; Mincer

*Only about 5 per cent of ameloblastomas contain granular cells and only about 1 per cent of all odontogenic tumours are ameloblastomas, so the granular cell ameloblastoma is a pretty rare tumour.

and McGinnis, 1972; Brocheriou *et al.*, 1975; Tandler and Rossi, 1977) (*Figures 93* and *94*); (2) congenital epulis, also known as the granular cell tumour of the gingiva of infants (Kay, Elzay and Willson, 1971); (3) ameloblastic fibroma (White *et al.*, 1977); (4) three cases of oligodendroglioma (out of ten cases studied) described by Takei, Mirra and Miles (1976); and (5) a unique ultrastructural variant of Wilms' tumour (Kurtz, 1979).

There is little doubt that the single membrane bound bodies found in the six types of granular cell tumours (including granular cell myoblastoma) described here are lysosomes. Despite the fact that some authors have called them 'autophagolysosomes', there is no hard evidence that they derive from sequestrated cytoplasmic structures. A probable exception may be the transplantable granular cell myoblastoma of the mouse, where a rare autophagic vacuole containing some rough endoplastic reticulum has been demonstrated in a welter of lysosomes (Mazzarella and DeBenedictis, 1967). Some of these lysosomes (e.g. *Figure 16* in Tandler and Rossi, 1977) contain numerous vesicles and, hence, resemble multivesicular bodies.

Whether the lysosomes in these granular cell tumours contain endocytosed material or endogenous material is not clear, but the very fact that such large numbers of quite large lysosomes occur suggests a defect in the digestive apparatus of the lysosome. Tandler and Rossi (1977) compare the situation here with the Chediak—Higashi syndrome, a disease with a genetic aetiology where large numbers of lysosomes occur. They state: '. . . the granular cell lesions here under consideration may also have undergone genetic alterations leading to a derangement in lysosomal production and function.'

References

ABRIKOSSOFF, A. (1926). Über Myome, ausgehend von der quergestreifter willkürlicher Muskulatur. *Virchows Arch. Path. Anat.*, **260**, 215

AHERNE, W. and HULL, D. (1966). Brown adipose tissue and heat production in the newborn infant. *J. Path. Bact.*, **91**, 223

ALLEGRA, S. R. (1971). Warthin's tumor: A hypersenssitivity disease? *Hum. Path.*, **2**, 404

APARICIO, S. R. and LUMSDEN, C. E. (1969). Light and electron-microscope studies on the granular-cell myoblastoma of the tongue. *J. Path.*, **97**, 339

ARCHER, R. and OMAR, M. (1969). Pink cell (oncocytic) metaplasia in a fibroadenoma of the human breast. Electron microscopic observations. *J. Path.*, **99**, 119

ARNOLD, B. M., KOVACS, K., HORVATH, E., MURRAY, T. M. and HIGGINS, H. P. (1974). Functioning oxyphil cell adenoma of the parathyroid gland: evidence for parathyroid secretory activity of oxyphil cells. *J. Clin. Endocr.*, **38**, 459

AZZOPARDI, J. G. (1956). Histogenesis of the granular cell 'myoblastoma'. *J. Path. Bact.*, **71**, 85

BANGLE, R., Jr. (1952). A morphological and histochemical study of granular cell myoblastoma. *Cancer*, **5**, 950

BAUSERMAN, S. C., HARDMAN, J. M., SCHOCHET, S. S. and EARL, K. M. (1978). Pituitary oncocytoma. *Archs Path. Lab. Med.*, **102**, 456

BLACK, W. C. III (1969). Pulmonary oncocytoma. *Cancer*, **23**, 1347

BROCHERIOU, C., HAUW, J. J., AURIOL, M., GUILBERT, F., CERNEA, P. and CHOMETTE, G. (1975). Étude ultrastructurale de 6 cas d'améloblastome. *Annls. Anat. Path.*, **20**, 231

CADOTTE, M. (1974). Malignant granular-cell myoblastoma. *Cancer*, **33**, 1417

DUNN, T. B. and GREEN, A. W. (1963). Cysts of the epididymis, cancer of the cervix, granular cell myoblastoma and other lesions after eostrogen injection in newborn mice. *J. Natn. Cancer Inst.*, **31**, 425

DUNN, T. B. and GREEN, A. W. (1965). A transplantable granular cell myoblastoma in strain C3H mice. *J. Natn. Cancer Inst.*, **34**, 389

FECHNER, R. E. and BENTINCK, B. R. (1973). Ultrastructure of bronchial oncocytoma. *Cancer*, **31**, 1451

FELDMAN, P. S., HORVATH, E. and KOVACS, K. (1972). Ultrastructure of three Hürthle cell tumors of the thyroid. *Cancer*, **30**, 1279

FISHER, E. R. and WECHSLER, H. (1962). Granular cell myoblastoma — a misnomer. Electron microscopic and histochemical evidence concerning its Schwann cell derivation and nature (granular cell Schwannoma). *Cancer*, **15**, 936

FUST, J. A. and CUSTER, R. P. (1949). On neurogenesis of so-called cell myoblastoma. *Am. J. Clin. Path.*, **19**, 522

GARANCIS, J. C., KOMOROWSKI, R. A and KUZMA, J. F. (1970). Granular cell myoblastoma. *Cancer*, **25**, 542

GHADIALLY, F. N. (1975). *Ultrastructural Pathology of the Cell*. London: Butterworths

GHADIALLY, F. N., DeCOTEAU, W. E., HUANG, S. and THOMAS, I. (1978). Ultrastructure of the skin of patients treated with sodium aurothiomalate. *J. Path.*, **124**, 77

GRAY, S. H. and GRUENFELD, G. E. (1937). Myoblastoma. *Am. J. Cancer*, **30**, 699

GULLINO, P. (1946). Sui cosidetti 'tumori di mioblasti' interpretati come granulomi die probabile origin parasitaria. *Tumori*, **20**, 102

HAMPERL, H. (1950). Onkocytes and the so-called Hürthle cell tumor. *Archs Path.*, **49**, 563

HEINMANN, P., HANSSON, G. and NILSSON, O. (1971). Primary hyperparathyroidism in a case of oxiphilic adenoma. *Acta Path. Microbiol. Scand. Sect. A.* **79**, 10

HÜBNER, G., KLEIN, H. J., KLEINSASSER, O. and SCHIEFER, H. G. (1971). Role of myoepithelial cells in the development of salivary gland tumors. *Cancer*, **27**, 1255

KAY, S., ELZAY, R. P. and WILLSON, M. A. (1971). Ultrastructural observations on a gingival, granular cell tumor (congenital epulis). *Cancer*, **27**, 674

KAY, S. and STILL, W. J. S. (1973). Electron microscopic observations on a parotid oncocytoma. *Archs Path.*, **96**, 186

KEYHANI, E. (1969). Anomalies de structure de mitochondries dans un adénocarcinome rénal spontané de la souris. *Archs Biol.*, **80**, 153

KLEMPERER, P. (1934). Myoblastoma of the striated muscle. *Am. J. Cancer*, **20**, 324

KOVACS, K. and HORVATH, E. (1973). Pituitary 'chromophobe' adenoma composed of oncocytes. *Archs Path.*, **95**, 235

KOVACS, K., HORVATH, E. and BILBAO, J. M. (1974). Oncocytes in the anterior lobe of the human pituitary gland. A light and electron microscopic study. *Acta Neuropath.*, **27**, 43

KURTZ, S. M. (1979). A unique ultrastructural variant of Wilms' tumor. *Am. J. Surg. Path.*, **3**, 257

LANDOLT, A. M. and OSWALD, U. W. (1973). Histology and ultrastructure of an oncocytic adenoma of the human pituitary. *Cancer*, **31**, 1099

LAUCHE, A. (1944). Sind die sog. 'Myoblastenmyome' Speicherzellgeschwülste? *Virchows Arch. Path. Anat.*, **312**, 335

LEROUX, R. and DELARUE, J. (1939). Sur trois cas de tumeurs à cellules granuleuses de la cavité buccale. *Bull. Assoc. Franc. Etude Cancer*, **28**, 427

LEVINE, G. D. (1972). Hibernoma. An electron microscopic study. *Hum. Path.*, **3**, 351

McGAVRAN, M. H. (1965). The ultrastructure of papillary cystadenoma lymphomatosum of the parotid gland. *Virchows Arch. Path. Anat.*, **338**, 195

McGREGOR, D. H., LOTUACO, L. G., RAO, M. S. and CHU, L. L. H. (1978). Functioning oxyphil adenoma of parathyroid gland. *Am. J. Path.*, **92**, 691

MARSHALL, R. B., ROBERTS, D. K. and TURNER, R. A. (1967). Adenomas of the human Parathyroid. Light and electron microscopic study following selenium 75 methionine scan. *Cancer*, **20**, 512

MAZZARELLA, L. and DeBENEDICTIS, G. (1967). Studio ultrastrutturale sul 'mioblastoma a cellule granulose' trapiantabile del topo. *Rivta Anat. Pat. Oncol.*, **31**, 1

MICHEL-BECHET, M., VALENTA, L. J. and ATHOUEL-HAON, A. M. (1971). *Bull. Assoc. Anat.*, **152**, 603

MINCER, H. H. and McGINNIS, J. P. (1972). Ultrastructure of thee histologic variants of the ameloblastoma. *Cancer*, **30**, 1036

MOSCOVIC, E. A. and AZAR, H. A. (1967). Multiple granular cell tumors ('myoblastomas'). Case report with electron microscopic observations and review of the literature. *Cancer*, **20**, 2032

NAVARRETE, A. R. and SMITH, M. (1971). Ultrastructure of granular cell ameloblastoma. *Cancer*, **27**, 948

PEARSE, A. G. E. (1950). Histogenesis of granular-cell myoblastoma (? granular-cell perineural fibroblastoma). *J. Path. Bact.*, **62**, 351

ROY, S. (1978). Ultrastructure of oncocytic adenoma of the human pituitary gland. *Acta Neuropath.*, **41**, 169

SCANARINI, M. and MINGRINO, S. (1974). Clinical, histological and ultrastructural observations upon the oncocytoma of the human pituitary gland. *J. Neurosurg. Sci.*, **18**, 263

SEEMAYER, T. A., KNAACK, J., WANG, N.-S. and AHMED, M. N. (1975). On the ultrastructure of hibernoma. *Cancer*, **36**, 1785

SELJELID, R. and ERICSSON, J. L. E. (1965). An electron-microscopic study of mitochondria in renal cell carcinoma. *J. Microsc.*, **4**, 759

SMALLELY, R. L. and DRYER, R. L. (1963). Brown fat: thermogenic effect during arousal from hibernation of the bat. *Science, N. Y.*, **140**, 1333

SMITH, R. E. and HOCK, R. J. (1963). Brown fat: thermogenic effector of arousal in hibernators. *Science, N. Y.*, **140**, 199

SOBEL, H. J. (1969). The nature of 'granular' cell myoblastoma. *Bull. Path.*, **10**, 238

SOBEL, H. J. and MARQUET, E. (1974). Granular cells and granular cell lesions. *Path. Ann.*, **9**, 43

SOBEL, H. J., MARQUET, E., AVRIN, E. and SCHWARZ, R. (1971). Granular cell myoblastoma. An electron microscopic and cytochemical study illustrating the genesis of granules and aging of myoblastoma cells. *Am. J. Path.*, **65**, 59

SOBEL, H. J., MARQUET, E. and SCHWARZ, R. (1973). Is schwannoma related to granular cell myoblastoma? *Archs Path.*, **95**, 396

SUN, C. N., WHITE, H. J. and THOMPSON, B. W. (1975). Oncocytoma (mitochondroma) of the parotid gland. *Archs Path.*, **99**, 208

SUN, C. N., WHITE, H. J. and THOMPSON, B. W. (1976). Warthin's tumor of the parotid gland. *Expl Path.*, **12**, 269

TAKEI, Y., MIRRA, S. S. and MILES, M. L. (1976). Eosinophilic granular cells in oligodendrogliomas. *Cancer*, **381**, 1968

TANDLER, B. (1966a). Fine structure of oncocytes in human salivary glands. *Virchows Arch. Path. Anat.*, **341**, 317

TANDLER, B. (1966b). Warthin's tumor. *Archs Otolar.* **84**, 68

TANDLER, B., HUTTER, R. V. P. and ERLANDSON, R. A. (1970). Ultrastructure of oncocytoma of the parotid gland. *Lab. Invest.*, **23**, 567

TANDLER, B. and ROSSI, E. P. (1977). Granular cell ameloblastoma: Electron microscopic observations. *J. Oral Path.*, **6**, 401

TANDLER, B. and SHIPKEY, F. H. (1964). Ultrastructure of Warthin's tumour. I. Mitochondria. *J. Ultrastruct. Res.*, **11**, 292

TONIETTI, G., BASCHIERI, L. and SALABE, G. (1967). Papillary and micro-follicular carcinoma of human thyroid. An ultrastructural study. *Archs Path.*, **84**, 601

VALENTA, L. J., MICHEL-BECHET, M., WARSHAW, J. B. and MALOOF, F. (1974). Human thyroid tumors composed of mitochondrion-rich cells: Electron microscopic and biochemical findings. *J. Clin. Endocr. Metab.*, **39**, 719

WHITE, D. K., CHEN, S.-Y., HARTMAN, K. S., GOMEZ, L. F. and MILLER, A. S. (1977). A clinical and ultrastructural study of the granular cell ameloblastic fibroma (Abstract). *Proceedings of the 31st Annual meeting of the American Academy of Oral Pathology*, 27

10
Is it a myosarcoma?*
(A study of intracytoplasmic filaments)

When one looks with the light microscope at a mesenchymal neoplasm that is difficult to classify, the presence of certain features such as 'cells that seem to be too plump and eosinophilic to be fibroblasts' may suggest the possibility that the tumour might be a myoma or myosarcoma of some sort.

This idea is then pursued by attempts to find striations and cross-striations with and without special stains. If the problem is not resolved, electron microscopic examination may prove helpful, because myofilaments and other intracytoplasmic filaments are too fine to be resolved with the light microscope but can be readily discerned with the electron microscope. However, more than a passing knowledge of the morphology and distribution of intracellular filaments is required because: (1) intracytoplasmic filaments are seen in quite a variety of normal cells; (2) they appear to be quite prominent in certain pathological states (*Figure 95*), including some neoplasms (*Figures 96* and *97*); and (3) identifying the correct type of filament is essential for the differential diagnosis of tumours (e.g. tonofilaments in squamous carcinoma, thin myofilaments in leiomyosarcoma, and thick and thin myofilaments in rhabdomyosarcoma).

Myofilaments

Myofilaments comprise a special class of intracytoplasmic filaments. Two types of filaments — thick (about 10 nm in diameter) and thin (about 5 nm in

diameter) — are recognized in striated muscle cells. The former contain myosin; the latter, actin and some tropomyosin. In striated muscle the two types of filaments are set side by side in a very orderly fashion and it is this which gives striated muscle its striated appearance (*Figures 98–100*).

In the usual preparations of vertebrate smooth muscle most of the filaments are very fine and only occasional thicker filaments are seen. However, there is now a mounting body of evidence that the thicker myosin filaments are present in substantial numbers in smooth muscle also, but special methods are required to preserve and demonstrate them. The characteristic feature of actin filaments in smooth muscle, as seen in routine preparations, is the occurrence of focal densities along their course. However, the presence of such filaments with focal densities is by no means the hall-mark of the smooth muscle cell and its tumours (*Figure 101*). One such exception, the myoepithelial cell (*Figure 8*), was well known to light microscopists, but electron microscopy has now shown many more cells containing myofilaments with focal densities. These include: (1) cells in the arterial wall where lipid accumulates in atherosclerosis (also called foam cells) (Flora, Dahl and Nelson, 1967; Peterson *et al.*, 1971; Wissler, 1967); (2) cells in the ganglion of the wrist (Ghadially and Mehta, 1971); (3) granulation tissue and repair tissue (Gabbiani *et al.*, 1976) (*Figure 15*); and (4) cells of Wharton's jelly (Parry, 1970).

Such cells bear a resemblance to smooth muscle cells in that they contain filaments with focal densities along their course, but there are also morphological and functional differences. Examples of morphological differences include the infrequency of plasmalemmal vesicles (as compared with true smooth muscle cells), and a relative abundance of elements of the Golgi complex and rough endoplasmic reticulum. Thus, these cells have some

*Largely as a result of electron microscopic studies, it has become apparent that myofilaments occur not only in tumours of smooth and striated muscle, but also in some other tumours. It is convenient to consider these here, although they cannot perhaps be strictly considered myomas or myosarcomas.

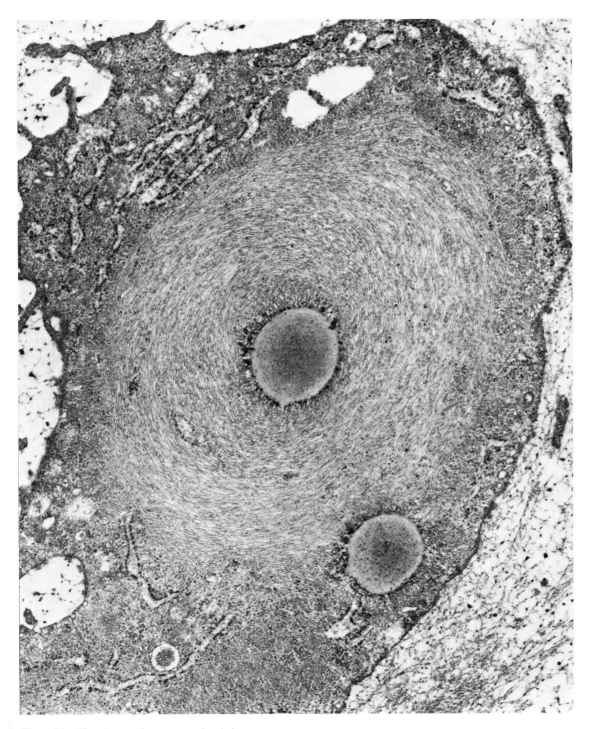

Figure 95   *Chondrocyte from osteoarthrotic human articular cartilage showing a whorl of intracytoplasmic filaments.* ×28 000

morphological features of both fibroblasts* and smooth muscle cells, so these cells are now called 'myofibroblasts'.

On the other hand, on the basis of functional characteristics such cells have been called 'multifunctional mesenchymal cells', for besides the power to contract they also have the capacity to trap lipoproteins (e.g. in atheroma) and synthesize the precursors of collagen fibrils, elastic fibres, and also glycosaminoglycans of the interfibrillary matrix and basement membrane material. (For references and details see Ghadially, 1975.)

*Fibroblasts are well endowed with rough endoplasmic reticulum but muscle cells are not. The external lamina (erroneously referred to as the basal lamina or basement membrane by some) is evident adjacent to smooth and striated muscle cells, but an external lamina is not seen around fibroblasts.

Other intracytoplasmic filaments

Intracytoplasmic filaments similar in thickness to myofilaments but of unknown chemical composition are of common occurrence in a variety of cells. A convenient term covering all such intracytoplasmic filaments has not yet been coined. Terms such as 'other intracytoplasmic filaments', 'cytoplasmic fine filaments', 'fine filamentous fibres (or fibrils)' and 'FFF' have been used for this purpose. In the text that follows the term 'intracytoplasmic filaments'†‡ is used in a restricted sense to mean all intracytoplasmic filaments except myofilaments.

†At times also referred to as 'intermediate filaments'; a not too sensible term, since some of them (e.g. tonofilaments) are about the same thickness as myosin filaments and others are thicker.

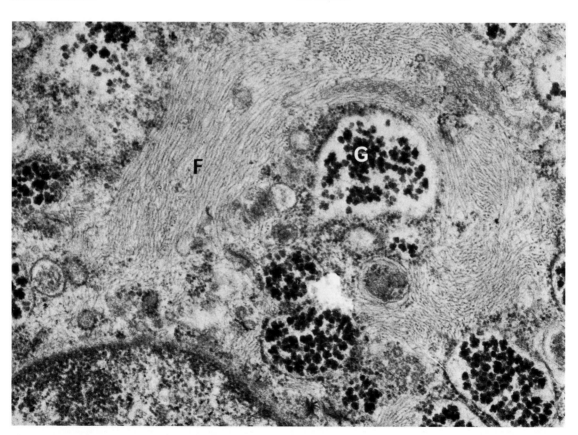

Figure 96   *Canine plasmacytoma. Cell showing intracytoplasmic filaments (F). The occurrence of glycogen (G) within vesiculated rough endoplasmic reticulum is an unusual phenomenon of unknown significance.* ×45 000. *from Ghadially, Lowes and Mesfin, 1977)*

118

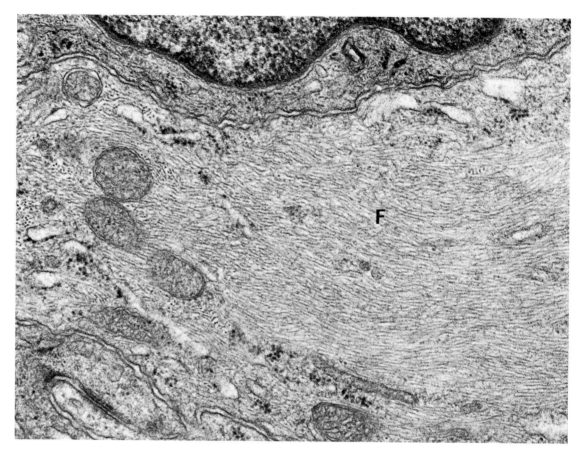

Figure 97   *Cardiac myxoma. Tumour cell containing*
intracytoplasmic filaments (F). ×*52 000*

It must, however, be realized that lack of knowledge about the chemical composition of these filaments and the suspicion that quite a few of them may be myofilaments after all precludes even a rough classification of the type sugggested above. The text that follows must be read with this limitation in mind.

The myofilaments of striated muscle are easily recognized by their highly ordered arrangement (as already noted, this is what produces the striated appearance). The myofilaments of smooth muscle are characterized by their orderly arrangement and the occurrence of focal densities along their course. But intracytoplasmic filaments possess no such constant or characteristic distinguishing feature. Some differences in orientation thickness and electron densities are, however, seen. For example, the filaments comprising the tonofibrils of squamous epithelia are usually arranged in bundles or sheaves (often electron-dense) which at times terminate or loop through the

plaques of desmosomes (Kelly, 1966) (*Figures 33* and *38*), while those in chondrocytes show a whorled fascicular arrangement (*Figure 95*).

The position of intracytoplasmic filaments in the cell is also quite variable. They may be scattered diffusely in the cell or they may show a perinuclear or juxtanuclear distribution. At times such filaments may appear to arise as bushy outgrowths from the nuclear envelope, a mitochondrion or a lipid droplet (Ghadially and Roy, 1969). Such images are explicable on the basis of sectioning geometry and superimposition, but the possibility that true continuity between the filaments and such structures exists cannot be ruled out.

An increase in the intracytoplasmic filament content of the cells has been noted in various experimental and pathological situations. Such an increase has been detected in cells that are often fairly well endowed with filaments (e.g. chondrocytes) and

119

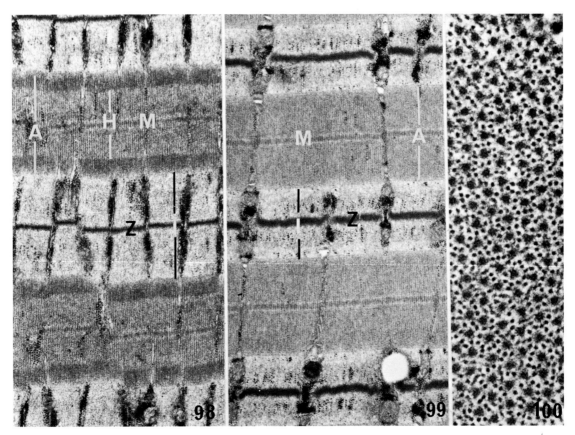

Figures 98 *and* 99   *Stretched and contracted skeletal muscle, respectively, are shown. Various details such as the A band (A), I band (I), H band (H), M line (M) and Z line (Z) are evident. ×17 000; ×17 000 (From Ghadially, 1975)*

Figure 100   *Transverse section through the A band, showing thick and thin filaments. Each myosin filament is surrounded by six actin filaments occupying the trigonal position — that is, equidistant from and shared by three myosin filaments. × 100 000*

also in others where no filaments are said to occur (e.g. lymphocytes from peripheral blood) or where only a few filaments are seen (e.g. vascular endothelial cells and synovial intimal cells).

An increase in the intracytoplasmic filament content of cells has been noted in the following cell types and conditions: (1) chondrocytes of rabbit articular cartilage as a result of ageing (Barnett, Cochrane and Palfrey, 1963), experimentally produced chronic haemarthrosis (Roy, 1968), experimentally produced lipoarthrosis (Ghadially, Mehta and Kirkaldy-Willis, 1970), after the production of superficial defects in articular cartilage (Fuller and Ghadially, 1972) and after intraarticular injections of sodium aurothiomalate (Ghadially and Lalonde, 1978); (2) synovial intimal cells in rheumatoid arthritis (for references see Ghadially and Roy, 1969) and villonodular synovitis (Ghadially, Lalonde and Dick, 1979); (3) vascular endothelial cells of synovial blood vessels in rheumatoid arthritis (Ghadially and Roy, 1967); (4) peritoneal macrophages in cases of malignant ascites (Ghadially, 1975); (5) human neurons in cases of sporadic motor neuron disease, infantile neuroaxonal dystrophy, vincristine neuropathy, Pick's disease and neurons of experimental animals in aluminium encephalopathy, spindle inhibitor encephalopathy, lathyrogenic encephalopathy, vitamin E deficiency, copper deficiency, and retrograde and Wallerian degeneration (Terry and Pena, 1965; Wisniewski, Terry and Hiraon, 1970; Terry, 1971); (6) human lymphocytes from thoracic duct (Zucker-Franklin, 1963); (7) activated lymphocytes from mixed lymphocyte cultures but not those activated by phytohaemagglutinin (Parker, Wakasa and Lukes, 1967); (8) lymphomas and leukaemias, including plasma cell and myeloid leukaemia (for references, see Rangan, Calvert and Vitols, 1971; Beltran and Stuckey, 1972; Ghadially, Lowes and Mesfin, 1977).

Intracytoplasmic filaments have been noted in a wide variety of experimentally produced and human tumours (*Figures 96* and *97*). Prominent juxtanuclear filamentous aggregates and psammoma bodies were found in a papillary adenocarcinoma of the endometrium by Hameed and Morgan (1972). These authors suggest that such aggregates of cytoplasmic filaments provide the scaffolding for calcification and psammoma body formation, not only in the tumour studied by them, but also in other tumours such as meningiomas. Furthermore, they and others who

have studied fine filaments in lymphomas and leukaemias have proposed that such an increase indicates a state of heightened metabolic activity associated with the neoplastic state.

However, many workers have taken a contrary view (for a critique see Ghadially, 1975) and suggested that the accumulation of intracytoplasmic filaments even in tumours is a sign of degeneration and impending necrosis. Such a view has been expressed about: (1) pituitary adenomas, where focal whorls of intracytoplasmic filaments occur (Cardell and Knighton, 1966; Peillon, Vila-Porcile and Olivier, 1970; Schochet, McCormick and Halmi, 1972); (2) Chang cells (hepatoma) cultured with activated lymphocytes (Biberfeld, 1971); and (3) human breast carcinoma cells in culture, where massive accumulation of 11 nm thick filaments occurs in declining cells in cultures no longer dividing (Tumilowicz and Sarkar, 1972).

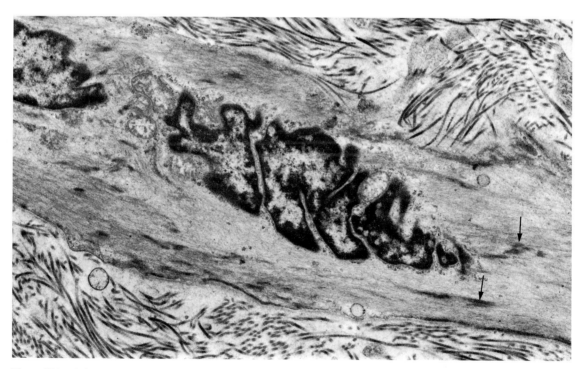

Figure 101   *Leiomyoma of uterus. Smooth muscle cell showing the characteristic folded nucleus. The actin filaments in smooth muscle cells and their tumours are so fine and arranged in such a manner that they are difficult to resolve or are only resolved in small areas within the cell. Thus, as Fawcett (1967) points out, '... the cytoplasm looks surprisingly homogeneous even at moderately high magnification'. The focal densities (arrows) are, however, easily seen. Note also the abundance of collagen fibrils in the matrix. ×16 000*

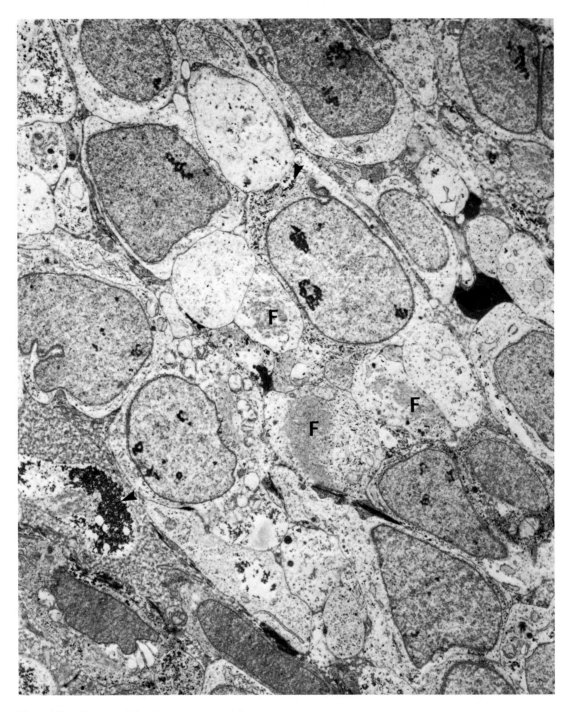

Figure 102 *Embryonal rhabdomyosarcoma of the orbit. The filamentous areas (F) are barely discernible in a few cells. The oval nuclei with a homogeneous appearance are quite typical of embryonal rhabdomyosarcoma. There is a* *fair amount of glycogen present in the tumour cells (arrow-heads) ×6000 (From a block of tissue supplied by Dr A. H. Cameron)*

Rhabdomyosarcoma*

Unequivocal establishment of the diagnosis of rhabdomyosarcoma is fraught with difficulties at both the light and the electron microscopic levels. If one insists that cross-striations be demonstrated (by light microscopy) before a tumour is labelled a rhabdomyosarcoma, then this would be a rather rare diagnosis and one would miss quite a few cases of rhabdomyosarcoma. On the other hand, if one is prepared to accept that the presence of strap-like cells with or without a fibrillar cytoplasm, tadpole cells or cells of tennis racquet shape with a markedly eosinophilic cytoplasm, nuclei in tandem or alveolar arrangement of cells as sufficient, then all sorts of other tumours are likely to be erroneously labelled rhabdomyosarcoma.

The electron microscopic diagnosis of rhabdomyosarcoma (*Figures 102–106*) is bedevilled by the same sort of problem — namely, that the tumour has to be sufficiently differentiated to form characteristic myofibrils containing thick and thin filaments (preferably with the formation of some bands and lines also). Demonstration of a few or even numerous nondescript filaments is just not good enough, because, as we have seen, intracytoplasmic filaments of various sorts including the thin actin filaments are common enough in a variety of cells and tumours and, hence, cannot be accepted as diagnostic of rhabdomyosarcoma.

With the light microscope one cannot visualize myofilaments or distinguish thick and thin filaments, but one can do this with the electron microscope. Hence, it follows that with the electron microscope one can at times unequivocally establish the diagnosis of rhabdomyosarcoma where the diagnosis was in doubt by light microscopy. Similarly, there are occasions where the diagnosis of rhabdomyosarcoma can be quite effectively refuted by electron microscopy, but experience shows that in a substantial number of cases (probably one-third to one-half) the electron microscope also fails to produce an unequivocal answer. This is because the tumour is just not differentiated enough or the rare well-differentiated cell with thick and thin filaments does not happen to be included in the minute amount of material that can be examined with the electron microscope (see page 10).

*The rare, benign rhabdomyoma poses no diagnostic problem, nor does it undergo malignant transformation. Hence, rhabdomyoma is not considered here. For an account of the ultrastructure of this tumour and references see Tandler *et al.* (1970).

These difficulties and the conceptual dilemma as to what is the minimum requirement for labelling a tumour a rhabdomyosarcoma is reflected in the numerous papers on the ultrastructure of rhabdomyosarcoma. Some authors have been quite happy to make the diagnosis of rhabdomyosarcoma on the basis of filaments alone or filaments with densities which could be construed as altered Z lines but could also equally well be focal densities of the type seen in smooth muscle; however, others have insisted (quite rightly) on much stricter criteria. A detailed list of references to this literature is not necessary, because in an excellent paper Morales, Fine and Horn (1972) describe the ultrastructure of '15 histologically malignant tumours in which a light microscope diagnosis of rhabdomyosarcoma had been rendered previously or was strongly suspected' and they also review past published cases in a most thorough and critical fashion, which is in accord with my own thinking about this matter.

They divide their tumours into two groups: Group A (six cases) where thin (6–8 nm) and thick (12–15 nm) filaments were present and at times I bands and Z lines were also seen. Group B (nine cases) lacked these features, but thin filaments (6–8 nm in diameter) were found distributed irregularly in the cytoplasm or arranged in bundles along the long axis of the cell. On this basis they considered the diagnosis of rhabdomyosarcoma as firmly established in the six cases in Group A but not in the nine cases in Group B. They accept the possibility that some of the tumours in Group B where only thin filaments were seen could have been rhabdomyosarcomas. In three of the tumours in Group B ultrastructural study clearly demonstrated that they were not rhabdomyosarcomas (two leiomyosarcomas, one osteogenic sarcoma).

Figure 103 shows a cell from an embryonal rhabdomyosarcoma of the orbit. The appearance seen here is diagnostic of rhabdomyosarcoma, because slender fibrils composed of quite straight, thick and thin filaments are clearly evident. A bonus here is that there are also some densities which are acceptable as attenuated Z lines, but this would not be absolutely necessary for diagnosing rhabdomyosarcoma. Also reassuring is the finding of ribosomes arranged in what is known as an 'Indian file' along some of the myofilaments, for such an appearance is thought to indicate that synthesis of new filaments is occurring. It is worth noting that this appearance has been seen in developing or regenerating striated muscle and rhabdomyomas and rhabdomyosarcomas.

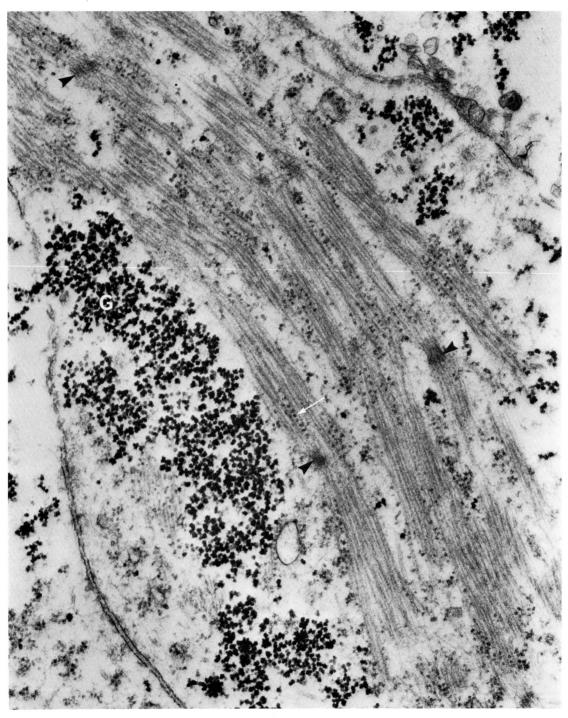

Figure 103   *Rhabdomyosarcoma. Same case as Figure 102, showing straight fibrils composed of thick and thin filaments. Note also the attenuated Z lines (arrowheads) and ribosomes (arrows) in Indian file arrangment. Larger,* *denser (as compared with ribosomes) glycogen particles (G) are also evident in the cytoplasmic matrix. ×52 000 (From a block of tissue supplied by Dr A. H. Cameron)*

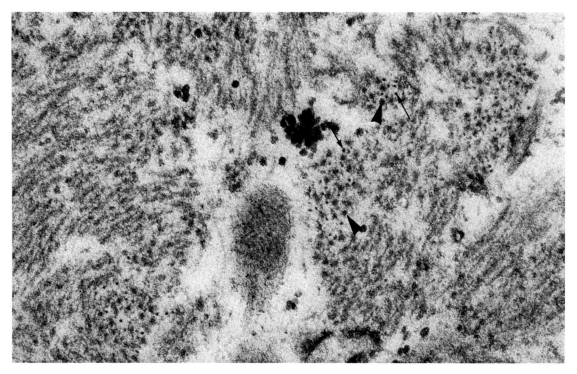

Figure 104　*Rhabdomyosarcoma. Same case as Figures 102 and 103, showing obliquely and transversely cut thick (arrowheads) and thin (arrows) filaments. The appearance is rather similar to that shown in Figure 100, except that far* *fewer thin filaments are present and an orderly arrangement is lacking. ×103 000 (From a block of tissue supplied by Dr A. H. Cameron)*

Thick and thin filaments can be readily identified in transverse sections through the A band (the I band contains thin filaments only) of normal muscle (*Figure 100*). Each myosin filament is surrounded by six actin filaments occupying the trigonal position — that is, equidistant from and shared by three myosin filaments. In rhabdomyosarcoma such a precise geometric arrangement can hardly be expected to occur, nor is the orientation of filaments likely to be so perfect that all of them will be transversely cut and, hence, well visualized. However, careful search does often reveal thick and thin filaments (*Figure 104*) mimicking the appearance seen in transverse sections of normal striated muscle (*Figure 100*). And this, too, is an appearance which can be confidently accepted as diagnostic of rhabdomyosarcoma.

Thus, on the basis of the appearance seen in *Figures 103* and *104* one could assert that this is a rhabdomyosarcoma, but at this stage one should pause to consider whether one is indeed looking at: (1) a neoplastic rhabdomyoblast containing myofila-ments in a rhabdomyosarcoma; or (2) an 'accidentally included' degenerating muscle fibre* in an infiltrating tumour; or (3) some quite different tumour in which rhabdomyoblasts occur.† To help solve this problem one should consider: (1) the accompanying cells, to see whether they fit in with the idea that they could be neoplastic rhabdomyoblasts (e.g. appearances seen in *Figures 105* and *106*), even though they cannot be unequivocally identified as such; and (2) the site from which the tumour came and from which portion the biopsy was collected.

---

*An excellent illustration of this is presented by Penney *et al*. (1978), who show (their *Figure 14*) a muscle fibre 'decomposed or degraded by one or more tumour cells' in a squamous cell carcinoma of the oral cavity.
†For example, some embryonal tumours (e.g. Wilms' tumour) contain rhabdomyoblasts showing varying stages of differentiation (Tremblay, 1971). The mere presence of some cells containing thick and thin filaments does not on its own establish the diagnosis of rhabdomyosarcoma.

Besides the diagnostically significant appearances shown in *Figures 103* and *104* there are other appearances which, although of little value on their own, constitute good supportive evidence (*Figures 105* and *106*). These include: (1) filaments of various sizes with or without structures resembling densities interpretable as altered Z lines; (2) dense rod-like structures similar to those seen in various myopathies, particularly nemaline myopathy (these are thought to be derived from Z line material); and (3) masses of tangled filaments reminiscent of that found in damaged muscle.

Vexatious though the problem of diagnosing rhabdomyosarcoma may be, it is possible to explain the appearance we find on the basis of past electron microscopic studies of cyto-differentiation of skeletal muscle (Hibbs, 1956; Price, Howes and Blumberg, 1964; Firket, 1967; Fischman, 1967; Ishikawa, Bischoff and Holtzer, 1968; Kelly, 1969). The primi-

tive mesenchymal cells from which striated muscle fibres arise are round or oval cells with abundant polyribosomes, but they contain only rare intracytoplasmic filaments (6 nm thick). Such cells may also be found in rhabdomyosarcoma, but if this is all that is present, then one cannot say that the tumour is a rhabdomyosarcoma, for the direction of differentiation is not evident at this stage.

Most investigators agree that in the developing myoblast thin filaments are laid down first, but there are a few dissenters who claim that thick and thin filaments form together or that the thick filaments come first. There is, however, general agreement that, of the various bands and lines, the Z lines form first. The rhabdomyosarcoma tends to recapitulate the process of normal development of the rhabdomyoblast, for, as can be seen in *Figure 103*, attenuated Z lines are discernible but no other variety of cross-striation is clearly evident.

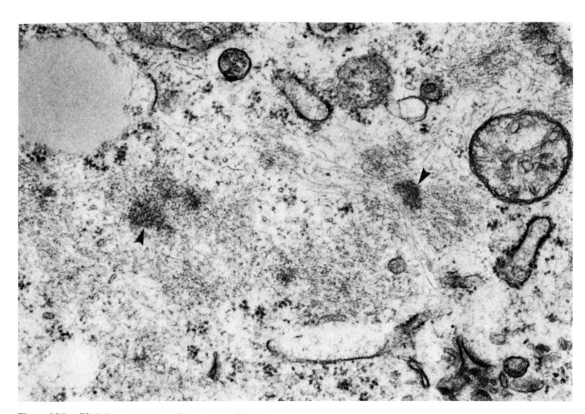

Figure 105 *Rhabdomyosarcoma. Same case as Figures 102–104. Only randomly scattered filaments and some dense areas probably representing altered Z line material (arrowheads) are evident. ×64 000 (From a block of tissue supplied by Dr A. H. Cameron)*

126

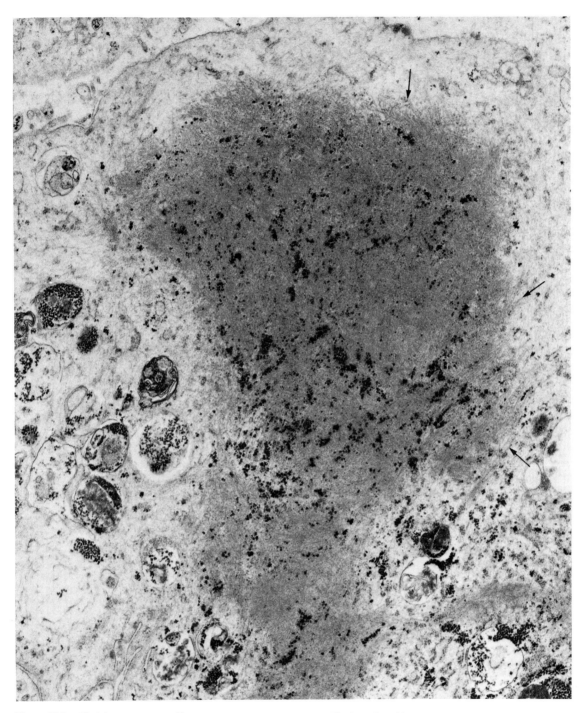

Figure 106 *Rhabdomyosarcoma. From same case as Figures 102–105. The large grey area comprises a tangle of extremely fine filaments and entrapped glycogen. The filamentous (arrows) nature of the aggregate may just be discerned by examining the peripheral parts of the grey area. The idea that this is a damaged cell is supported by the autolysosomes (arrowheads) containing glycogen and membranous material. ×25 000 (From a block of tissue supplied by Dr A. H. Cameron)*

Our views on the unequivocal diagnosis of rhabdomyosarcoma can now be summarized as follows: (1) the finding of haphazardly arranged filaments (they can be thin or quite thick; up to about 10 nm or more) is a finding of very limited diagnostic value, because intracytoplasmic filaments can be found in a variety of normal and neoplastic cells; (2) the finding of well-aligned filaments with what might appear like focal densities or altered Z lines* along their course is, again, of very limited value, for such an appearance is seen in smooth muscle and its tumours, in other tumours such as cardiac myxoma and also in myofibroblasts; and (3) it is mandatory to show fibrils comprising thick and thin filaments to establish the diagnosis of rhabdomyosarcoma. These concepts are in accord with those enunciated by Ishikawa, Bischoff and Holtzer (1968) Kelly (1969) and Morales, Fine and Horn (1972).

Leiomyoma and Leiomyosarcoma

The unequivocal establishment of the histogenesis of a neoplasm with the electron microscope often rests upon the demonstration of some specific organelle or feature which occurs in a particular cell line and its tumour but in no other. Such examples include melanosomes in melanoma, beta cell granules in insulinoma and also the example we have just noted in this chapter, viz. the characteristic myofibrils composed of thick and thin filaments which are found in rhabdomyosarcoma.

There is, alas, no such single specific trait which distinguishes the smooth muscle cell from all others. However, this cell can usually be distinguished by a combination of features, which include: (1) a nucleus which is often folded (concertina fashion) or notched or shows many invaginations; (2) a cytoplasm which is packed with thin actin filaments with focal densities along their course; (3) a few mitochondria and sparse elements of endoplasmic reticulum and Golgi complex situated adjacent to the poles of the nucleus; (4) abundant micropinocytotic vesicles; (5) dense plaques on the cytoplasmic aspects of the cell membrane into which some of the myofilaments appear

to be anchored; and (6) a thin but usually distinct external lamina.†

Myosin filaments (thick filaments) are not totally absent from smooth muscle and, indeed, a few such filaments or groups of such filaments can at times be discerned, even in routine preparations, but they do not show the highly ordered arrangment found in striated muscle. It is thought that in the relaxed smooth muscle myosin exists in a dispersed or soluble form but during contraction aggregates into filaments which interact with the actin filaments to produce muscle contraction.

The cells of leiomyomas bear a close resemblance to normal smooth muscle cells (Meyer *et al.*, 1968; Welsh and Meyer, 1969; Ferenczy, Richart and Okagaki, 1971). Virtually all the features of normal smooth muscle, such as a folded nucleus, filaments with densities, dense plaques and an external lamina, can be detected in these tumours (*Figure 101*). However, some slight variations may also be noted, the most common ones being a relative paucity§ of pinocytotic vesicles and an external lamina that is not quite so well developed and continuous as in the normal state.

Ultrastructural differences between leiomyoma and leiomyosarcoma (*Figures 107–109*) depend upon the degree of differentiation. In the markedly anaplastic versions of leiomyosarcoma filaments may be sparse, and even when a fair number are present, one has to look around for focal densities to convince oneself that we have myofilaments and not just 'other intracytoplasmic filaments'. In the better-differentiated examples thin filaments are plentiful

*In smooth muscle the spindle-shaped or oval densities lie parallel to the filaments but the Z lines of striated muscle lie at right angles to the filaments. Unfortunately, this distinction is often not maintained in the rather slender fibrils in rhabdomyosarcoma. Therefore, at times it can be quite difficult to decide whether one is looking at a focal density or a short altered segment of the Z line.

†This is often referred to as a 'basal lamina' or, worse still, 'basement membrane'. The basal lamina lies at the base of various epithelia. A similar but thinner lamina invests cells such as smooth muscle cells and Schwann cells. There is nothing 'basal' about this lamina. It should, therefore, be called an 'external lamina'. In electron microscopy the term 'membrane' is restricted to describe only those structures where the characteristic trilaminar appearance is evident – e.g. plasma membrane, cytomembranes, mitochondrial membranes and lysosomal membranes. For this reason and also because of the fact that the basement membrane of the light microscopist includes not only the basal lamina of the electron microscopist, but also some underlying collagen fibrils, it would be erroneous to call the 'basal lamina' 'basement membrane'. It is, of course, quite legitimate to continue using the term 'basement membrane' in light microscopy.

§As noted earlier, normal smooth muscle cells are usually well endowed with micropinocytotic vesicles, but this does depend to some extent on the physiological activity of the cell at a given moment.

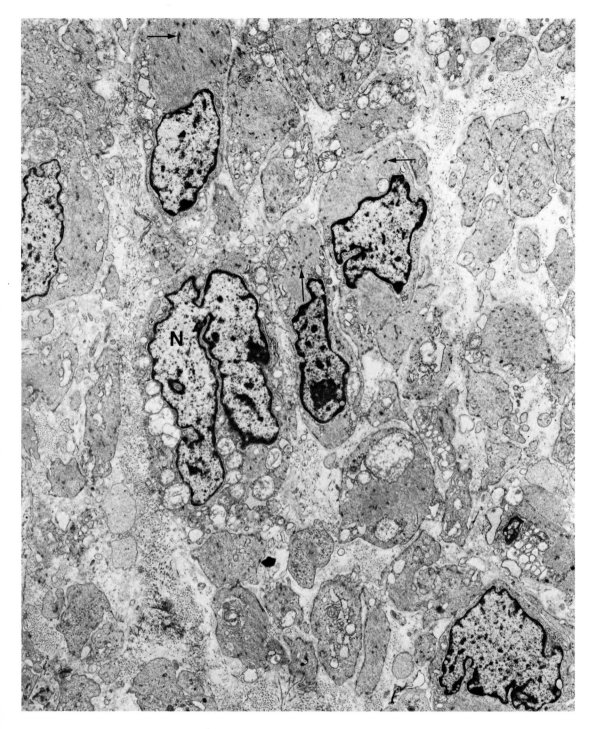

Figure 107   *Leiomyosarcoma of the ankle. Note nuclear and cellular pleomorphism, particularly the cell with the bizarre nucleus (N) and numerous swollen mitochondria.*

The cytoplasm is packed with filaments, as evidenced by the homogeneous appearance of the cytoplasm. Focal densities may just be discerned (arrows). ×3000

129

and so are focal densities, which can at times be quite large and prominent (*Figure 109*).

Irregularity of nuclear form is of limited value, since this is a normal feature in this cell type, but bizarre grossly enlarged nuclei are of some value. Other features in leiomyosarcoma may be summarized by the following points: (1) the filaments show a much greater degree of disorientation than in leiomyoma; (2) quite large areas of the cell may be devoid of filaments (filaments only at the periphery of the cell) and such areas are occupied by various other organelles such as polyribosomes, atypical mitochondria, rough endoplasmic reticulum and Golgi complex; (3) paucity of pinocytotic vesicles; (4) paucity of dense plaques; and (5) aberrations and discontinuities of the external lamina.

The recognition of malignancy in smooth muscle tumours can be quite difficult by light microscopy. Correlation of light and electron microscopic findings may be of some value here, for Morales *et al.* (1975) have found that while the presence of well-developed and abundant structures such as myofilaments, focal densities, dense plaques and pinocytotic vesicles is no assurance that a tumour is benign, the converse situation — that is to say, a paucity or atypia of one or more of these features — is highly likely to be an indicator of malignancy, even in cases where the tumour appears benign by light microscopic examination. This seems to be an important observation (although as yet based on only a few cases) worthy of further thought and study.

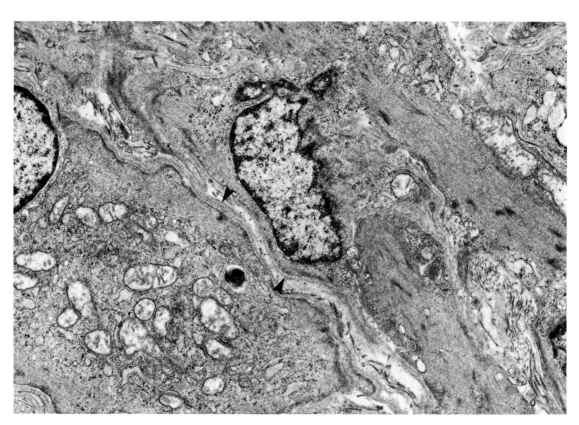

Figure 108   *Leiomyosarcoma. Higher-power view from same case as Figure 107. The cell in the bottom left-hand corner contains numerous mitochondria and some rough endoplasmic reticulum; the other cells are better-endowed with filaments and focal densities. An external lamina (arrowheads) invests the tumour cells.* ×17 000

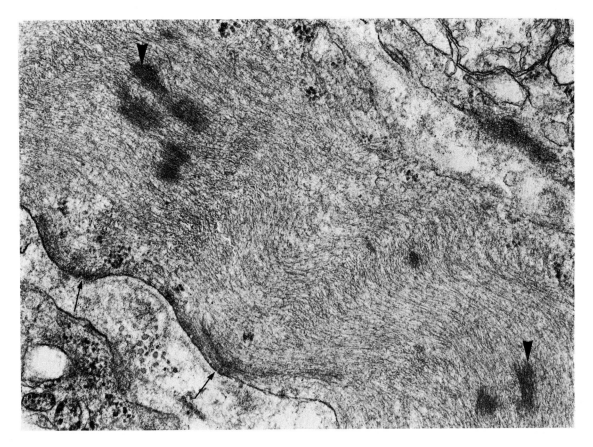

Figure 109 *Leiomyosarcoma. Same case as Figures 107 and 108. Note fine filaments with large focal densities (arrowheads) along their course and dense plaques (arrows) on the cell membrane.* ×45 000

Myofilaments in other tumours

Cells containing myofilaments with focal densities (as seen in smooth muscle) have been found not only in leiomyomas and leiomyosarcomas, but also in other tumours and tumour-like conditions. Examples of this will now be presented.

Myoepithelial cells are found in the normal acini of some glands, the best-known example being the breast. They are involved in a variety of pathological conditions (e.g. sclerosing adenosis and fibro-adenoma) (*Figure 8*) affecting the breast and also cancer (*Figures 110* and *111*) (Murad and Scarpelli, 1967; Murad and Von Haam, 1968; Carter, Yardley and Shelley, 1969; Schafer and Bässler, 1969; Tannenbaum, Weiss and Marx, 1969; Harris and Ahmed, 1977).

The glomus cell has been regarded as either a modified smooth muscle cell or a modified pericyte. The former view appears to be closer to the truth, because glomus cells contain myofilaments with focal densities, dense plaques and numerous micro-pinocytotic vesicles. Glomangiomas of the skin and stomach have been shown to contain these structures also (Harris, 1971; Morales *et al.*, 1975).

The filaments in pericytes are well oriented and form a band beneath the surface of the cell facing the vascular endothelium. However, focal densities and dense plaques are absent. The pericyte contains a fair amount of rough endoplasmic reticulum; in this it more resembles a fibroblast than a smooth muscle cell. In keeping with these features is the observation

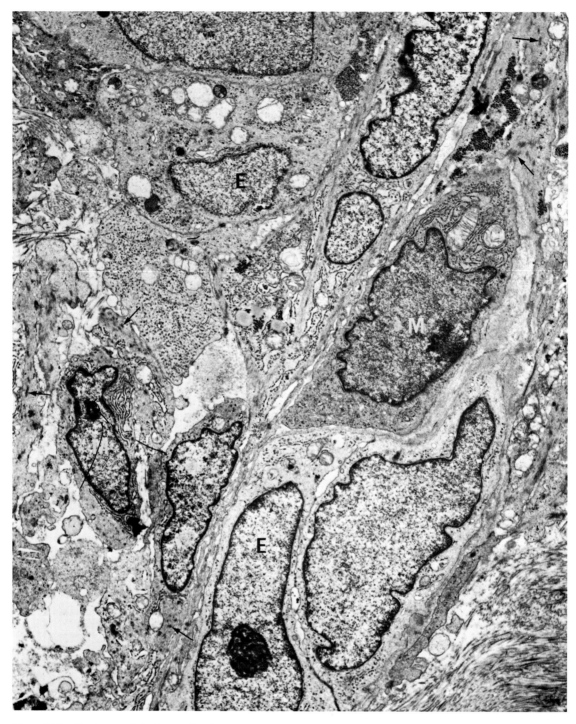

Figure 110   *Carcinoma of the breast, showing neoplastic epithelial cells (E) and myoepithelial cells (M). The latter are recognizable by a more electron-dense cytoplasm and* *some focal densities (arrows) which are just discernible at this low magnification.* ×*9000*

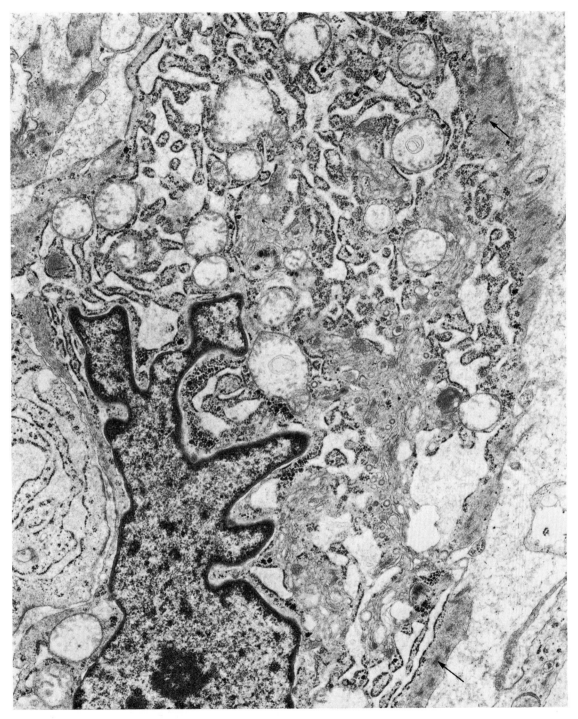

Figure 111   *Carcinoma of the breast. Same case as Figure 110, showing details of a myoepithelial cell. Note the irregular nucleus, abundant rough endoplasmic reticulum, Golgi complex and filaments with focal densities (arrows).*

Compare also with myoepithelial cell from fibroadenoma of breast shown in Figure 8. There the filamentous areas are more prominent. ×22 000

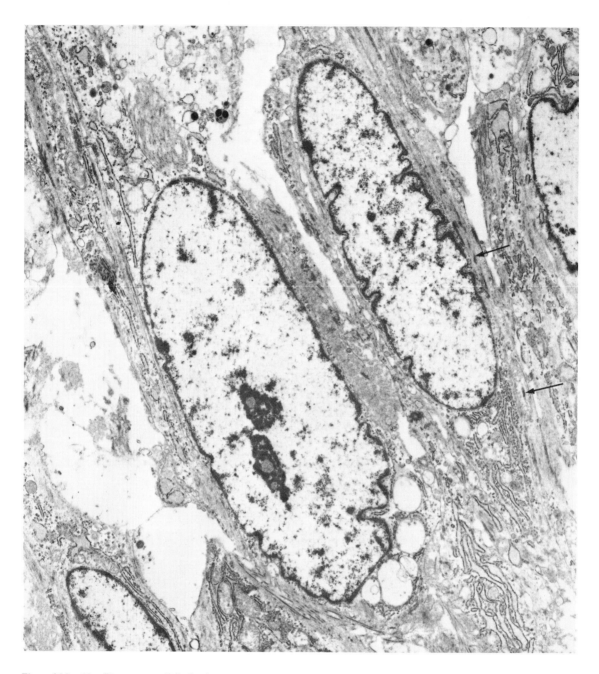

Figure 112   *Myofibrosarcoma. Spindle-shaped tumour cells
(neoplastic myofibroblasts) containing indented nuclei,
rough endoplasmic reticulum and zones of myofilaments
with focal densities (arrows).* × *7500 (From Vasudev and
Harris, 1978)*

that myofilaments with focal densities along their course are not found in haemangiopericytomas (for references see Morales *et al.*, 1975).

We noted (p. 116) that the cells (myofibroblasts) in the myxomatous tissue of the umbilical cord (Wharton's jelly) contain myofilaments with focal densities. A review of the literature and my personal experience with cardiac myxomas seem to indicate that in some examples of this tumour or tumour-like lesion one can find cells containing filaments with focal densities but in others only filaments of the type we refer to as 'other intracytoplasmic filaments' are found (*Figure 97*). (For references and critique see Kelly and Bhagwat, 1972; Stovin, Heath and Khaliq, 1973; Morales *et al.*, 1975.)

Kaposi's sarcoma is now thought to arise from a primitive mesenchymal cell which has the ability to differentiate into a variety of cell types. The list of cell types is quite long, but ultrastructural studies have confirmed the presence of endothelial cells, fibroblasts, perithelial cells, histiocytes, undifferentiated mesenchymal cells, smooth muscle cells and also quite characteristic myofibroblasts (Pepler and Theron, 1962; Yodaiken, 1962; Hashimoto and Lever, 1964; Niemi and Mustakallio, 1965; Mottaz and Zelickson, 1966; Barbera and Mazzarella, 1967; Martinez-Penuela *et al.*, 1970; Domagala *et al.*, 1975; Harrison and Kahn, 1978).

Numerous fibroblastic tumours and tumour-like lesions once thought to be composed of fibroblasts have now been shown to contain a few or many myofibroblasts. Such examples include: (1) desmoid fibromatosis (Stiller and Katenkamp, 1975); (2) nodular fasciitis (Wiseman, 1976); (3) circumscribed

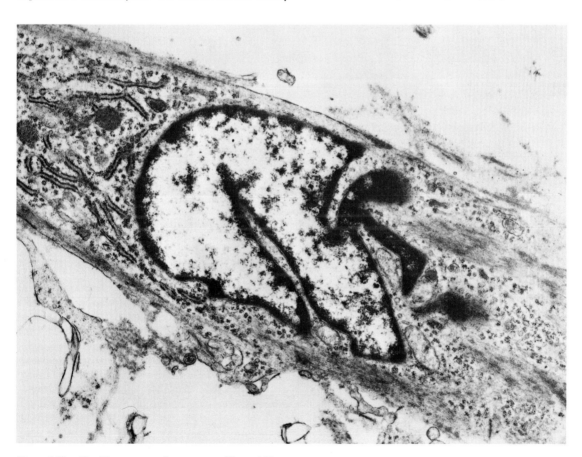

Figure 113 *Myofibrosarcoma. Same case as Figure 112, showing a neoplastic myofibroblast. Note the irregular nucleus and myofilaments with focal densities.* ×15 000 *(From Vasudev and Harris, 1978)*

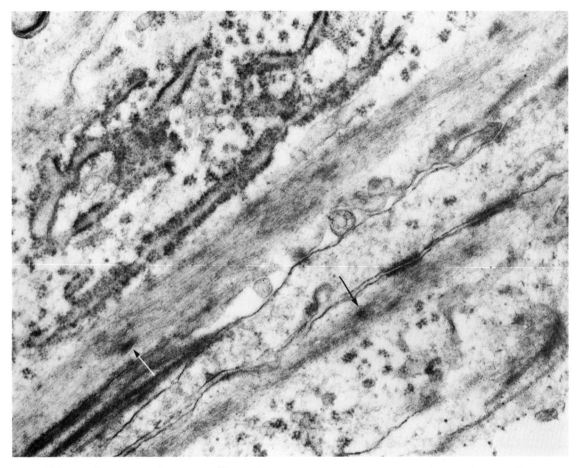

Figure 114   *Myofibrosarcoma. Same case as Figures 112 and 113. Desmosome-like junctions are seen between two myofibroblasts. Note the rough endoplasmic reticulum,* *polyribosomes lying free in the cytoplasm and filaments with focal densities (arrows). ×41 000 (From Vasudev and Harris, 1978)*

fibromatosis (Feiner and Kaye, 1976); (4) dermato-fibroma (Katenkamp and Stiller, 1975); (5) giant cell fibroma of the oral mucosa (Weathers and Campbell, 1974) (dubious because study carried out on material retrieved from paraffin block); and (6) tumours that histologically were considered to be fibrosarcomas of a low-grade malignancy (*Figures 112–114*) (Crocker and Murad, 1969; Stiller and Katenkamp, 1975; Vasudev and Harris, 1978).

Some six cases (i.e. fibrosarcomas containing myofibroblasts) have been described, and since myofibroblasts are more numerous in desmoid fibro-matosis than in fibrosarcomas, it has been suggested (Stiller and Katenkamp, 1975) that the presence of numerous myofibroblasts may be an indicator of a low level of malignancy and a better prognosis.

It is worth noting that not all fibrosarcomas are found to contain myofibroblasts, even when this feature has been specifically searched for (Jakobiec and Tannenbaum, 1974), and they were not described in seven cases of dermatofibrosarcoma protuberans in the report by Hashimoto, Braunstein and Jakobiec (1974). The data available to date are too scant to form any firm opinion as to whether a distinct and different sarcoma of myofibroblasts* exists or whether fibroblasts can synthesize myofila-ments under appropriate stimuli. Be that as it may,

*It seems that the time has come to coin some names. I would suggest that a benign tumour of myofibroblasts be called a 'myofibroma' and a malignant one 'myofibrosarcoma'; these terms would be in keeping with 'fibroma' and 'fibrosarcoma' designating benign and malignant tumours of fibroblasts.

from the diagnostic and prognostic point of view it is now important to study a series of such cases correlating the presence or absence of myofibroblasts with the biological behaviour of the tumour so as to confirm or refute the growing notion that the presence of myofibroblasts is an indicator of a more 'differentiated', less aggressive lesion.

It will now be apparent to the reader that the finding of filaments and focal densities in some cells in a tumour biopsy is not in itself sufficient to establish the diagnosis of leiomyoma or leiomyosarcoma, for these features have been seen in quite a few tumours (e.g. myofibrosarcoma and cardiac myxoma) and cells containing myofilaments form a part of the tumour mass in others (e.g. myoepithelial cells in carcinoma of the breast).

Ignorance of such matters has no doubt led to some erroneous diagnoses in the past, but this need no longer be the case. In competent hands the electron microscope can often assist in unequivocally establishing the diagnosis of a rhabdomyosarcoma or leiomyosarcoma when the diagnosis is uncertain by light microscopy. Conversely, it can at times effectively refute such a diagnosis made with the light microscope. Furthermore, for distinguishing myofibrosarcoma from fibrosarcoma the electron microscope is obviously essential.

References

BARBERA, V. and MAZZARELLA, L. (1967). Caratteristiche ultrastrutturali del sarcoma di Kaposi. *Tumori*, 53, 379

BARNETT, C. H., COCHRANE, W. and PALFREY, A. J. (1963). Age changes in articular cartilage of rabbits. *Ann. Rheum. Dis.*, 22, 389

BELTRAN, G. and STUCKEY, W. J. (1972). Nuclear lobulation and cytoplasmic fibrils in leukemic plasma cells. *Am. J. Clin. Path.*, 58, 159

BIBERFELD, P. (1971). Cytotoxic interaction of phytohemagglutin-stimulated blood lymphocytes with monolayer cells. A study by light and electron microscopy. *Cell. Immunol.*, 2, 54

CARDELL, R. R. Jr. and KNIGHTON, R. S. (1966). The cytology of a human pituitary tumour: an electron microscopic study. *Trans. Am. Microsc. Soc.*, 85, 58

CARTER, D., YARDLEY, J. H. and SHELLEY, W. M. (1969). Lobular carcinoma of the breast. An ultrastructural comparison with certain duct carcinomas and benign lesions. *Johns Hopkins Med. J.*, 125, 25

CROCKER, D. J. and MURAD, T. M. (1969). Ultrastructure of fibrosarcoma in a male breast. *Cancer*, 23, 891

DOMAGALA, W., CZERNIAK, B., MIETKIEWSKI, J. and SZYROKI, L. (1975). Ultrastruktura miȩsaka Kaposiego. *Pat. Pol.*, 26, 517

FAWCETT, D. W. (1967). *An Atlas of Fine Structure. The Cell, its Organelles and Inclusions.* Philadelphia and London: Saunders

FEINER, H. and KAYE, G. I. (1976). Ultrastructural evidence of myofibroblasts in circumscribed fibromatosis. *Archs Path. Lab. Med.*, 100, 265

FERENCZY, A., RICHART, R. M. and OKAGAKI, T. (1971). A comparative ultrastructural study of leiomyosarcoma, cellular leiomyoma and leiomyoma of the uterus. *Cancer*, 28, 1004

FIRKET, H. (1967). Ultrastructural aspects of myofibrils formation in cultured skeletal muscle. *Z. Zellforsch.*, 78, 313

FISCHMAN, D. A. (1967). An electron microscope study of myofibril formation in embryonic chick skeletal muscle. *J. Cell Biol.*, 32, 557

FLORA, G., DAHL, E. and NELSON, E. (1967). Electron microscopic observations on human intracranial arteries. Changes seen with aging and atherosclerosis. *Archs Neurol., Chicago.*, 17, 162

FULLER, J. A. and GHADIALLY, F. N. (1972). Ultrastructural observations on surgically produced partial-thickness defects in articular cartilage. *Clin. Orthop. Rel. Res.*, 86, 193

GABBIANI, G., LE LOUS, M., BAILEY, A. J., BAZIN, S. and DELAUNAY, A. (1976). Collagen and myofibroblasts of granulation tissue. A chemical, ultrastructural and immunologic study. *Virchows Arch. Abt. B. Zellpath.*, 21, 133

GHADIALLY, F. N. (1975). *Ultrastructural Pathology of the Cell.* London: Butterworths

GHADIALLY, F. N. and LALONDE, J.-M.A. (1978). Long term effects of myochrysine on articular cartilage. *Virchows Arch. Abt. B. Zellpath.*, 28, 31

GHADIALLY, F. N., LaLONDE, J.-M.A. and DICK, C. E. (1979). Ultrastructure of pigmented villonodular synovitis. *J. Path.*, 127, 19

GHADIALLY, F. N., LOWES, N. R. and MESFIN, G. M. (1977). Atypical glycogen deposits in a plasmacytoma: An ultrastructural study. *J. Path.*, 122, 157

GHADIALLY, F. N. and MEHTA, P. N. (1971). Multifunctional mesenchymal cells resembling smooth muscle cells in ganglia of the wrist. *Ann. Rheum. Dis.*, 30, 31

GHADIALLY, F. N., MEHTA, P. N. and KIRKALDY-WILLIS, W. H. (1970). Ultrastructure of articular cartilage in experimentally produced lipoarthrosis. *J. Bone Jt Surg.*, 52A, 1147

GHADIALLY, F. N. and ROY, S. (1967). Ultrastructure of synovial membrane in rheumatoid arthritis. *Ann. Rheum. Dis.*, 26, 426

GHADIALLY, F. N. and ROY, S. (1969). *Ultrastructure of Synovial Joints in Health and Disease.* London: Butterworths

HAMEED, K. and MORGAN, D. A. (1972). Papillary adenocarcinoma of endometrium with psammoma bodies. Histology and fine structure. *Cancer*, 29, 1326

HARRIS, M. (1971). Ultrastructure of a glomus tumour. *J. Clin. Path.*, 24, 520

HARRIS, M. and AHMED, A. (1977). The ultrastructure of tubular carcinoma of the breast. *J. Path.*, 123, 79

HARRISON, A. C. and KAHN, L. B. (1978). Myogenic cells in Kaposi's sarcoma. An ultrastructural study. *J. Path.*, 124, 157

HASHIMOTO, K., BRAUNSTEIN, M. H. and JAKOBIEC, F. A. (1974). Dermatofibrosarcoma protuberans: A tumor with perineural and endoneural cell features. *Archs Derm.,* **110,** 874

HASHIMOTO, K. and LEVER, W. F. (1964). Kaposi's sarcoma. Histochemical and electron microscopic studies. *J. Invest. Derm.,* **43,** 593

HIBBS, R. G. (1956). Electron microscopy of developing cardiac muscle in chick embryos. *Am. J. Anat.,* **99,** 17

ISHIKAWA, H., BISCHOFF, R. and HOLTZER, H. (1968). Mitosis and intermediate-sized filaments in developing skeletal muscle. *J. Cell Biol.,* **38,** 538

JAKOBIEC, F. A. and TANNENBAUM, M. (1974). The ultrastructure of orbital fibrosarcoma. *Am. J. Ophthal.,* **77,** 899

KATENKAMP, D. and STILLER, D. (1975). Cellular composition of the so-called dermatofibroma (histiocytoma cutis). *Virchows Arch. Path. Anat. Hist.,* **367,** 325

KELLY, D. E. (1966). Fine structure of desmosomes, hemidesmosomes and an adepidermal globular layer in developing newt epidermis. *J. Cell Biol.,* **28,** 51

KELLY, D. E. (1969). Myofibrillogenesis and Z-band differentiation. *Anat. Rec.,* **163,** 403

KELLY, M. and BHAGWAT, A. G. (1972). Ultrastructural features of a recurrent endothelial myxoma of the left atrium. *Archs Path.,* **93,** 219

MARTINEZ-PENUELA, J. M., ANTON, M. A. L., HERRERO, R. T. and ERICE, J. G. (1970). The ultrastructure of Kaposi's sarcoma. *Archo Ital. Patol. Clin. Tum.,* **13,** 79

MEYER, S. L., FINE, B. S., FONT, R. L. and ZIMMERMAN, L. E. (1968). Leiomyoma of the ciliary body-electron microscopic verification. *Am. J. Ophthal.,* **66,** 1061

MORALES, A. R., FINE, G. and HORN, R. C., Jr. (1972). Rhabdomyosarcoma: An ultrastructural appraisal. *Path. Ann.,* **7,** 81

MORALES, A. R., FINE, G., PARDO, V. and HORN, R. C. (1975). The ultrastructure of smooth muscle tumors with a consideration of the possible relationship of glomangiomas hemangiopericytomas and cardiac myxomas. *Path. Ann.,* **10,** 65

MOTTAZ, J. H. and ZELICKSON, A. S. (1966). Electron microscope observations of Kaposi's sarcoma. *Acta Derm. Venereol.,* **46,** 195

MURAD, T. M. and SCARPELLI, D. G. (1967). The ultrastructure of medullary and scirrhous mammary duct carcinoma. *Am. J. Path.,* **50,** 335

MURAD, T. M. and VON HAAM, E. (1968). Ultrastructure of myoepithelial cells in human mammary gland tumors. *Cancer,* **21,** 1137

NIEMI, M. and MUSTAKALLIO, K. K. (1965). The fine structure of the spindle cell in Kaposi's sarcoma. *Acta Path. Microbiol. Scand.,* **63,** 567

PARKER, J. W., WAKASA, H. and LUKES, R. J. (1967). Cytoplasmic fibrils in mixed lymphocyte cultures. *Blood,* **29,** 608

PARRY, E. W. (1970). Some electron microscope observations on the mesenchymal structures of full term umbilical cord. *J. Anat.,* **107,** 505

PEILLON, F., VILA-PORCILE, E. and OLIVIER, L. (1970). L'action des oestrogenes sur les adenomas hypophysaires chez l'homme. *Ann. Endocr.,* **31,** 259

PENNEY, D. P., JOHANSEN, E., RUBIN, P., AVERILL, K. and WALKER, S. (1978). Fine structural studies of radiation-resistant human squamous cell carcinomas. *J. Oral Path.,* **7,** 111

PEPLER, W. J. and THERON, J. J. (1962). An electron microscope study of Kaposi's haemangiosarcoma. *J. Path. Bact.,* **83,** 521

PETERSON, M., DAY, A. J., TUME, R. K. and EISENBERG, E. (1971). Ultrastructure, fatty acid content and metabolic activity of foam cells and other fractions separated from rabbit atherosclerotic lesions. *Expl Molec. Path.,* **15,** 157

PRICE, H. M., HOWES, E. L. and BLUMBERG, J. H. (1964). Ultrastructural alterations in skeletal muscle fibers injured by cold II cells of the sarcolemmal tubes: observations on 'discontinuous' regeneration and myofibril formation. *Lab. Invest.,* **13,** 1279

RANGAN, S. R. S., CALVERT, R. C. and VITOLS, K. (1971). Fibrillar bundles in canine lymphomas: An ultrastructural study. *J. Ultrastruct.,* **36,** 425

ROY, S. (1968). Ultrastructure of articular cartilage in experimental haemarthrosis. *Archs Path.,* **86,** 69

SCHAFER, A. and BÄSSLER, R. (1969). Vergleichende elektronenmikroskopische Untersuchungen am Drüsenepithel und am sog. lobulären Carcinom de Mamma. *Virchows Arch. Path. Anat.,* **346,** 269

SCHOCHET, S. S., McCORMICK, W. F. and HALMI, N. S. (1972). Acidophil adenomas with intracytoplasmic filamentous aggregates. A light and electron microscope study. *Archs Path.,* **94,** 16

STILLER, D. and KATENKAMP, D. (1975). Cellular features in desmoid fibromatosis and well-differentiated fibrosarcomas: An electron microscopic study. *Virchows Arch. Path. Anat. Hist.,* **369,** 155

STOVIN, P. G. I., HEATH, D. and KHALIQ, S. U. (1973). Ultrastructure of the cardiac myxoma and the papillary tumour of heart valves. *Thorax,* **28,** 273

TANDLER, B., ROSSI, E. P., STEIN, M. and MATT, M. M. (1970). Rhabdomyoma of the lip. Light and electron microscopical observations. *Archs Path.,* **89,** 118

TANNENBAUM, M., WEISS, M. and MARX, A. J. (1969). Ultrastructure of the human mammary ductile. *Cancer,* **23,** 958

TERRY, R. D. (1971). Presidential address — Neuronal fibrous protein in human pathology. *J. Neuropath. Expl Neurol.,* **30,** 8

TERRY, R. D. and PENA, C. (1965). Experimental production of neurofibrillary degeneration. 2. Electron microscopy, phosphatase histochemistry and electron probe analysis. *J. Neuropath. Expl Neurol.,* **24,** 200

TREMBLAY, M. (1971). Ultrastructure of a Wilms' tumour and myogenesis. *J. Path.,* **105,** 269

TUMILOWICZ, J. J. and SARKAR, N. H. (1972). Accumulating filaments and other ultrastructural aspects of declining cell cultures derived from human breast tumors. *Expl Molec. Path.,* **16,** 210

VASUDEV, K. S. and HARRIS, M. (1978). A sarcoma of myofibroblasts. *Archs Path. Lab. Med.,* **102,** 185

WEATHERS, D. R. and CAMPBELL, W. G. (1974). Ultrastructure of the giant cell fibroma of the oral mucosa. *Oral Surg. Path. Med.,* **38,** 550

WELSH, R. A. and MEYER, A. T. (1969). Ultrastructure of gastric leiomyoma. *Archs Path.,* **87,** 71

138

WISEMAN, J. A. (1976). Nodular fasciitis, a lesion of myo-fibroblasts: An ultrastructural study. *Cancer,* **38,** 2378

WISNIEWSKI, H., TERRY, R. D. and HIRANO, A. (1970). Neurofibrillary pathology. *J. Neuropath. Expl Neurol.,* **29,** 163

WISSLER, R. W. (1967). Editorial: the arterial medial cell, smooth muscle, or multifunctional mesenchyme?. *Circulation,* **36,** 1

YODAIKEN, R. E. (1962). Features of the fine structure of the Kaposi sarcoma. *S. Afr. Med. J.,* **36,** 989

ZUCKER-FRANKLIN, D. (1963). The ultrastructure of cells in human thoracic duct lymph. *J. Ultrastruct. Res.,* **9,** 325

11
Is it a schwannoma or a fibroblastic* neoplasm?

When histological examination shows a mesenchymal tumour composed of spindle-shaped cells arranged in fascicles, with suggestion of nuclear palisading, the question that arises in one's mind is whether the tumour is of Schwann cell rather than fibroblastic lineage.† There are various light microscopic criteria which are used to distinguish such tumours (e.g. Antoni type A and type B areas in schwannomas), but at times it is difficult to arrive at a firm decision. In such instances electron microscopy may assist in establishing a diagnosis, for Schwann cells have quite a prominent external lamina but fibroblasts virtually lack an external lamina; only rare small foci of basal lamina-like material may be found adjacent to the cell membrane of the fibroblast. The abundance or otherwise of collagen fibrils in the matrix is a relatively minor consideration, since both cell types can produce and secrete the precursors of matrical collagen (Nathaniel and Pease, 1963a,b; Thomas, 1964). However, the normal fibroblast is more generously endowed with rough endoplasmic reticulum than the Schwann cell.

The WHO classification (Enzinger, Lattes and Torloni, 1969) splits benign peripheral nerve tumours into neurofibromas and schwannomas (neurilemmomas), but the malignant versions are lumped together as malignant schwannomas. Further, it is widely held that both neurofibromas and schwannomas originate from Schwann cells (Harkin and Reed, 1969). However, the old idea that neurofibromas and neurofibrosarcomas derive from fibroblasts, while benign and malignant schwannomas derive from Schwann cells, has been revived by electron microscopy.

Thus, for example, regarding neurofibromas, Oota and Takahama (1962) state: '...the tumour was diagnosed without doubt as neurofibroma on the basis of experiences with classical optical study, though electron microscope revealed all the characteristics of a purely fibroblastic tumour and not a Schwann cell proliferation.' Johannessen, Stenwig and Brennhovd (1976) state: '...our ultrastructural experience is, however, that the neurofibromas or neurofibrosarcomas are composed chiefly of fibroblast-like cells, in contrast to the numerous Schwann-like cells seen in benign schwannomas or in the more cellular ones with higher mitotic rates and a possible malignant potential.'

The idea that neurofibromas derive from a proliferation of nerve sheath connective tissue cells (i.e. fibroblasts), while benign and malignant schwannomas derive from Schwann cells, is also supported by a recent scanning electron microscopic study, for in neurofibromas collagen sheets similar to those in the normal nerve sheath were found but in schwannomas the neoplastic cells produced tube-like columns surrounding 'empty' spaces comparable in diameter to nerve axons (Jones and Strafuss, 1978).

In this chapter we will not concern ourselves any further about the histogenesis of peripheral nerve tumours; but we shall address ourselves to the much wider issue of distinguishing tumours of Schwann cells from fibroblastic tumours.

Schwannoma

Quite a few studies depicting the ultrastructural morphology of schwannomas have been published (Cravioto and Lockwood, 1968; Fisher and Vuzevski, 1968; Sun and White, 1974; Alvira, Mandybur and Menefee, 1976; Johannessen, Stenwig and Brennhovd, 1976; Silverman, Leffers and Kay, 1976; Kemmann *et al.*, 1977).

---

*By this we mean a tumour containing neoplastic fibroblasts and not one that just contains collagen fibres.
†There would also be the possibility that it could be a smooth muscle tumour, but this has already been considered in Chapter 10.

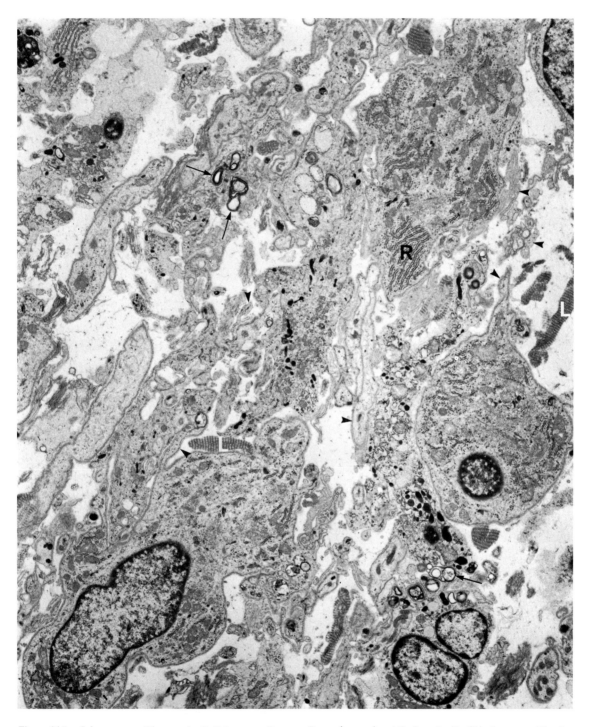

Figure 115   *Schwannoma. The neoplastic Schwann cells have a modest amount of rough endoplasmic reticulum (R) and numerous cell processes (arrowheads). Note the myelin figures (arrows) and the Luse bodies (L). An external lamina invests the cells and cell processes but this is difficult to appreciate at this low magnification.* ×6500

141

The ultrastructual features (*Figures 115—120*) may be summarized as follows: (1) a prominent external lamina envelops Schwann cells in benign schwannoma and this feature persists, albeit in an attenuated and interrupted form, even in the metastasizing malignant epitheloid schwannoma (Alvira, Mandybur and Menefee, 1976); (2) elongated cytoplasmic processes ensheathed in an external lamina are seen extending into the matrix, or wrapping around the main cell body or around collagen fibrils; (3) desmosome-like junctions may develop between such processes or between such processes and the main body of the Schwann cell or between the opposing membranes of the mesaxon;* (4) myelinated and non-myelinated axons are sometimes seen encased in the Schwann cell; (5) myelin figures and lysosomal bodies presumably derived from these are also often seen in the cell cytoplasm;† and (6) Luse bodies (fibrous long-spacing collagen) are found in the matrix. Long-spacing collagen has been seen in normal tissues and many pathological states; even so, this is quite a constant feature of schwannomas, and, hence, taken with other findings it is of some diagnostic value.

*The cell membrane is infolded at a site on the surface of the Schwann cell. The opposing infolded membranes and the intervening space comprise the mesaxon, which spirals around the axon. Fusion of the outer lamina of the opposing infolded membrane produces the inter-period of intermediate line of the myelin sheath.
†In this connection it is worth recalling that Schwann cells are capable of phagocytosing damaged axons and resorbing their own myelin (Nathaniel and Pease, 1963c).

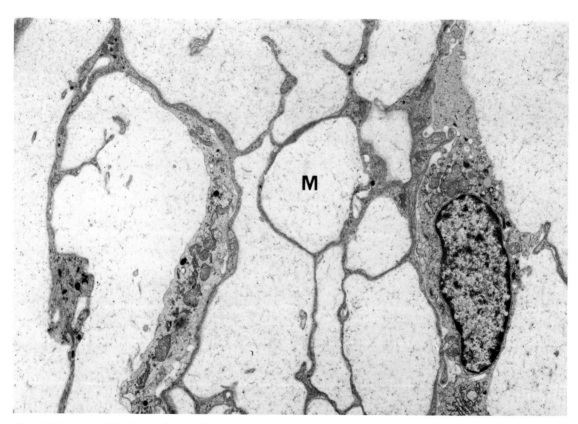

Figure 116   *Antoni Type B area from a schwannoma. Same case as Figure 115. Schwann cells and their cell processes have formed a laciform network; enmeshed within it is an abundant proteoglycan-rich matrix (M). The peppered appearance of the matrix is due to the presence of innumerable electron-dense protein-polysaccharide particles. ×6500*

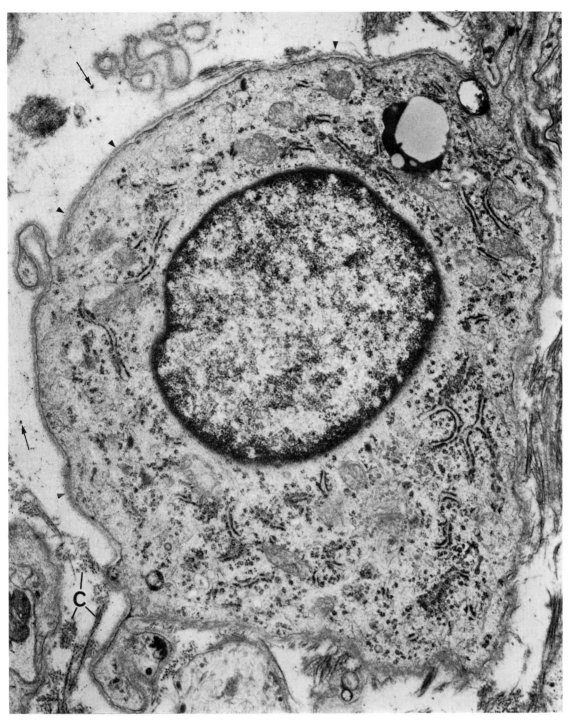

Figure 117   *Schwannoma. Same case as Figures 115 and 116. The neoplastic Schwann cell shown here contains a modest amount of rough endoplasmic reticulum; hence, it bears some resemblance to the fibroblast. However, the* *feature which distinguishes the Schwann cell from the fibroblast is the presence of an external lamina (arrowheads). Note also the collagen fibrils (C) and protein-polysaccharide particles (arrows) in the matrix. ×20 000*

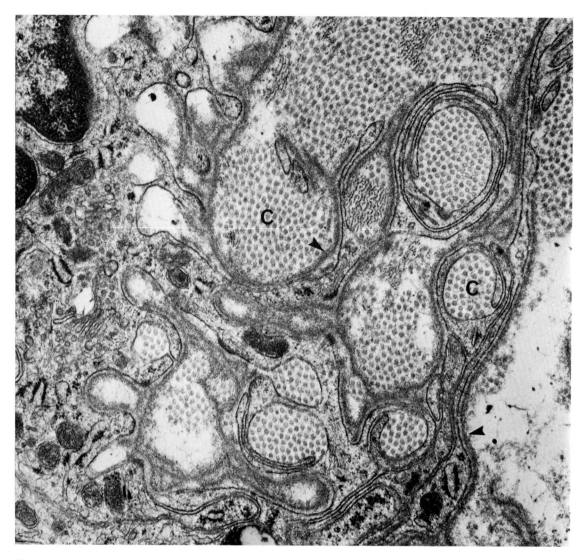

Figure 118 *Schwannoma. Same case as Figures 115—117.*
Complex folds of the cell membrane (invaginations and/or
cell processes) of the Schwann cell are seen wrapping around
collagen fibres (C). A well-developed external lamina (arrow-
heads) is evident. ×34 000

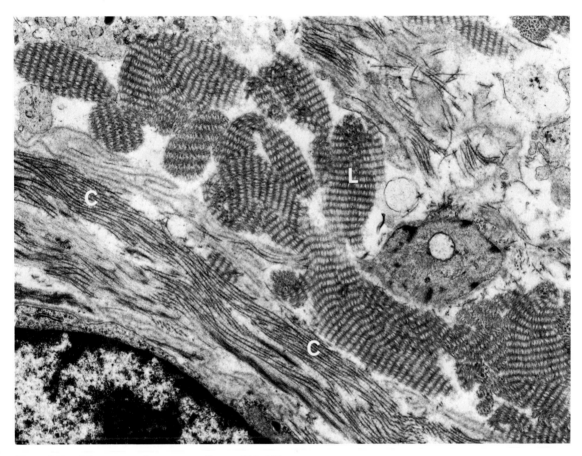

Figure 119   *Schwannoma. Same case as Figures 115–118.*
Collagen fibres (C) and Luse bodies (L) are seen in the
matrix. ×16 000

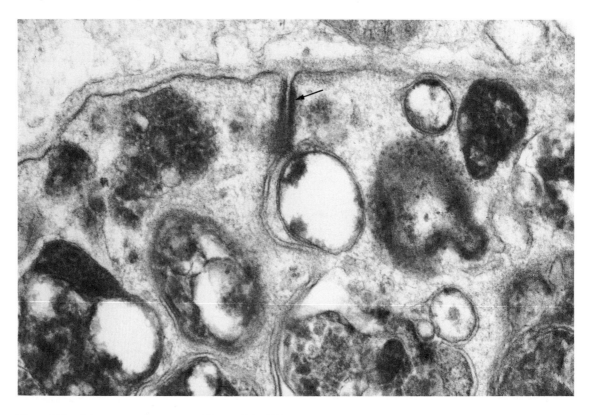

Figure 120   *Schwannoma. Same case as Figures 115—119.*
A desmosome-like structure (arrow) is seen between the in-
folded membranes of the mesaxon. ×57 000

Figure 121   *Fibroadenoma of breast. A fibroblast with*
three cell processes, profiles of rough endoplasmic
reticulum (R) and Golgi complex (G). Note banded collagen
fibrils (arrowheads), collagen fibres (F) and protein poly-
saccharide particles (arrows) in the interfibrillary matrix.
×14 500. (Ghadially and Yong, unpublished electron
micrograph)

Figure 122   *Non-ossifying fibroma of bone. A fibroblast*
showing abundant rough endoplasmic reticulum. ×22 000

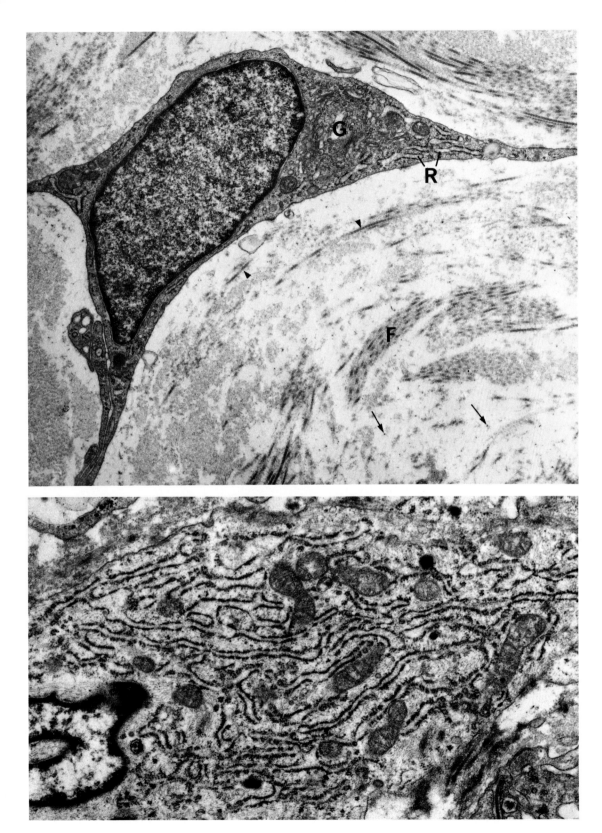

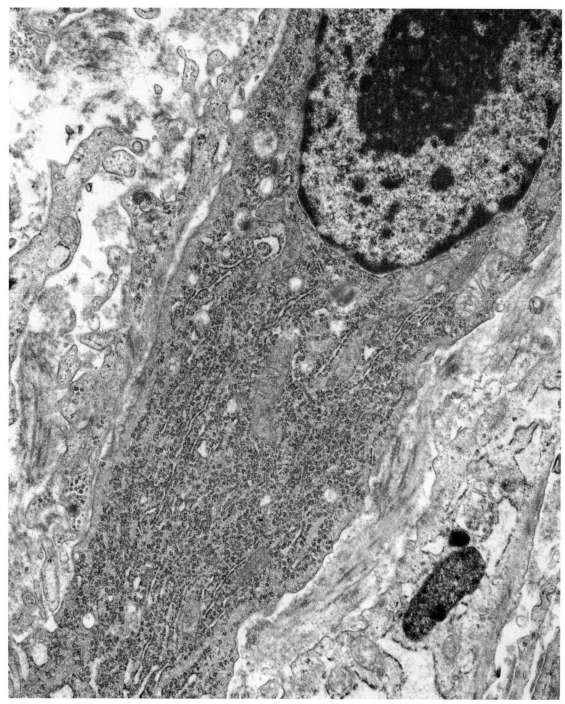

Figure 123 *Non-ossifying fibroma of bone. Same case as Figure 122. Fibroblast showing an enlarged nucleolus, strands of rough endoplasmic reticulum and numerous polyribosomes; most of them are almost certainly lying on the surface of tangentially cut membranes of the rough endoplasmic reticulum rather than lying free in the cytoplasmic matrix. At higher magnifications it was evident that the dense appearance of the cytoplasmic matrix is due to the presence of numerous filaments, but no focal densities were detected.* ×22 000

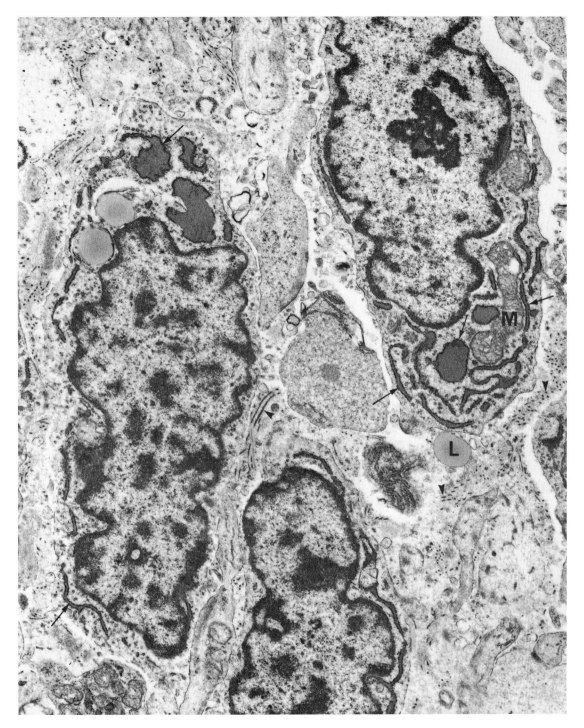

Figure 124   *Fibrosarcoma from the pelvis of a 2-month-old boy (6.5 cm in maximum diameter). Exact site of origin not known. Light microscopy revealed a spindle cell tumour with barely detectable collagen in the matrix. This electron micrograph shows neoplastic fibroblasts with much enlarged irregular nuclei. Dilated and vesiculated cisternae of the rough endoplasmic reticulum (arrows) and rare bizarre mitochondria (M) are evident. Only a few collagen fibrils (arrowheads) but much cellular debris and a liberated lipid droplet (L) are seen in the matrix. ×19 000 (From a block of tissue supplied by Dr A. H. Cameron)*

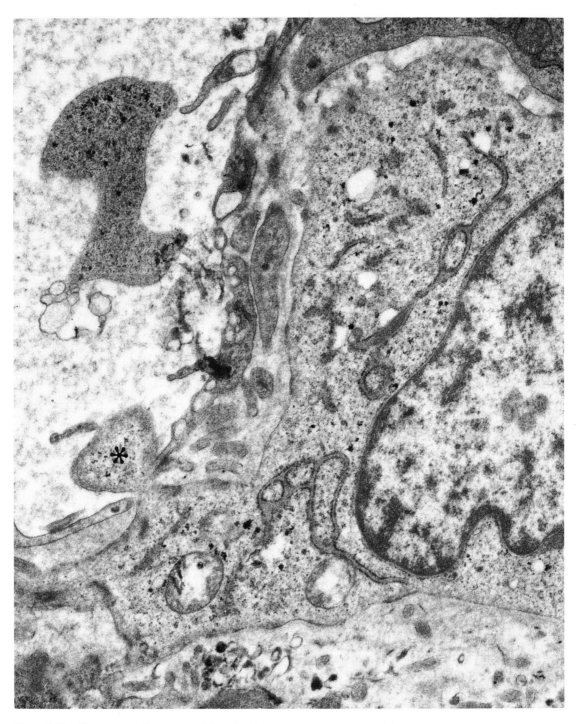

Figure 125   *Fibrosarcoma. Same case as Figure 124. Appearances seen here suggest that a neoplastic fibroblast is commencing to invade a vessel (probably lymphatic). Note the cell processes (*) insinuated between endothelial cells. ×28 000 (From a block of tissue supplied by Dr A. H. Cameron)*

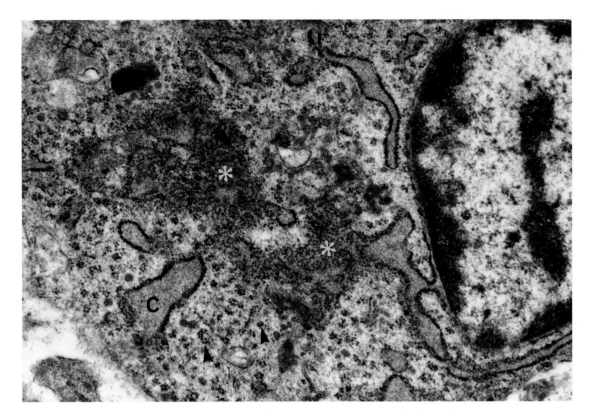

Figure 126 *Fibrosarcoma. Same case as Figures 124 and 125. Cell showing numerous polyribosomes lying free in the cytoplasm (arrowheads). Note dilated cisternae of the rough endoplasmic reticulum (C) and polyribosomes lying* *on the surface of tangentially cut cisternae (*) of the rough endoplasmic reticulum. ×18 000 (from a block of tissue supplied by Dr A. H. Cameron)*

Fibroblastic neoplasms*

Fibroblasts

Neoplastic fibroblasts occur not only in fibromas and fibrosarcomas, but also in various other benign and malignant tumours (e.g. fibroadenoma, elastofibroma, neurofibroma, neurofibrosarcoma, fibrous histiocytoma, synovioma, synovial sarcoma, benign and malignant mesenchymoma, osteosarcoma and chondrosarcoma). Thus, the finding of fibroblasts or fibroblast-like cells is not diagnostic of any particular tumour or tumour-like lesion; nevertheless it is important to learn to recognize this cell type. Usually this is easily accomplished, because, as pointed out

*This section should be read in conjunction with pp. 135–137, where the occurrence of myofibroblasts in some fibroblastic tumours (including some fibrosarcomas) and tumour-like lesions is dealt with and references pertaining to the ultrastructure of these lesions are presented.

earlier, fibroblasts virtually lack an external lamina but they are well endowed with rough endoplasmic reticulum.

However, there are morphological variations worth noting. Some of the fibroblasts found in benign lesions such as fibroma and fibroadenoma (*Figure 121*) show the characteristic spindle shape and two or three long cell processes. There is usually an increase in the nuclear–cytoplasmic ratio, but the scant cytoplasm still shows a few profiles of rough endoplasmic reticulum and a Golgi complex. On the other hand, even in benign tumours or tumour-like lesions such as the non-ossifying fibroma of bone† (*Figures 122* and *123*) quite plump fibroblasts, singularly well endowed with rough endoplasmic reticulum, may be

†Probably not a true tumour but a cellular proliferation due to local developmental abberations at the epiphyseal region of long bones (Jaffe, 1958; Dahlin, 1970; Steiner, 1974).

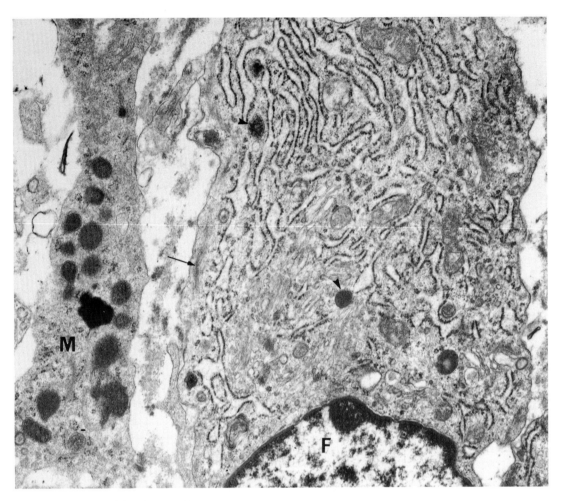

Figure 127 *Non-ossifying fibroma of bone. Same case as Figures 122 and 123. This electron micrograph shows a macrophage (M) containing little besides some lysosomes and a fibroblast (F) well endowed with rough endoplasmic reticulum and a juxtanuclear Golgi complex. Some dense bodies acceptable as lysosomes (arrowheads) are present. A few intracytoplasmic filaments (arrows) are also evident. ×23 000*

found. A juxtanuclear Golgi complex is evident when the plane of sectioning is favourable. Hypertrophy of the nucleolus is also seen, but here it is not an indicator of cell division and rapid growth (evidenced by paucity of polyribosomes lying free in the cytoplasm) but rather an indicator of synthesis of export proteins (e.g. collagen precursors and protein part of proteoglycans).

The malignant fibroblast of fibrosarcoma is somewhat different in appearance (*Figures 124–126*). The nucleus is larger and more irregular and often shows a prominent nucleolus. The rough endoplasmic reticulum is not quite as abundant but is often distended, with moderately electron-dense to quite dense material. Polyribosomes are plentiful in the cytoplasm of some of the cells. As discussed in Chapter 4 (pp. 41–46) such changes indicate a proliferating population of cells rather than a well-differentiated one engaged in functional (secretory) activity.

Macrophages

A few non-neoplastic macrophages or histiocytes* may be encountered in a variety of human tumours (e.g. melanophages in melanomas: Chapter 7), this being particularly so in some mesenchymal tumours.† It therefore behoves us to examine the ultrastructural differences between macrophages and fibroblasts.

Macrophages are rounded cells with few or many cell processes.* In contrast to this, the fibroblast is

*In the fibrous histiocytoma many histiocytes or macrophages are present and it is thought that both the fibroblasts and histiocytes are neoplastic and that they probably derive from a common mesenchymal stem cell. In most other tumours the macrophages are non-neoplastic.
†In some mouse and rat fibrosarcomas up to 65 per cent of the cells may be macrophages (Haskill, Proctor and Yamamura, 1975). In human tumours, even mesenchymal ones, macrophages are quite rare, except near obviously necrotic regions.
*Abundance of cell processes is thought to be an indicator of heightened phagocytic activity.

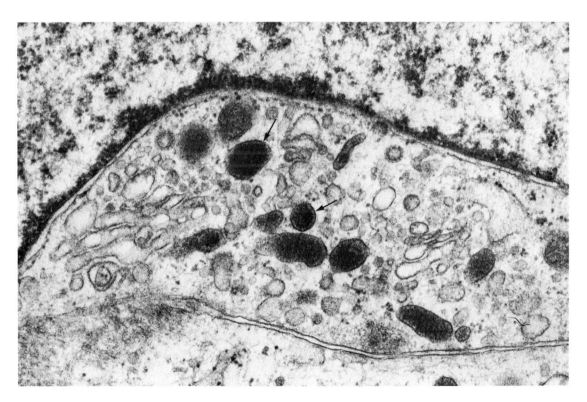

Figure 128 *Macrophage from a fibrosarcoma. These electron-dense bodies (arrows) are thought to be the primary lysosomes of the macrophage; only a rare small profile of rough endoplasmic reticulum was evident in this macrophage. ×49 000*

elongated or spindle-shaped and usually has only two or three long cell processes. Electron-dense bodies acceptable as lysosomes are rare in fibroblasts,* but they are an essential and important part of the macrophage (*Figure 127*). Thus, one finds fairly homogeneous electron-dense bodies (with a thin lucent halo between the contents and lysosomal membrane) which are probably the primary lysosomes of the macrophage (*Figure 128*) and also larger more pleomorphic lysosomes (heterolysosomes) stemming from phagocytosis of red blood cells and/or haemoglobin† and/or other materials such as cell fragments and fibrin (*Figures 129–131*).

*Fibroblasts adjacent to areas of haemorrhage may contain quite a few siderosomes, but the abundant rough endoplasmic reticulum distinguishes them from macrophages.

An important point of distinction is that macrophages are as a rule poorly endowed with rough endoplasmic reticulum, but stimulated macrophages (i.e. ones actively engaged in phagocytosis) are somewhat better endowed with rough endoplastic

†The phagocytosis of intact erythrocytes, lysed erythrocytes and haemoglobin leads to the formation of three types of lysosomal bodies: (1) myelinosomes containing whorled osmiophilic membranes; (2) siderosomes containing haemosiderin; and (3) myelinosiderosomes containing osmiophilic membranes and haemosiderin. Since haemorrhage is not rare in tumours, one frequently encounters such lysosomal bodies in tumours. For details of morphology, atomic composition and mode of evolution of these bodies the reader is referred to some of our recent papers (e.g. Ghadially, Ailsby and Yong, 1976; Ghadially, Lalonde and Oryschak, 1976; Lalonde and Ghadially, 1977; Lalonde, Ghadially and Massey, 1978; Ghadially, 1979).

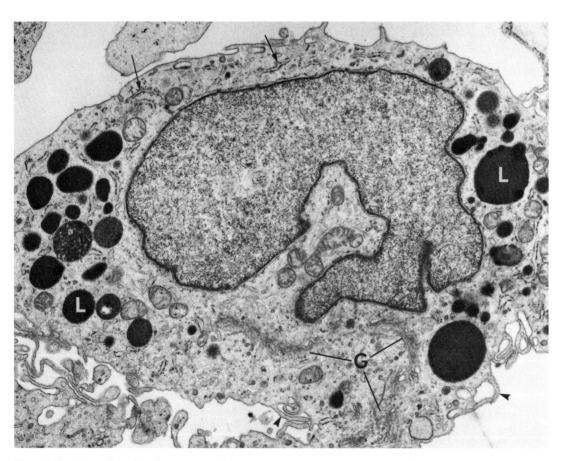

Figure 129 *Macrophage from hamartoma of lung. Most of the heterolysosomes (L) seen here are derived from phagocytosed erythrocyte fragments or haemoglobin. Note the cell processes (arrowheads), small but numerous profiles of rough endoplasmic reticulum (arrows) and the prominent Golgi complex (G). ×13 500 (Ghadially and Dick, unpublished electron micrograph)*

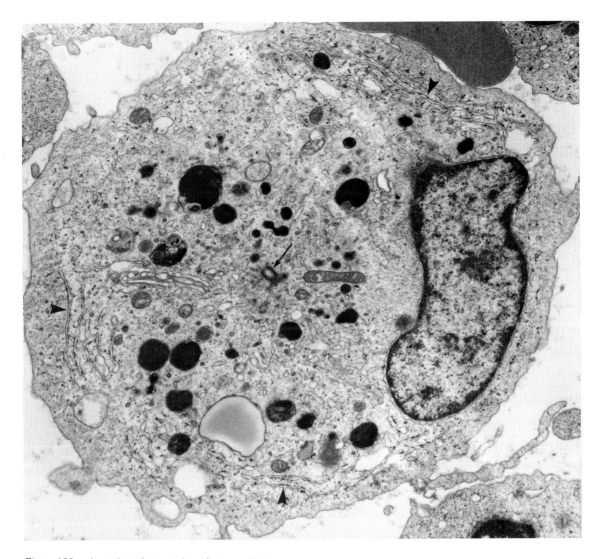

Figure 130 *An activated macrophage from a malignant ascites. The cell shows numerous lysosomes containing membranous and electron-dense material (which at higher magnification has the particular structure of haemosiderin deposits), stacks of rough endoplasmic reticulum (arrowheads), a large Golgi zone with a centriole (arrow) in the middle and some cell processes.* × 14 000

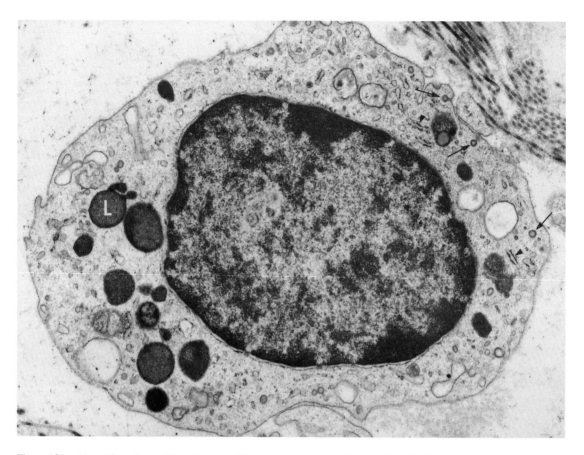

Figure 131 *Macrophage from a fibroadenoma of the breast. Although this cell contains some lysosomal bodies (L) with a particulate content (morphologically acceptable as siderosomes), it is not noticeably 'activated', for the rough endoplasmic reticulum (arrowheads) is scant, the Golgi* *complex is not evident (at least in this plane or sectioning) nor are the cell processes. The cell, however, does seem to be picking up some proteinaceous material, as suggested by the presence of coated vesicles (arrows). ×18 000*

reticulum, presumably necessary for the synthesis of lysosomal enzymes and new primary lysosomes. These facts are well known and supported by many studies and observations, including studies on macrophages in tissue culture, collagen resorption in

*One of these (*Figure 1.6* in Carr *et al.*, 1977) shows a macrophage with so few and such minute strands of rough endoplasmic reticulum that it could more aptly be labelled as 'poorly endowed with rough endoplasmic reticulum'; the other macrophage (*Figure 1.5* in Carr *et al.*, 1977) contains some heterolysosomes, and, in keeping with this, it has slightly more rough endoplasmic reticulum. If cells such as these are described as having 'prominent rough endoplasmic reticulum', one wonders what term one would use to describe the rough endoplasmic reticulum in fibroblasts and plasma cells?

involuting uterus (for references see Parakkal, 1968) and wound healing (Ross and Odland, 1968). However, a contrary view has also been expressed (Carr *et al.*, 1977). These authors repeatedly assert that macrophages have a 'prominent granular endoplasmic reticulum'. Fortunately, the two illustrations presented to support this statement effectively belie such a contention.*

Matrix

As a rule the matrix in benign lesions tends to be more abundant and better organized than in the malignant ones, but there are exceptions. Two main components may be discerned in the matrix: (1) the fibrous component (also called the fibrillary matrix), comprising characteristically banded collagen fibrils and fibres and also other finer fibrils and filaments which, too, are presumably collagenous in nature (in some tumours elastic fibres may also be encountered); and (2) mucopolysaccharide-containing (glycosaminoglycans) interfibrillary matrix.

At times collagen fibrils lie very close to the cell membrane of the fibroblast and, owing to vagaries of sectioning geometry, appearances suggesting a sprouting of fibrils from the cell surface or from within the cell are seen. On rare occasions, however, banded collagen fibrils have been seen within tubular membrane bound spaces lying in the cell cytoplasm (referred to as 'intracellular collagen'), and it has been suggested that this indicates that synthesis and polymerization of collagen can at times occur within the cell. Such instances include tumours or tumour-like lesions such as: (1) infantile fibroma of kidney (Tannenbaum, 1971); and (2) desmoid fibromatosis (Welsh, 1966; Allegra and Broderick, 1973).

There has been much resistance to accepting the idea that at times collagen fibrils can form in an intracellular location. We (Ghadially *et al.*, 1978) have recently seen this phenomenon in normal semilunar cartilages and reviewed the literature on this subject, so this will not be repeated here. Nevertheless, much caution is needed, for in a majority of instances collagen lying in tubular or vacuolar spaces is likely to represent phagocytosis and degradation of collagen by macrophages (for illustrations and review see Ghadially, 1975) rather than collagen synthesis and polymerization in fibroblasts.

References

ALLEGRA, S. R. and BRODERICK, P. A. (1973). Desmoid fibroblastoma. Intracytoplasmic collagensynthesis in a peculiar fibroblastic tumour light and ultrastructural study of a case. *Human. Path.*, 4, 419

ALVIRA, M. M., MANDYBUR, T. I. and MENEFEE, M. G. (1976). Light microscopic and ultrastructural observations of a metastasizing malignant epithelioid schwannoma. *Cancer*, 38, 1977

CARR, I., HANCOCK, B. W., HENRY, L. and MILFORD WARD, A. (1977). *Lymphoreticular Disease.* Oxford: Blackwell Scientific

CRAVIOTO, H. and LOCKWOOD, R. (1968). Long spacing fibrous collagen in human acoustic nerve tumors: In vivo and in vitro observations. *J. Ultrastruct Res.*, 24, 70

DAHLIN, D. C. (1970). *Bone Tumors.* Springfield, Illinois: Thomas

ENZINGER, F. M., LATTES, R. and TORLONI, H. (1969). *Histological Typing of Soft Tissue Tumours.* Geneva: World Health Organization

FISHER, E. R. and VUZEVSKI, V. D. (1968). Cytogenesis of schwannoma (neurilemoma), neurofibroma, dermatofibroma and dermatofibrosarcoma as revealed by electron microscopy. *Am. J. Clin. Path.*, 49, 141

GHADIALLY, F. N. (1975). *Ultrastructural Pathology of the Cell.* London: Butterworths

GHADIALLY, F. N. (1979). Haemorrhage and haemosiderin. *J. Submier. Cytol.* In press

GHADIALLY, F. N., AILSBY, R. L. and YONG, N. K. (1976). Ultrastructure of haemophilic synovial membrane and electron probe x-ray analysis of haemosiderin. *J. Path.*, 120, 201

GHADIALLY, F. N., LALONDE, J.-M.A. and ORYSCHAK, A. F. (1976). Electron proble x-ray analysis of siderosomes in the rabbit haemarthrotic synovial membrane. *Virchows Arch. Abt. B. Zellpath.*, 22, 135

GHADIALLY, F. N., THOMAS, I., YONG, N. and LALONDE, J.-M.A. (1978). Ultrastructure of rabbit semilunar cartilages. *J. Anat.*, 125, 499

HARKIN, J. C. and REED, R. J. (1969). Tumours of the peripheral nervous system. In: *Atlas of Tumour Pathology*, 2nd Series, Fascicle 3. Washington, D. C.: Armed Forces Institute of Pathology

HASKILL, J., PROCTOR, J. W. and YAMAMURA, Y. (1975). Host responses within solid tumors. I. Monocytic effector cells within rat sarcomas. *J. Natn. Cancer Inst.*, 54, 387

JAFFE, H. L. (1958). *Tumors and Tumourous Conditions of the Bones and Joints.* Philadelphia: Lea and Febiger

JOHANNESSEN, J. V., STENWIG, A. E. and BRENNHOVD, I. O. (1976). Schwannoma with uncertain degree of malignancy. *Case Histories in Medicine,* No. 12 (Philips Electronics)

JONES, A. and STRAFUSS, A. C. (1978). Scanning electron microscopy of nerve sheath neoplasms. *Am. J. Vet. Res.*, 39, 1069

KEMMANN. E., CONRAD, P., CHEN, C. K. and NICASTRI, A. D. (1977). Pelvic neurilemmoma. *Gynec. Oncol.*, 5, 387

LALONDE, J.-M.A. and GHADIALLY, F. N. (1977). Ultrastructure of experimentally produced subcutaneous haematomas in the rabbit. *Virchows Arch. Abt. B. Zellpath.*, 25, 221

LALONDE, J.-M.A., GHADIALLY, F. N. and MASSEY, K. L. (1978). Ultrastructure of intramuscular haematomas and electron-probe x-ray analysis of extracellular and intracellular iron deposits. *J. Path.*, 125, 17

NATHANIEL, E. J. H. and PEASE, D. C. (1963a). Collagen and basement membrane formation by Schwann cells during nerve regeneration. *J. Ultrastruct. Res.*, 9, 550

NATHANIEL, E. J. H. and PEASE, D. C. (1963b). Regenerative changes in rat dorsal roots following Wallerian degeneration. *J. Ultrastruct. Res.*, 9, 533

NATHENIEL, E. J. H. and PEASE, D. C. (1963c). Degenerative changes in rat dorsal roots during Wallerian degeneration. *J. Ultrastruct. Res.*, 9, 511

PARAKKAL, P. F. (1968). Involvement of macrophages in collagen resorption. Brief Notes Publication, No. 365. *J. Cell Biol.*, 41, 345

OOTA, K. and TAKAHAMA, M. (1962). Electron microscopic study of human non-epithelial malignant tumors. *J. Electronmicrosc.*, 11, 85

ROSS, R. and ODLAND, G. (1968). Human wound repair. II. Inflammatory cells, epithelial-mesenchymal interrelations and fibrogenesis. *J. Cell Biol.,* **39,** 152

SILVERMAN, J. F., LEFFERS, B. R. and KAY, S. (1976). Primary pulmonary neurilemoma. *Archs Path. Lab. Med.,* **100,** 644

STEINER, G. C. (1974). Fibrous cortical defect and non-ossifying fibroma of bone. *Archs Path.,* **97,** 205

SUN, C. N. and WHITE, H. J. (1974). An electron-microscopic study of a schwannoma with special reference to banded structures and peculiar membranous multiple-chambered spheroids. *J. Path.,* **114,** 13

TANNENBAUM, M. (1971). Ultrastructural pathology of human renal cell tumors. *Path. Ann.,* **6,** 249

THOMAS, P. K. (1964). The deposition of collagen in relation to Schwann cell basement membrane during peripheral nerve regeneration. *J. Cell Biol.,* **23,** 375

WELSH, R. A. (1966). Intracytoplasmic collagen formations in desmoid fibromatosis. *Am. J. Path.,* **49,** 515

12
Differential diagnosis of Ewing's tumour, neuroblastoma and lymphoma

The difficulties at times encountered in sorting out the tumours dealt with in this chapter are now legend (Colville and Willis, 1933; Willis, 1940; Barden, 1943; Nakayama *et al.*, 1975). They belong to the group of tumours variously referred to as 'small round-cell tumours of childhood', 'small round-cell tumours of bone' or just 'small round-cell neoplasms'. These tumours can occur in osseous or extra-osseous sites and the clinical history and roentgenographic and histological appearances can be so similar as to make it impossible to arrive at a definitive diagnosis. It is, therefore, gratifying to note that there are quite a few ultrastructural differences between these tumours which often permit one to resolve this diagnostic dilemma.

Ewing's tumour

Despite numerous light microscopic and electron microscopic studies, the histogenesis of Ewing's tumour remains an enigma. However, the ultrastructural features have been well documented (Friedman and Gold, 1968; Kadin and Bensch, 1971; Hou-Jensen, Priori and Dmochowski, 1972; Rice, Cabot and Johnston, 1973; Szakacs, Carta and Szakacs, 1974; Nakayama *et al.*, 1975; Povýšil and Matějovský, 1977), and there is general agreement that the main diagnostic feature here is the abundance of glycogen and the manner of its disposition in this neoplasm (*Figures 132* and *133*). Glycogen occurs in this tumour principally as small and large focal deposits within the cytoplasm of the tumour cells, although some is also scattered about in a diffuse fashion in the cytoplasmic matrix. A peculiar feature which can be discerned in many published electron micrographs is the occurrence of a 'hole' within the glycogen deposits. Some authors ignore them, even though this feature is evident in their electron micrographs, while others have looked for the limiting membrane of these 'vacuoles'. My own view about the matter is that these 'holes' reflect sites from which lipid was lost

during tissue preparation, for not all such lipid is totally extracted and careful search does reveal an occasional quite characteristic medium-density lipid droplet in this position. Such a situation is by no means unique, for I have on occasions seen a lipid droplet surrounded by glycogen in hepatocytes and also chondrocytes of articular cartilage. Even so, this is quite a frequent feature seen in Ewing's tumour and, hence, of some diagnostic value when taken in conjunction with other findings.

A peculiar feature frequently noted in Ewing's tumour is the occurrence of glycogen between the tumour cells (*Figure 133*). This matrical or stromal glycogen could reflect an *in vivo* situation or it could be a handling artefact or both. Ewing's tumour is a friable neoplasm, with a scant stroma; collagen fibrils are rarely seen except near blood vessels. One may therefore argue that extracellular glycogen is probably the result of mechanical trauma inflicted during surgical manipulations or in chopping up the specimen for fixation.

On the other hand, one may argue that excess glycogen is liberated from the cells probably when the cells suffer necrosis. The concept that extracellular glycogen occurs *in vivo* is supported by *Figure 9* in Nakayama *et al.* (1975). Here a cell acceptable as a macrophage (which the authors describe as a second type of Ewing's sarcoma cell) containing numerous lysosomal bodies is shown; some appear to contain erythrocyte fragments, while others contain glycogen, but no focal cytoplasmic glycogen deposits characteristic of Ewing's tumour cells are present in this cell. What is even more intriguing is that this cell has abundant cell processes and they appear to be trapping glycogen lying in the intercellular matrix. Thus, it seems likely that glycogen does occur in the matrix of Ewing's tumour during life, but some more may well be liberated during manipulation of the specimen during surgery or after removal. Be that as it may, glycogen is seen in the matrix of Ewing's tumour quite constantly; hence, this, too, is a feature of some diagnostic import.

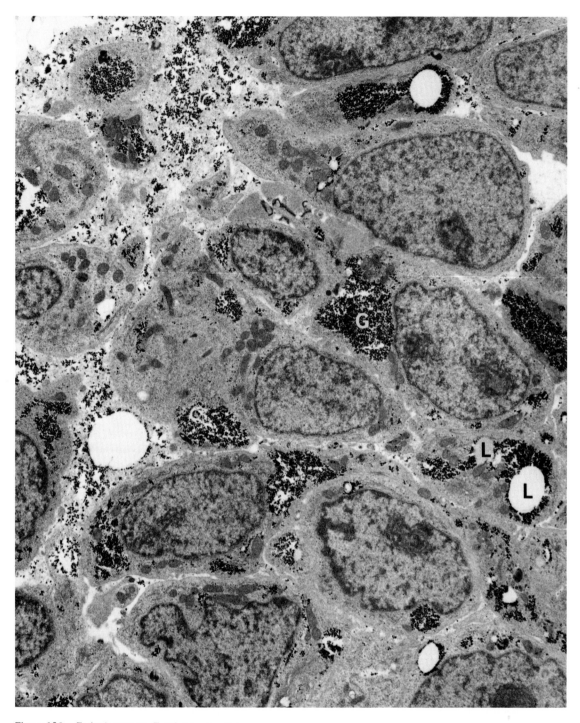

Figure 132 *Ewing's tumour. Focal deposits of glycogen
(G) are seen in the tumour cells. Some deposits are
associated with lipid droplets (L). ×9000 (From a block of
tissue supplied by Dr A. H. Cameron)*

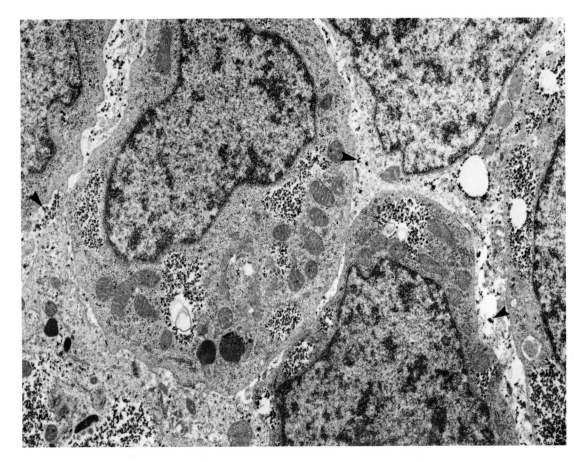

Figure 133 *Ewing's tumour. Same case as Figure 132. Besides the focal deposits of glycogen there are also glycogen particles (arrowheads) between the tumour cells. ×16 500 (From a block of tissue supplied by Dr A. H. Cameron)*

The cells of this tumour are poorly endowed with organelles, save the occasional mitochondrion and abundant polyribosomes attesting the rapid growth rate of this tumour. Some controversy exists as to whether desmosomes or desmosome-like structures are seen in Ewing's tumour. Published electron micrographs lead me to conclude that at least in some instances desmosome-like structures do develop in tumours acceptable on every ground as Ewing's tumour. True desmosomes, however, have not so far been depicted. Desmosome-like structures occur also in neuroblastomas, so this finding is of no diagnostic value in distinguishing Ewing's tumour from neuroblastoma but it is of value in distinguishing these two from lymphoma. Cell processes are sparse and slender or virtually absent in Ewing's tumour, and they do not contain microtubules or mitochondria as do the plumper more numerous cell processes of neuroblastoma. Cell processes are seen in some lymphomas also (e.g. Hodgkin's disease and follicular lymphoma) but they do not contain microtubules.

Neuroblastoma

A feature of considerable diagnostic import which distinguishes neuroblastoma from Ewing's tumour is the paucity of glycogen; what little is present does not form focal aggregates. The ultrastructural morphology of neuroblastoma (*Figures 134–136*) varies somewhat, depending on the degree of differentiation (Misugi, Misugi and Newton, 1968; Yanagisawa, 1970;

161

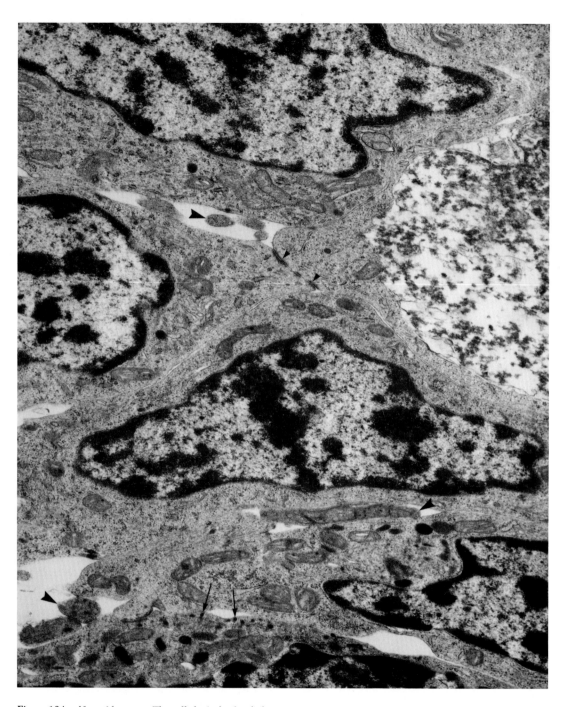

Figure 134   *Neuroblastoma. The cells lack the focal glyco-*
gen deposits seen in Ewing's tumour. The cell processes
(large arrowheads) are plump and some contain mito-
chondria. Neurosecretory granules are just discernible
(arrows). Note also the desmosome-like structures (small
arrowheads). ×25 000

162

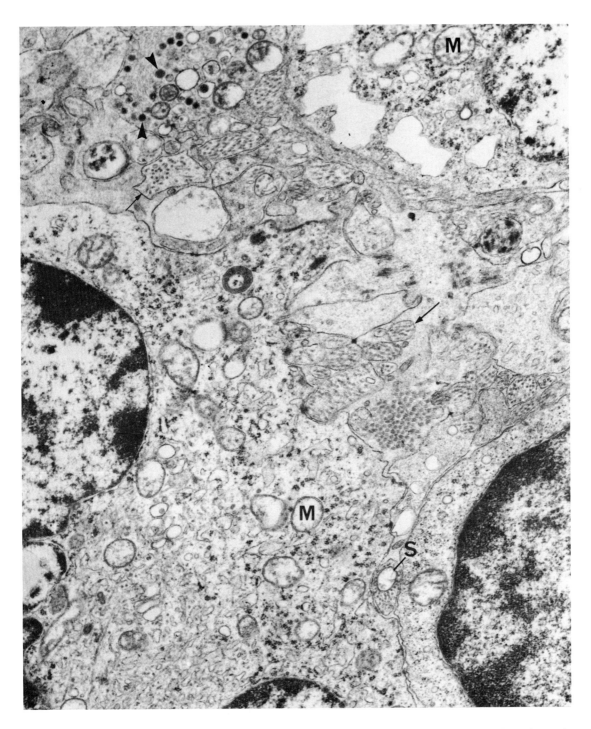

Figure 135　*A better differentiated, rosette-forming neuro-blastoma than the one illustrated in Figure 134. Glycogen is absent but numerous polyribosomes and swollen mito-chondria (M) are seen in the tumour cells. One cell contains numerous neurosecretory granules (arrowheads). Note also the neurites (arrows) containing microtubules and a neurite which contains a swollen mitochondria (S) and micro-tubules. ×19 000*

Tazawa, Soga and Ito, 1971; Nakayama *et al.*, 1975; Azzarelli *et al.*, 1977; Rhodes *et al.*, 1978).

The better-differentiated rosette-forming type of neuroblastoma is characterized by the presence of numerous plump cylindrical processes (axons or dendrites, collectively referred to as 'neurites') which contain microtubules (also called 'neurotubules'), intracytoplasmic filaments (also called 'neurofilaments'), neurosecretory granules and mitochondria. Multiple synaptic junctions (desmosome-like structures) are seen between the neurites and between the neurites and adjacent cells.

The nucleus is unremarkable and shows little more than the usual features of neoplasia. The cytoplasm is scant and contains little besides mitochondria and numerous polyribosomes. Other features of diagnostic import include: (1) numerous microtubules and intracytoplasmic filaments; and (2) dense granules or dense core granules about 150 nm in diameter (also called neurosecretory granules or catecholamine granules) and also a few larger pleomorphic granules which could be lysosomes.

The poorly differentiated non-rosette-forming neuroblastoma is characterized by: (1) greater irregu-

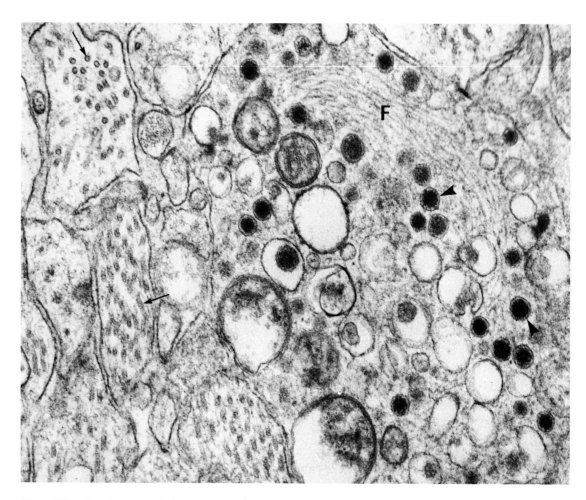

Figure 136 *Neuroblastoma. A high-power view from the top left-hand corner of Figure 135 showing the microtubles (arrows) in the neurites, neurosecretory granules (arrowheads) and intracytoplasmic filaments (F). ×56 000 (From a block of tissue supplied by Dr A. H. Cameron)*

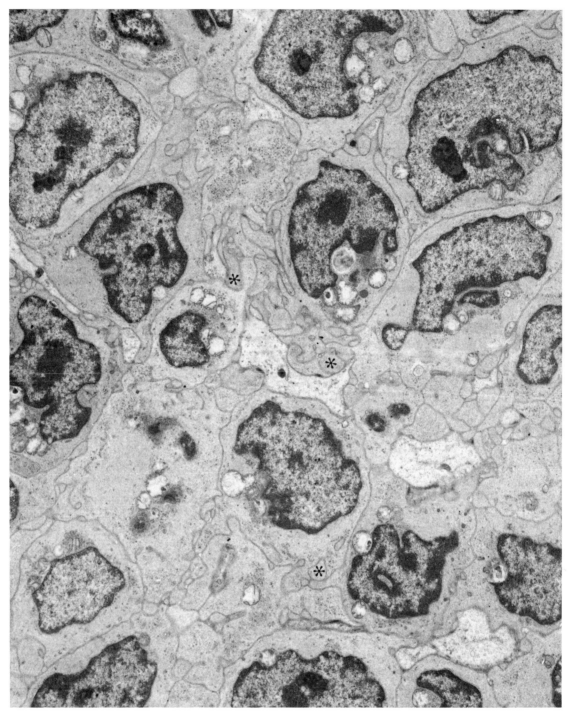

Figure 137   *Follicular lymphoma. Numerous cell processes. (*) are seen among the closely packed tumour cells. No cell junctions are present. Except for a few swollen mitochondria the cytoplasm is featureless. At higher power, however, polyribosomes were found lying free in the cytoplasm. The nuclear pockets one expects to see in this type of tumour are not seen in this field of view but they were present in other areas. ×8000 (Skinnider, unpublished electron micrograph)*

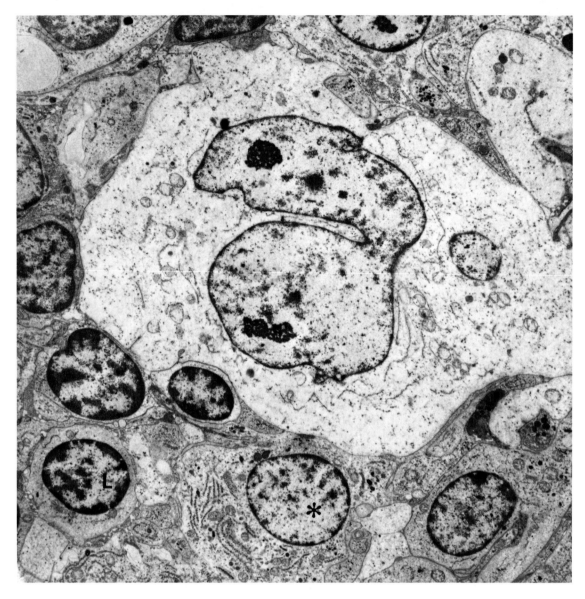

Figure 138 *Hodgkin's disease. The large cell in the centre of the picture is a Sternberg–Reed cell. Also evident are small lymphocytes (L) and a plasmacytoid cell (*). Note the absence of cell junctions. ×13 000 (Skinnider, unpublished electron micrograph)*

larity of nuclear form and more numerous mitoses, (2) paucity of microtubules but usually not intra-cytoplasmic filaments; (3) a relative paucity of neurites, but they still tend to be quite plump and contain mitochondria but fewer microtubules; (4) paucity or total absence of synaptic junctions; (5) absence of glycogen, but presence of numerous polyribosomes in the cytoplasmic matrix; and (6) paucity of neurosecretory granules.

A diligent search for these granules should be made, for this is an important point in differential diagnosis; neither Ewing's tumour nor other tumours such as reticulum cell sarcoma, small cell osteogenic sarcoma, embryonal rhabdomyosarcoma and eosinophilic granuloma which at times cause diagnostic confusion contain such granules. There are, of course, other features which distinguish these tumours, most of which have been dealt with under appropriate headings in other chapters of this book.

Lymphomas

Bonikos, Bensch and Kempson (1976) state: '. . .with regard to the differential diagnosis of neoplastic disorders of the lymphorecticular system, it seems that electron microscopy has little to offer.' There is some truth in this, for electron microscopy has not as yet proved to be quite as useful as in the differential diagnosis of some other neoplasms, but, by and large, this is too pessimistic a view. For example, electron microscopy has something to offer in the differential diagnosis of leukaemias (Chapter 13) and multiple myeloma (Chapter 14), not to mention various other small points and observations of diagnostic interest, such as the nucleus in Sezary's syndrome, the abundance of nuclear pockets in follicular lymphoma, the lysosomes in histiocytic lymphoma and glycogen in erythroleukaemia (Chapter 15).

However, at the moment perhaps the most important contribution that electron microscopy can make with regard to this group of neoplasms is that one can distinguish lymphomas as a group (e.g. lymphosarcoma, reticulum cell sarcoma and Hodgkin's disease) from other classes of neoplasms.

Lymphomas, as a group, are characterized by a lack of specific features rather than the presence of certain specific identifiable traits (*Figures 137* and *138*; see also illustrations in Chapter 13). Thus: (1) the absence of cell junctions,* basal lamina, tonofilaments and intracellular and intercellular lumina distinguishes them from carcinomas: (2) the absence of an external lamina distinguishes them from schwannoma and the absence of myofilaments from myosarcomas; (3) the absence or paucity of glycogen† distinguishes them from Ewing's tumour: and (4) the absence of neurosecretory granules and neurites containing microtubules distinguishes them from neuroblastoma.

*This is the majority view but see also Chapter 5 for a detailed discussion on this point.
†An exception here is erythroleukaemia, where glycogen does occur (Chapter 15), but not as focal deposits found in Ewing's tumour.

References

AZZARELLI, B., RICHARDS, D. E., ANTON, A. H. and ROESSMANN, U. (1977). Central neuroblastoma: electron microscopic observations and catecholamine determinations. *J. Neuropath. Expl Neurol.*, 36, 384

BARDEN, R. P. (1943). The similarity of clinical and roentgen findings in children with Ewing's sarcoma (endothelial myeloma) and sympathetic neuroblastoma. *Am. J. Roentgen.* 50, 575

BONIKOS, D. S., BENSCH, K. G. and KEMPSON, R. L. (1976). The contribution of electron microscopy to the differential diagnosis of tumours. *Beitr. Path.*, 158, 417

COLVILLE, H. C. and WILLIS, R. A. (1933). Neuroblastoma metastasis in bones, with criticism of Ewing's endothelioma. *Am. J. Path.*, 9, 421

FRIEDMAN, B. and GOLD, H. (1968). Ultrastructure of Ewing's sarcoma of bone. *Cancer*, 22, 307

HOU-JENSEN, K., PRIORI, E. and DMOCHOWSKI, L. (1972). Studies on ultrastructure of Ewing's sarcoma of bone. *Cancer*, 29, 280

KADIN, M. E. and BENSCH, K. G. (1971). On the origin of Ewing's tumor. *Cancer*, 27, 257

MISUGI, K., MISUGI, N. and NEWTON, W. A., Jr. (1968). Fine structural study of neuroblastoma, ganglioneuroblastoma and pheochromocytoma. *Archs Path.*, 86, 160

NAKAYAMA, I., TSUDA, N., MUTA, H., FUJII, H., TSUJI, K., MATSUO, T. and TAKAHARA, O. (1975). Fine structural comparison of Ewing's sarcoma with neuroblastoma. *Acta Path. Jap.*, 25, 251

POVÝŠIL, C. and MATĚJOVSKÝ, Z. (1977). Ultrastructure of Ewing's tumour. *Virchows Arch. Path. Anat. Hist.*, 374, 303

RHODES, R. H., DAVIS, R. L., KASSEL, S. H. and CLAGUE, B. H. (1978). Primary cerebral neuroblastoma: A light and electron microscopic study. *Acta Neuropath.*, 41, 119

RICE, R. W., CABOT, A. and JOHNSTON, A. D. (1973). The application of electron microscopy to the diagnostic differentiation of Ewing's sarcoma and reticulum cell sarcoma of bone. *Clin. Orthop.*, 91, 174

SZAKACS, J. E., CARTA, M., and SZAKACS, M. R. (1974). Ewing's sarcoma, extraskeletal and of bone. Case report with ultrastructural analysis. *Ann. Clin. Lab. Sci.*, 4, 306

TAZAWA, K., SOGA, J. and ITO, H. (1971). Fine structure of neuroblastoma — a case report. *Acta Path. Jap.*, 21, 257

WILLIS, R. A. (1940). Metastatic neuroblastoma in bone presenting the Ewing syndrome, with a discussion of 'Ewing's sarcoma'. *Am. J. Path.*, 16, 317

YANAGISAWA, M. (1970). Electron microscopic study of neuroblastoma. *Pediatria Universitatis Tokyo*, 17, 30

13
Differential diagnosis of acute leukaemias

Opinion varies as to the value of electron microscopy in establishing the cell line of an acute leukaemia in cases that are difficult to diagnose by light microscopy. Certainly, there are no unique ultrastructural features which can unequivocally distinguish the 'blasts' of various cell lines. However, one has to agree with Bessis (1973) when he states that '. . .electron microscopy may occasionally be useful in identifying the cell line of an acute leukaemia when light microscopy fails to do so'. He amplifies this by pointing out that in about 75 per cent of the cases one can easily determine by routine light microscopy which cell line has undergone malignant transformation but in the remaining cases cytochemical and ultrastructural studies can usually but not invariably establish a diagnosis.

The problems in diagnosing these difficult cases stem from: (1) the complete or near-complete lack of differentiation and, hence, an obliteration of the very characteristics or hall-marks by which we classify these cells; (2) confusion arising from features which are found in more than one cell line and; (3) deciding whether two separate cell lines are neoplastic or whether only one is neoplastic and the other is showing a reactive or non-neoplastic proliferation.

For the purpose of our discussion in this chapter, we will exclude certain rare leukaemias which usually do not create the kind of diagnostic problem we are dealing with here or have been described in other chapters in this book. These include: (1) erythroleukaemia (Di Guglielmo's disease) (Chapter 15). It would appear that in both acute and chronic forms of this condition the neoplastic cells are sufficiently distinctive for one to be able to distinguish this leukaemia from other leukaemic states. The problem here is distinguishing this leukaemia from other conditions such as polycythaemia rubra vera (Vaquez-Osler's disease), acute haemolytic anaemias, sideroblastic refractory anaemias and aplastic anaemias. It must, however, be remembered that in erythroleukaemia the myeloid series of cells are often abnormal and that quite a few cases of this condition evolve

into a frank myeloid leukaemia, so confusion may arise on this account. (2) Plasma cell neoplasms (Chapter 14). Here various laboratory findings and the ultrastructural appearances are sufficiently characteristic, so that confusion with other acute leukaemias is unlikely.

Thus, after light microscopy the main question that usually remains, in the difficult cases, is whether a given acute leukaemia should be assigned to the lymphoid, myeloid or monocytic series of cells. The differential diagnosis of these leukaemias rests heavily but not entirely on deciding whether granules are present in the neoplastic cells and whether they are azurophilic granules or not. The advantage which the electron microscope has over the light microscope is that fewer and/or smaller granules can be detected and their morphology and staining characteristic (i.e. peroxidase reactivity) more clearly appreciated. In order to understand these matters it is essential to recall some of the features of the granules seen in leucocytes.

Granules in normal myeloid, lymphoid and monocytic series of cells

It is now universally accepted that neutrophils contain at least two (probably three) distinct types of granules, a primary or azurophilic granule and a secondary or a specific granule (Bainton and Farquhar, 1966, 1968; Wetzel, Horn and Spicer, 1967; Wetzel, Spicer and Horn, 1967; Dunn, Hardin and Spicer, 1968). It is clear that they are formed quite independently at different periods of cell maturation (*Figures 139–141*). The primary granule is formed in the promyelocyte phase, while the secondary granules are produced during the later stages of neutrophil maturation (metamyelocyte, myelocyte and band form) after primary granule formation has virtually ceased.

Ultrastructural, cytochemical and biochemical studies now show the existence of a tertiary granule

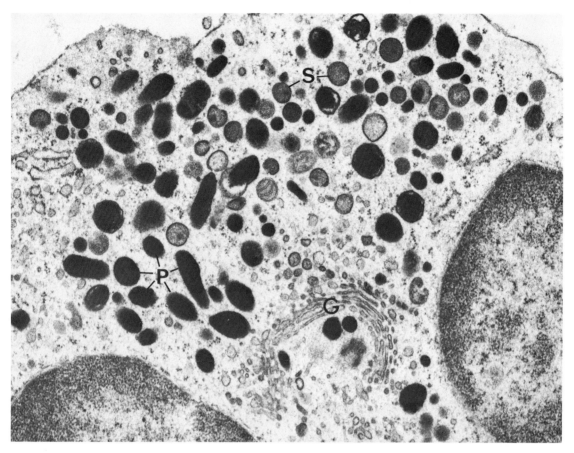

Figure 139 *Immature neutrophil leucocyte from human bone marrow. Fixed in osmium (cacodylate buffer), stained with uranium and lead. The primary granules (P) are easily distinguished from the smaller, less dense secondary granules (S). The presence of a well-defined Golgi complex (G) and very small granules (arrows) of a density similar to that of the secondary granules suggests that the cell is at a stage of development where secondary granule production is in progress. ×28 000 (From Ghadially, 1975)*

which develops at a relatively late stage of neutrophil development (segmented forms) (Baggiolini, Hirsch and DeDuve, 1969; Scott and Horn, 1970). Only the primary granules (azurophilic granules) contain myeloperoxidase (Dunn *et al.*, 1968) and thus are peroxidase-positive. Ultrastructurally the primary granule presents as a round or oval electron-dense body about 0.3 μm in diameter. The secondary granule is electron-dense after osmium fixation. In glutaraldehyde-fixed preparations of the buffy coat from human blood they are often slightly or markedly extracted, and in such instances they present as electron-lucent bodies or as moderately dense granules with a lucent periphery. The tertiary granules are small pleomorphic bodies (usually bacilliform) seen

mainly in mature circulating neutrophils (Daems, 1968).

Azurophilic granules occur also in the lymphocytic and monocytic series of cells. When entire cells are examined (as in smears), some 5—30 per cent of lymphocytes are seen to contain one to six azurophilic granules which measure 0.3—0.6 μm in diameter (Bessis, 1973). The possibility of these granules being included in an ultrathin section is therefore small. Thus, granules are rarely seen in the lymphocytic series of cells in sectioned material. In the monocytic series the granules are quite numerous, but they are usually fine and powdery and some of them are rod-shaped. At the ultrastructural level, except for size and frequency of occurrence, there is nothing that

169

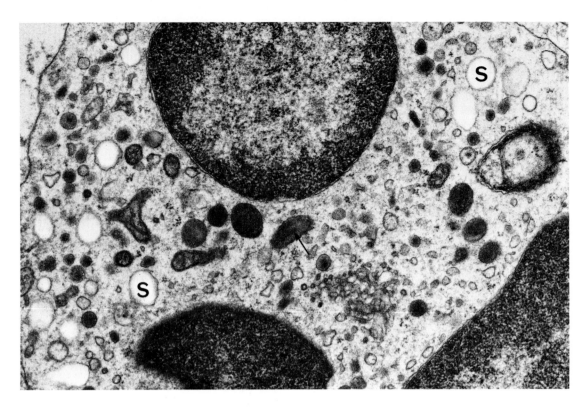

Figure 140 *Neutrophil leucocyte from peripheral blood of man. Fixed in glutaraldehyde (cacodylate buffer), post-fixed in osmium, stained with uranium and lead. The secondary granules (S) are markedly extracted and appear electron-lucent. The primary granules are electron-dense. A crystalloid (arrow) difficult to discern is present in some of the primary granules.* ×28 000 *(From Ghadially, 1975)*

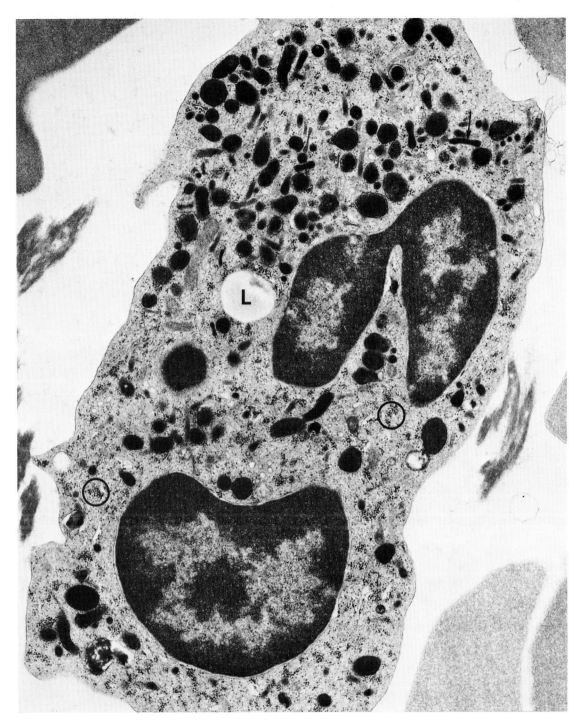

Figure 141   *Neutrophil leucocyte from peripheral blood of man. Fixed in osmium (cacodylate buffer), stained with uranium and lead. The primary and secondary granules cannot be confidently identified. It is worth noting that this is not infrequently the case. However, numerous bacilliform tertiary granules (arrow) are easily recognized. These together with the segmented nucleus, numerous glycogen particles (in circles) and an atrophic Golgi complex, represented by a few vesicles in the juxtanuclear position, are indicative of maturity in this leucocyte. Also seen is a lipid droplet (L). × 20 000 (From Ghadially, 1975)*

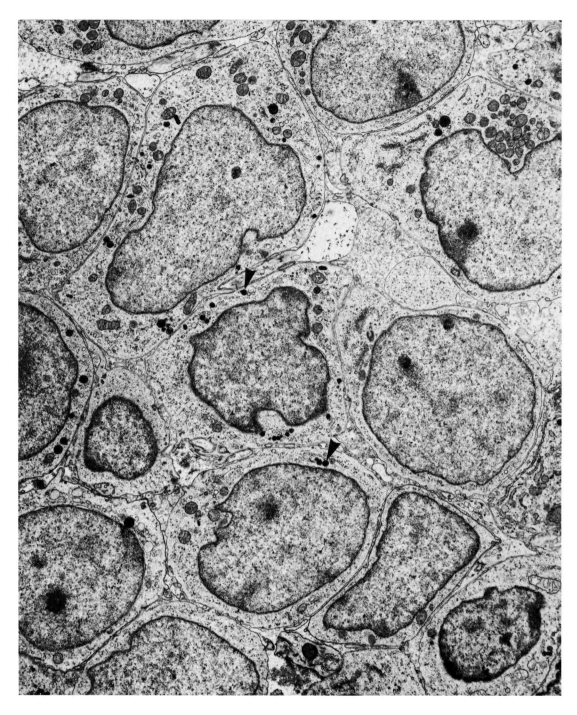

Figure 142   *Bone marrow from a case of acute myeloid leukaemia showing myeloblasts with scant primary granules (arrowheads). Note absence of cell junctions.* ×7500

unequivocally distinguishes these granules in the three cell lines, but, generally speaking, the granules in the myeloid cells tend to be homogeneously electron-dense, while those in the monocytic series tend to be more pleomorphic and variable in electron density.

Leukaemic cells

In acute myeloid leukaemia (*Figures 142* and *143*) the neoplastic myeloblasts usually lack secondary granules, but such granules are found in the better-differentiated cells of chronic myeloid leukaemia*

---

*Interestingly enough, in some myeloid leukaemias secondary granules are present but primary granules are sparse or virtually absent, as if the stage of primary granule production had been skipped or aborted.

(*Figure 144*). It stands to reason that when a case is difficult to diagnose, the degree of differentiation will be so poor that secondary granules are unlikely to be produced. Hence, in the diagnosis of difficult cases of acute myeloid leukaemia our interest focuses on the demonstration of primary or azurophilic granules. If such granules are reasonably large and not too sparse, the diagnosis of acute myeloid leukaemia can be established with the light microsope, but if they are small and few, the diagnosis may be more confidently established with the electron microscope. When one is examining difficult cases with the electron microscope, one tries to assure oneself that: (1) the cells one is assessing belong to the neoplastic clone; and (2) at least some of them contain granules of a morphology acceptable as that belonging to the

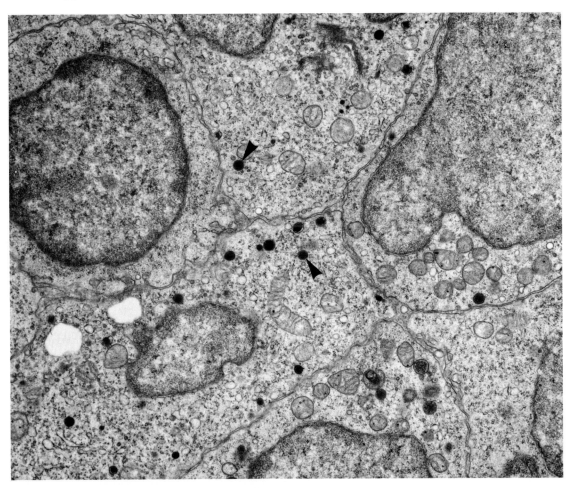

Figure 143   *Acute myeloid leukaemia. Same case as Figure 142, showing primary granules (arrowheads) in neoplastic myeloblasts.* ×14 500

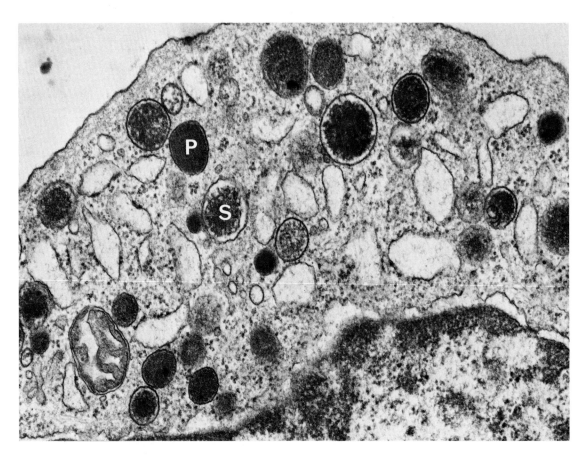

Figure 144 *Chronic myeloid leukaemia. Buffy coat from peripheral blood fixed in osmium (cacodylate buffer), stained with uranium and lead. Leukaemic cell showing primary (P) and secondary (S) granules. Tertiary granules are absent. ×22 000*

primary granules of the neutrophil series. It is the overall impression that is important here, not the finding of a rare dense little granule in one or two cells.

Consider now the situation where one has found a few electron-dense granules (presumably azurophilic granules) in a number of neoplastic cells where light microscopy has revealed no azurophilic granules or only a rare or doubtful one. Since azurophilic granules are found in monocytes and a few also occur in lymphocytes, one may argue, and quite rightly, that the finding of a few electron-dense granules does not necessarily mean that one is looking at the myeloid series of cells.

Similarly, the total absence of azurophilic granules (*Figure 145*), while arguing very strongly in favour of a lymphocytic derivation, would still leave one

wondering whether it might be a highly anaplastic myeloid or monocytic leukaemia (stem cell leukaemia).

The discovery of an Auer body would go a long way towards establishing the diagnosis of myeloid leukaemia, but such bodies are rare (approximately 5 per cent of cases) and the chances of encountering one in ultrathin sections even rarer. These rod-like structures (Auer bodies) are thought to arise by the enlargement and/or fusion of primary granules, and up to now they have not been seen in the monocytic or lymphocytic series of cells (Bessis, 1973). Auer bodies usually show a characteristic crystalline structure with repeats at 11 nm intervals, but this depends also on the quality of preservation and a favourable plane of sectioning.

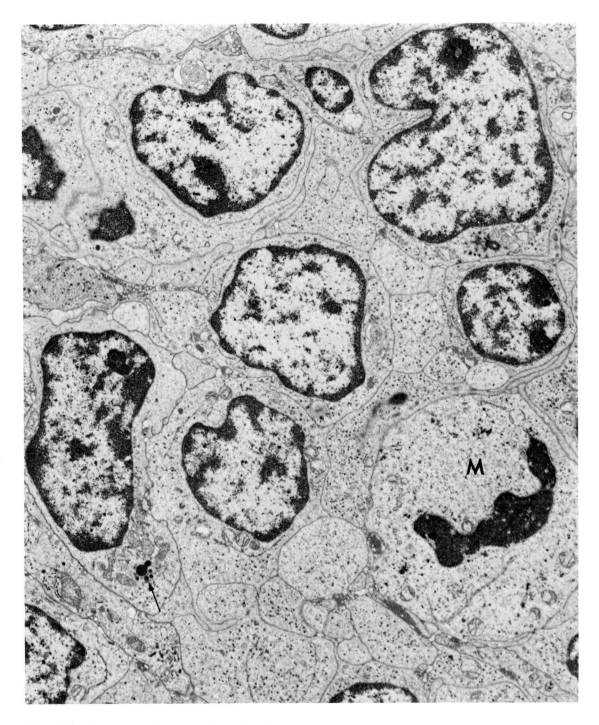

Figure 145   *Bone marrow from a case of acute lympho-*
blastic leukaemia. Most of the leukaemic blasts lack
granules but a cluster of granules (arrow) of unknown
nature is seen in one cell. Note a cell in mitosis (M),
and lack of cell junctions. ×8000

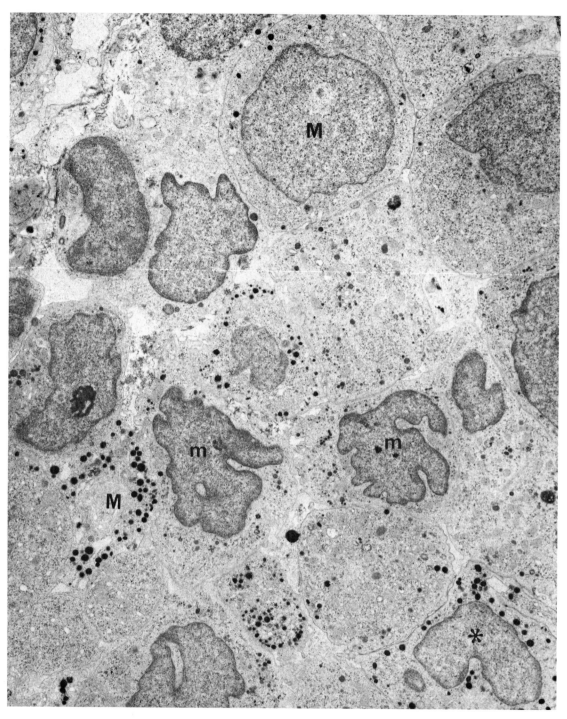

Figure 146   *Bone marrow from a case of acute myelo-monocytic leukaemia. One can identify myeloid cells (M) with quite large electron-dense granules and monocytoid cells (m) by their irregular nuclei and fine not so dense granules. Also present are cells difficult to classify, such as the one (*) in the bottom corner of the picture, which has a notched nucleus and quite large dense granules. ×7000*

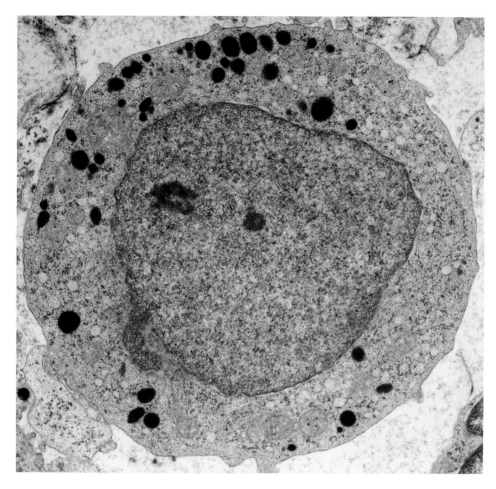

Figure 147 *Acute myelomonocytic leukaemia. From same block of tissue as Figure 146, showing a myeloblast with numerous large round and oval uniformly electron-dense primary granules. Not a single granule acceptable as a secondary granule is present.* ×15 000

Conditions in which neoplastic monocytic or monocytoid cells circulate in the peripheral blood in any number are monocytic leukaemia (Schilling type), myelomonocytic leukaemia (Naegali type), histiocytic medullary reticulosis and the leukaemic phase of reticulum cell sarcoma (Cline and Golde, 1973; Schnitzer and Kass, 1973; Schumacher *et al.*, 1973; Williams, 1973; Skinnider and Ghadially, 1977).

There are no morphological differences which are constant or characteristic enough to distinguish un-equivocally the circulating histiocytic or monocytic cells in these conditions. The monocytic nature of the cells in these conditions is no longer in doubt, except in the case of myelomonocytic leukaemia (*Figures 146–149*), where it is not too clear whether these cells* are: (1) neoplastic cells of monocytic lineage; (2) a reactive proliferation of the monocytic series of cells; or (3) altered or atypical myeloblasts that look like monocytes and monoblasts. Intermediate forms difficult to classify as either monocytic or myelocytic are also found. Therefore, the idea that the mono-

---

*Often called 'monocytoid' rather than 'monocytic', to register the element of doubt which exists regarding their true nature.

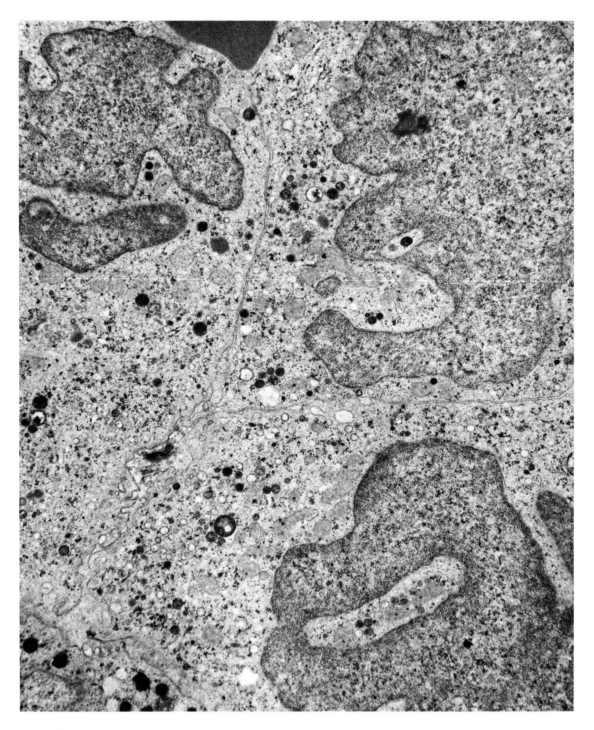

Figure 148   *Acute myelomonocytic leukaemia. Same
block of tissue as Figures 146 and 147. A group of leukaemic
monocytoid cells showing bizarre nuclei and pleomorphic
granulation.* ×15 000

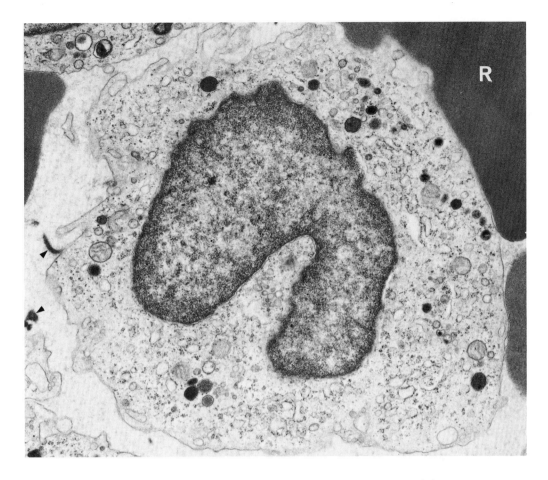

Figure 149 *Acute myelomonocytic leukaemia. Although this monocytoid cell comes from the same block of tissue (bone marrow) as Figures 146—148, it is almost certainly a cell from the circulating blood rather than the bone marrow proper. This is evidenced by the fibrin (arrowheads) and mature red blood cells (R) that surround it and the more mature appearance when compared with the monocytoid cells in the bone marrow (Figure 148). Note the horseshoe-shaped nucleus and the pleomorphic granulation.*
×15 000

cytic and myelocytic series of cells derive from a common stem cell is attractive (Skinnider, Card and Padmanabh, 1977).

The monocytic (*Figure 150*) or monocytoid (*Figures 146—149*) cells in the above-mentioned conditions are characterized by the presence of clusters of a few to fairly numerous quite small rounded (an occasional rod-shaped granule is also present) granules. The granules are quite pleomorphic in size and electron density. This distinguishes them from the myelocytic series, where the granules are larger, more uniform in shape and usually also more uniformly electron-dense. But these are broad generalizations which are helpful in many but not in all

cases, particularly when one is dealing with a 'blast' containing only a few granules.

Differences of diagnostic import exist also in the nucleus, but once again these are not absolute differences. The nucleus of the leukaemic monocytic or monocytoid cell may be round or only slightly notched, and then it is indistinguishable from any other stem cell nucleus. It may, however, have quite a characteristic appearance, which has been variously described as 'contorted', 'convoluted', 'lumpy', 'U-shaped', 'horseshoe-shaped' and 'deeply notched'.

Collections of filaments, at times compact enough to be designated fibrils and on much rarer occasions deployed in an orderly manner to form a crystalloid,

179

have been seen in the nucleus of various cell types (for a review see Ghadially, 1975), but as far as leukaemic cells are concerned, at one stage it appeared that intranuclear filaments occurred only in leukaemic monocytes (Bessis, 1973), but they have now been seen in the lymphoblasts of follicular lymphoma (Skinnider, personal communication), plasma cell of multiple myeloma (Smetana et al., 1973, and the myelocytic cells of myeloid leukaemia (Glick, 1976). In any case, this is a rare phenomenon and one that is of little diagnostic value but of some theoretical interest, because the occurrence of filaments in nuclei has frequently been linked with virus infections.

Of the haematogenous cell lines, the monocytic cells are better endowed with intracytoplasmic filaments; in fact, normal lymphocytes contain virtually no filaments. In the monocyte the filaments are usually found in the juxtanuclear position within the 'hollow' of the U-shaped nucleus. In keeping with this is the fact that one is more likely to find intracytoplasmic filaments in neoplastic monocytoid and monocytic series of cells than in lymphoid or myeloid cells. This is generally accepted as a point of diagnostic value, even though intracytoplasmic filaments occur in other types of leukaemias and, indeed, in a variety of other neoplasms (Chapter 10; Ghadially, 1975; Ghadially, Lowes and Mesfin, 1977).

Other features of interest

Blisters, blebs and vermipodia

Recently we (Ghadially and Skinnider, 1976; Skinnider and Ghadially, 1977) had the opportunity to study with the transmission and scanning electron

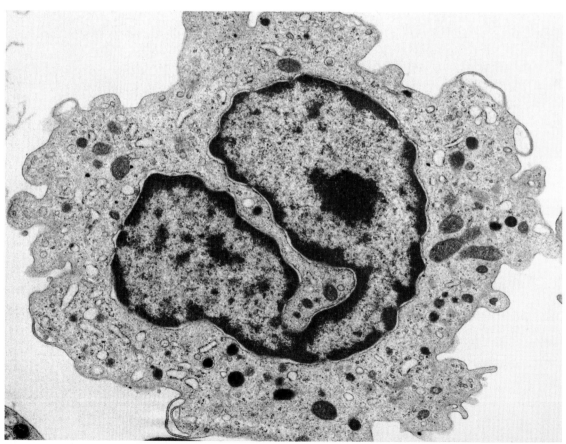

Figure 150 *Malignant histiocytosis. A neoplastic monocyte from peripheral blood showing characteristic nucleus and* *pleomorphic granules.* ×*18 000 (Skinnider and Ghadially, unpublished electron micrograph)*

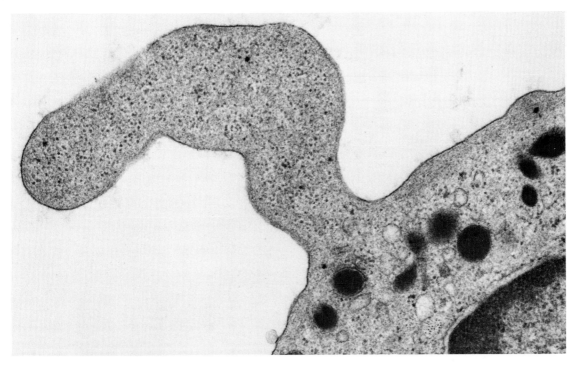

Figure 151   *Malignant histiocytosis. Same case as Figure 150, showing the vermipodium of a leukaemic cell found* *in peripheral blood.* ×*40 000 (From Skinnider and Ghadially 1977)*

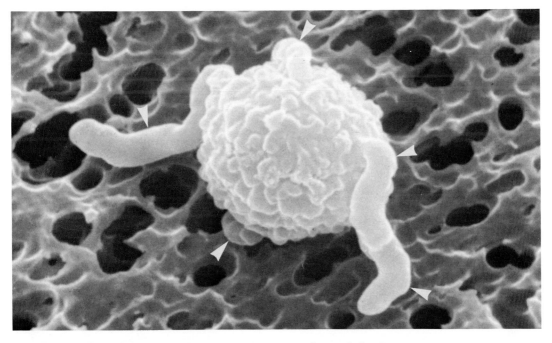

Figure 152   *Malignant histiocytosis. Different case from that shown in Figures 150 and 151. Scanning electron* *micrograph showing a leukaemic cell with five vernipodia (arrowheads).* ×*7500 (From Ghadially and Skinnider, 1976)*

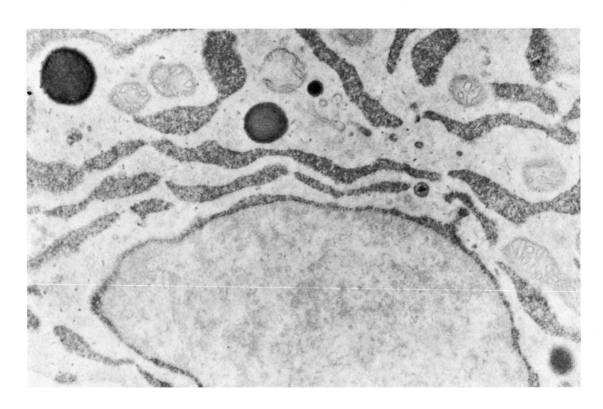

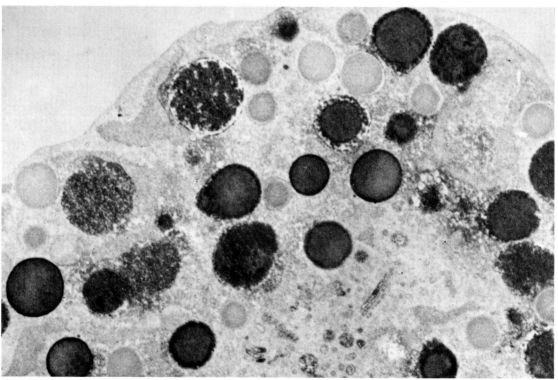

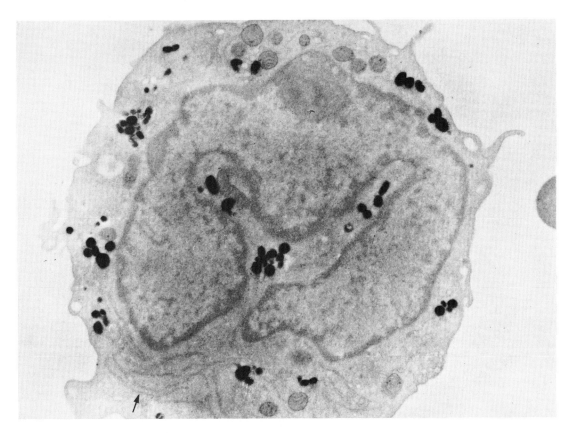

Figure 155   *Monoblastic leukaemia. Buffy coat subjected to the peroxidase reaction to demonstrate myeloperoxidase. The convoluted nucleus, groups of peroxidase-positive granules and absence of peroxidase-positivity in the perinuclear cistern and endoplasmic reticulum (arrow) identify this as a monocytic cell. ×13 000 (From Lambertenghi-Deliliers et al., 1978)*

Figure 153   *Myeloblastic leukaemia. Buffy coat subjected to the peroxidase reaction to demonstrate myeloperoxidase. The peroxidase-positivity is evident in the granules, cisternae of the rough endoplasmic reticulum and perinuclear cistern. This identifies the cell as belonging to the myeloid series. ×27 000 (From Lambertenghi-Deliliers et al., 1978)*

Figure 154   *Myeloblastic leukaemia. Buffy coat subjected to the peroxidase reaction to demonstrate myeloperoxidase. Same case as Figure 153. Peroxidase-positive reaction is evident in some but not all the granules of this leukaemic cell. ×22 000 (From Lambertenghi-Deliliers, et al., 1978)*

microscope two cases of malignant histiocytosis and a case of leukaemic reticulum cell sarcoma. Work-like cell processes (vermipodia) and blisters and blebs were seen in the malignant cells of these cases (*Figures 150–152*). The blisters (containing clear fluid) appear to develop by a single membrane bound vacuole approaching the cell membrane and acquiring another membrane on discharging from the cell. The blebs (containing cytoplasmic material) appear to correspond to the already well-known processes of zeiosis, and these, too, appear to be discharged from the cell. Since then blisters and blebs have been noted in two cases of lymphoblastic leukaemia (Skinnider, personal communication), so this does not appear to be of diagnostic value.

However, far more intriguing are the peculiar vermipodia (*Figures 151* and *152*). The idea that they are a preparative artefact may be ruled out, because we (Ghadially and Skinnider, 1976; Skinnider and Ghadially, 1977) have seen them in: (1) wet preparations of peripheral blood; (2) blood films stained with Wright–Giemsa stain; (3) transmission electron microscopic preparations from the buffy coat; and (4) scanning electron microscopic preparations of leucocyte-rich fraction of freshly collected blood. The underlying factors responsible for these phenomena are not clear, nor is the diagnostic value of these observations (because of the small number of cases studied), but to date we have seen vermipodia only in circulating neoplastic histiocytic or monocytic

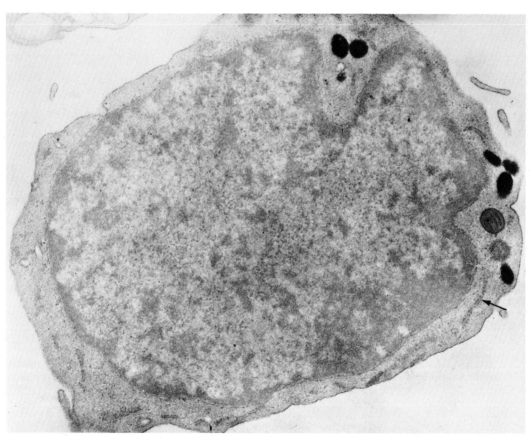

Figure 156 *Monoblastic leukaemia. Buffy coat subjected to the peroxidase reaction to demonstrate myeloperoxidase. The cells were peroxidase-negative by light microscopy. Here we see a cell that can on morphological grounds be mistaken as belonging to the myeloid series, because the nucleus is only slightly indented and quite large granules* *are present. However, the fact that the granules are peroxidase-positive but there is no reaction product in the perinuclear cisterna and in the few strands of rough endoplasmic reticulum (arrows) present, establishes this as a cell of the monocytic series. ×19 000 (From Lambertenghi-Deliliers et al., 1978)*

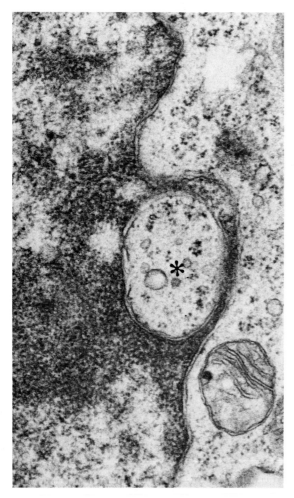

Figure 157   *Stem cell leukaemia, probably lymphoblastic. A leukaemic cell from bone marrow showing a nuclear pocket containing cytoplasmic material (*).* ×*51 000*

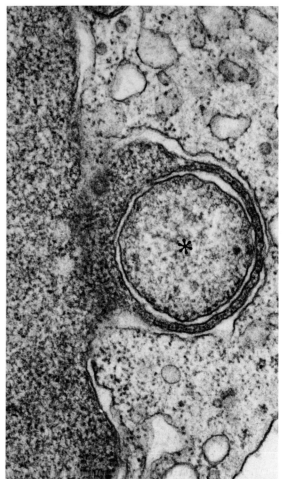

Figure 158   *Acute lymphoblastic leukaemia. A leukaemic cell from peripheral blood showing a nuclear pocket containing nuclear material (*).* ×*52 000*

cells but not in hundreds of other haematological disorders (including various leukaemias) which we have studied.

Peroxidase positivity

The peroxidase test has long been used to distinguish the myeloid series of cells at the light microscopic level. An extension of this is the peroxidase reaction performed at the ultrastructural level (*Figures 153–156*). Myeloperoxidase is synthesized by the polyribosomes on the cisternae of rough endoplasmic reticulum and the perinuclear cistern. Bessis and Maigné (1970) state that '. . .peroxidase positivity in the perinuclear cistern and in the ergastoplasm can

occasionally be identified by electron microscopy in myeloblasts that are peroxidase negative by light microscopy. This may be the only indication of the myeloblastic nature of a leukaemia.' Such a contention is supported by other studies (for references and discussion see Lambertenghi-Deliliers *et al.*, 1978) which show that by this technique cells thought to be neoplastic lymphoblasts by light microscopy have at times had to be reclassified as myeloblasts because of peroxidase positivity demonstrated at the ultrastructural level in the perinuclear cistern and the cisternae of the rough endoplasmic reticulum (*Figure 153*). Needless to say, if any azurophilic granules are present, they too, will be peroxidase-positive (*Figure 154*).

The usefulness of this cytochemical reaction has also been demonstrated in cases of monocytic leukaemia (Lambertenghi-Deliliers *et al.*, 1978), which may be peroxidase-negative (because the granules may be too small and/or too few) at the light microscopic level but peroxidase-positive at the ultrastructural level. In such cases only the granules give a positive reaction but not the contents of the perinuclear cistern or the cisternae of the rough endoplasmic reticulum (*Figures 155* and *156*). Further, one can confidently distinguish the peroxidase-positive azurophilic granules from others. In myelomonocytic leukaemia, cells showing the staining reaction of myeloblasts (i.e. positive reaction seen in granules, perinuclear cistern and cisternae of the rough endoplasmic reticulum) and cells showing the staining reaction of monocytic cells (i.e. positive granules only) are found.

*It is best to call these structures 'nuclear pockets', because terms such as 'blisters', 'blebs' and 'projections' have been used to designate various other alterations of nuclear morphology (see Ghadially, 1975, for details).

Nuclear pockets*

These peculiar formations (*Figures 157* and *158*), referred to as 'blebs', 'projections' or 'pockets', may on rare occasions be found in a variety of normal and neoplastic cells, but then only a rare cell shows a pocket. If many cells show such formations, it is likely that one is looking at a lymphoma or leukaemia. A detailed description of the morphology of these pockets and the instances in which they have been seen will not be repeated here (see Ghadially, 1975). Suffice to say that nuclear pockets have been seen in myeloid, monocytic and lymphoid series of cells,† so this feature is not particularly useful for the differential diagnosis of leukaemias. However, a review of our own material and published electron micrographs shows that there are at least two varieties of

†A rare pocket is seen in normal leukocytes (e.g. about 1 per cent of circulating neutrophils in normal individuals), but many more are seen in leukaemic cells.

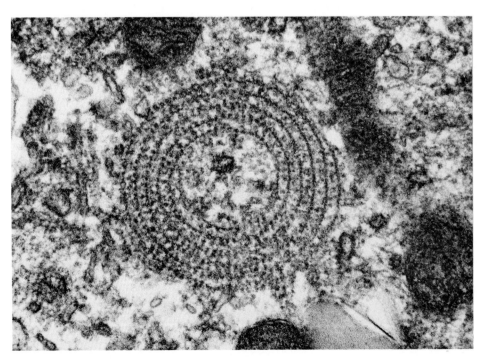

Figure 159 *Lymphosarcoma cell leukaemia. Ribosome lammellae complex found in a leukaemic cell.* ×69 000 (*From Djaldetti et al., 1974*)

186

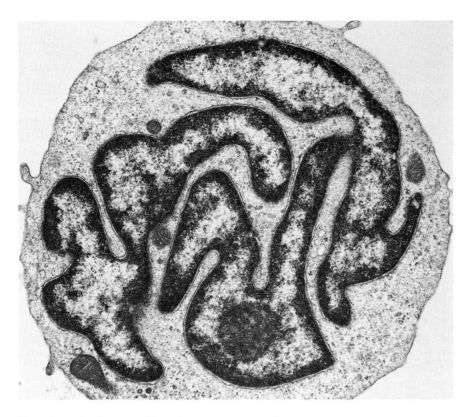

Figure 160 *Leukaemic cell from Sezary's syndrome. The Sézary cell nuclei show a cerebriform appearance in blood smears, but appear serpentine or drawn out into narrow ribbons in ultrathin sections. ×21 000 (Djaldetti, unpublished electron micrograph)*

nuclear pockets — those that contain cytoplasmic material and those that contain nuclear material — but this point has so far been ignored. I have seen both types of pockets in a single case of stem cell leukaemia (probably lymphoblastic), so this distinction may not be of diagnostic value. It is more likely that we are witnessing stages of evolution of a single basic morphological lesion. Even so, this is a point worth studying in greater detail, if for no other reason than to learn more about these peculiar formations whose significance eludes us.

Ribosome—lamella complex

This term is employed to describe tubular structures which on section present as circular (concentric) oval or linear arrays of lamellae studded with ribosomes (*Figure 159*). It is important to note that these are lamellae and not membranes, in that they do not have the characteristic trilaminar structure of cytomembranes. This distinguishes them from other somewhat similar structures such as the 'ergatroplasmic Nebenkern', composed of membranes studded with ribosomes, and the glycogen body, where membranous whorls interspersed with glycogen particles occur (for a fuller description and situations in which such structures are found see Ghadially, 1975).

Ribosome—lamella complexes have on rare occasions been seen in tumours such as adrenal cortical adenoma (Hoshino, 1966) and paraganglionoma (Nabarra, Sonsino and Andrianarison, 1977), but the large majority of sightings have been in leukaemic cells, notably the hairy cells of hairy cell leukaemia (Zucker-Franklin, 1963; Katayama, Li and Yam, 1972; Anday, Goodman and Tishkoff, 1973; Daniel and Flandrin, 1974; Djaldetti *et al.*, 1974; Schnitzer and Kass, 1974; Brunning and Parkin, 1975). In view of the prevailing chaos in the nomenclature and classification of lymphomas and leukaemias and the innumerable terms used to describe just about every single condition, it is difficult to sort out in which particular condition these structures occur. The diagnostic value of these inclusions is therefore small, but one should first think of hairy cell leukaemia if these structures are sighted.

It must be noted that ribosome—lamella complex are not found in all cases of hairy cell leukaemia. We (Ghadially and Skinnider, 1972, and subsequent unpublished observations) did not find them in the four cases that we have studied, and on reviewing the published reports of hairy cell leukaemia, it seems that at the most only about half (probably much less) of the cases show ribosome—lamella complexes.

Sézary cell nucleus

The nuclei of most leukaemic cells tend to be somewhat more irregular in form than their normal counterparts, and at times a few cells may be found where the nucleus is beset by numerous invaginations, so that the nuclear form is quite irregular. However, the nuclei of leucocytes in Sézary's syndrome are so bizarre that they are almost in a class by themselves (*Figure 160*). This is a point of considerable diagnostic value. In smears of blood these nuclei show a cerebriform appearance, but they appear serpentine or drawn out into a mass of overlapping narrow ribbons in ultrathin sections examined with the electron microscope (Lutzner and Jordan, 1968; Djaldetti *et al.*, 1975).

It is, however, worth stressing that while the finding of a substantial number of cells with nuclei of the kind shown in *Figure 160* is of value in establishing the diagnosis of Sézary's syndrome, one should not fall into the trap of making such a diagnosis on the basis of a few irregular nuclei.

References

ANDAY, G. J., GOODMAN, J. R. and TISHKOFF, G. H. (1973). An unusual cytoplasmic ribosomal structure in pathologic lymphocytes. *Blood, 41*, 439

BAGGIOLINI, M., HIRSCH, J. G. and DeDUVE, C. (1969). Resolution of granules from rabbit heterophil leukocytes into distinct populations by zonal sedimentation. *J. Cell Biol., 40*, 529

BAINTON, D. F. and FARQUHAR, M. G. (1966). Origin of granules in polymorphonuclear leukocytes. Two types derived from opposite faces of the Golgi complex in developing granulocytes. *J. Cell Biol., 28*, 277

BAINTON, D. F. and FARQUHAR, M. G. (1968). Differences in enzyme content of azurophil and specific granules of polymorphonuclear leukocytes. I. Histochemical staining of bone marrow smears. *J. Cell Biol., 39*, 286

BESSIS, M. (1973). *Living Blood Cells and their Ultrastructure*. New York, Berlin: Springer

BESSIS, M. and MAIGNÉ, J. (1970). Le diagnostic des variétés de leucémies aiguës par la réaction des peroxydases au microscope électronique. Son intérêt et ses limites. *Rev. Europ. Et. Clin Biol., 15*, 691

BRUNNING, R. D. and PARKIN, J. (1975). Ribosome-lamella complexes in neoplastic hematopoietic cells. *Am. J. Path., 79*, 565

CLINE, M. J. and GOLDE, D. W. (1973). A review and re-evaluation of the histiocytic disorders. *Am. J. Med., 55*, 49

DAEMS, W. T. (1968). On the fine structure of human neutrophilic leukocyte granules [Letter to the Editor]. *J. Ultrastruct. Res., 24*, 343

DANIEL, M. T. and FLANDRIN, G. (1974). Fine structure of abnormal cells in hairy cell (tricholeukocytic) leukemia with special reference to their *in vitro* phagocytic capacity. *Lab. Invest., 30*, 1

DJALDETTI, M., BESSLER, H., FISHMAN, P. and MACTEY, I. (1975). Functional and ultrastructural studies of Sézary cells. *Nouv. Revue. Fr. Hémat., 15*, 567

DJALDETTI, M., LANDAU, M., MANDEL, E. M., HARZAAV, L. and LEWINSKI, U. (1974). Electron microscopic study of lymphosarcoma cell leukaemia. *Blut, 29*, 210

DUNN, W. B., HARDIN, J. H. and SPICER, S. S. (1968). Ultrastructural localization of myeloperoxidase in human neutrophil and rabbit heterophil and eosinophil leukocytes. *Blood, 32*, 935

GHADIALLY, F. N. (1975). *Ultrastructural Pathology of the Cell*. London: Butterworths

GHADIALLY, F. N., LOWES, N. R. and MESFIN, G. M. (1977). Atypical glycogen deposits in a plasmacytoma: an ultrastructural study. *J. Path., 122*, 157

GHADIALLY, F. N. and SKINNIDER, L. F. (1972). Ultrastructure of hairy cell leukaemia. *Cancer, 29*, 444

GHADIALLY, F. N. and SKINNIDER, L. F. (1976). Vermipodia — a new type of cell process. *Experientia, 32*, 1061

GLICK, A. D. (1976). Acute leukemia: electron microscopic diagnosis. *Seminars in Oncology, 3*, 229

HOSHINO, M. (1969). 'Polysome—lamellae complex' in the adenoma cells of the human adrenal cortex. *J. Ultrastruct. Res., 27*, 205

KATAYAMA, I., LI, C. Y. and YAM, L. T. (1972). Ultrastructural characteristics of the 'hairy cells' of leukemic reticuloendotheliosis. *Am. J. Path., 76*, 361

LAMBERTENGHI-DELILIERS, G., POZZOLI, E., ZANON, P. and MAIOLO, A. T. (1978). Ultrastructural study of myeloperoxidase activity in acute leukaemia cells. *J. Submicrosc. Cytol., 10*, 239

LUTZNER, M. A. and JORDAN, H. W. (1968). The ultrastructure of an abnormal cell in Sézary's syndrome. *Blood, 31*, 719

NABARRA, B., SONSINO, E. and ANDRIANARISON, I. (1977). Ultrastructure of a polysome-lamellae complex in a human paraganglioma. *Am. J. path., 86*, 523

SCHNITZER, B. and KASS, L. (1973). Leukaemic reticulum cell sarcoma. *Cancer,* **31,** 547

SCHNITZER, B. and KASS, L. (1974). Hairy cell leukemia: A clinicopatholgic and ultrastructural study. *Am. J. Clin. Path.,* **61,** 176

SCHUMACHER, H. R., SZEKELY, I. E., PARK, S. A. and FISHER, D. R. (1973). Ultrastructural studies on the acute leukemic lymphoblast. *Blut,* **27,** 396

SCOTT, R. E. and HORN, R. G. (1970). Ultrastructural aspects of neutrophil granulocyte development in humans. *Lab. Invest.,* **23,** 202

SKINNIDER, L. F., CARD, R. T. and PADMANABH, S. (1977). Chronic myelomonocytic leukemia: An ultrastructural study by transmission and scanning electron microscopy. *Am. J. Clin. Path.,* **67,** 339

SKINNIDER, L. F. and GHADIALLY, F. N. (1977). Ultrastructure of cell surface abnormalities in neoplastic histiocytes. *Br. J. Cancer,* **35,** 657

SMETANA, K., GYORKEY, F., GYORKEY, P. and BUSCH, H. (1973). Ultrastructural studies on human myeloma plasmacytes. *Cancer Res.,* **33,** 2300

WETZEL, B. K., HORN, R. G. and SPICER, S. S. (1967). Fine structural studies on the development of heterophil, eosinophil and basophil granulocytes in rabbits. *Lab. Invest.,* **16,** 349

WETZEL, B. K., SPICER, S. S. and HORN, R. G. (1967). Fine structural localization of acid and alkaline phosphatases in cells of rabbit blood and bone marrow. *J. Histochem. Cytochem.,* **15,** 311

WILLIAMS, W. J. (1973). *Haematology.* Toronto: McGraw-Hill

ZUCKER-FRANKLIN, D. (1963). Virus-like particles in the lymphocytes of a patient with chronic lymphocytic leukemia. *Blood,* **21,** 509

14
Is it plasma cell hyperplasia or neoplasia?

Opinion varies as to whether the plasma cells of patients with multiple myeloma are significantly and demonstrably different from normal plasma cells or those found in reactive plasmacytosis (plasma cell hyperplasia) (Brecher *et al.*, 1964; Snapper and Kahn, 1964; Zucker-Franklin, 1964; Maldonado *et al.*, 1966; Fisher and Zawadzki, 1970; Waldenstrom, 1970; Osserman, 1971). There are those who contend that there are no constant morphological alterations of diagnostic import, while others hold that quite specific ultrastructural alterations, which can be correlated with malignancy and clinical condition, are detectable (Graham and Bernier, 1975).

On theoretical grounds alone it is hard to believe that the plasma cell is so unique that its neoplastic form is identical and indistinguishable from normal. One would, for example, expect to find: (1) signs of lack of differentiation in the nucleus, evidenced by loss of the characteristic clock-face pattern (i.e. heterochromatin aggregates abutting the nuclear envelope); and (2) signs of a lack of differentiation in the cytoplasm, such as a diminution and/or aberrations in the morphology of the abundant rough endoplasmic reticulum found normally in this cell type. It will be noted from the above that a study of the distribution and size of heterochromatin aggregates is of some importance. Therefore, it is worth recalling (see Chapter 4 for details) that in tissues fixed in osmium (collidine- or veronal acetate-buffered) and stained with lead, nuclei have a somewhat homogeneous appearance and condensations of heterochromatin with the pattern familiar to light microscopists is either absent or barely discernible (*Figure 161*). However, the characteristic heterochromatin pattern is seen when tissues are either: (1) fixed in osmium (cacodylate buffer) and stained with uranium and lead; or (2) fixed in glutaraldehyde, post fixed in osmium and stained with uranium and lead (*Figure 162*).

It is worth noting that all the earlier major electron microscopic studies on plasma cells and myeloma were carried out on osmium-fixed material and before uranium staining came into common use. Little wonder, then, that the nuclear differences were missed* and a somewhat fictitious controversy as to whether there are ultrastructural differences between normal and neoplastic plasma cells developed in the subsequent literature.

Reactive plasmacytosis (plasma cell hyperplasia)

An increase in the number of plasma cells (*Figures 161* and *162*) in tissues and/or bone marrow occurs in a variety of disorders (e.g. chronic infections, rheumatoid arthritis, cirrhosis of the liver, periarteritis nodosa and a variety of tumours). The salient morphological features of such plasma cells may be summarized as follows: (1) eccentrically placed nucleus with a low nuclear/cytoplasmic ratio; (2) heterochromatin aggregates occurring as fair-sized masses mainly adjacent to the nuclear envelope; (3) nucleoli not too prominent and seen only in a small percentage of cells (because of small size they are not often included in the section); (4) abundant rough endoplasmic reticulum: cisternae may be flattened or slightly dilated, with flocculent, proteinaceous contents; and (5) occasional cells with dilated or vesiculated cisternae of the rough endoplasmic reticulum are found, as also cells with a few or many Russell bodies† (*Figure 163*). Besides cells of the

*Light microscopists knew better, for they could discern the presence or absence of the clock-face pattern in formaldehyde-fixed material.

†These present as rounded electron-dense bodies within dilated or vesiculated cisternae of the rough endoplasmic reticulum. Sometimes the rough endoplasmic reticulum breaks up to form large vacuoles and the proteinaceous secretion (glycoprotein) condenses to form numerous Russell bodies. A cell 'stuffed' with numerous Russell bodies is the equivalent of the 'Mott cell' of the light microscopist.

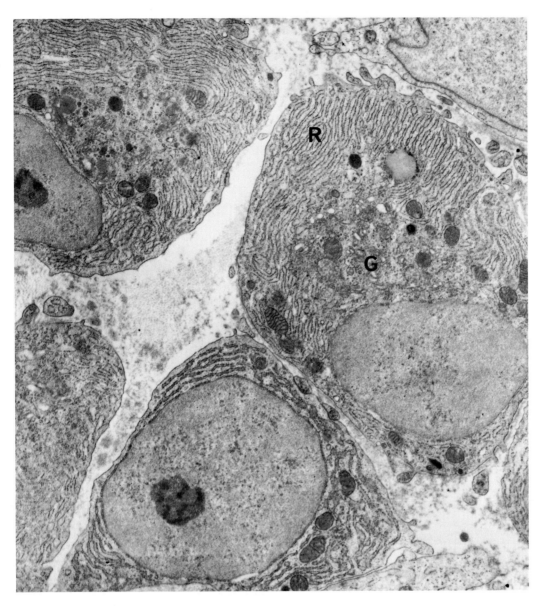

Figure 161 *Plasma cells from rheumatoid synovial membrane. In this material fixed in osmium (phosphate buffer) and stained with lead the nuclei have a bland appearance; the characteristic clock-face arrangement of heterochromatin masses is not demonstrated. Note the abundant arrays of rough endoplasmic reticulum (R) which produces the cytoplasmic basophilia characteristic of this cell type and the well-developed juxtanuclear Golgi complex (G) which presents at light microscopy as a clear crescentic area called the 'hof'.* ×11 500 *(From Ghadially and Roy, 1969)*

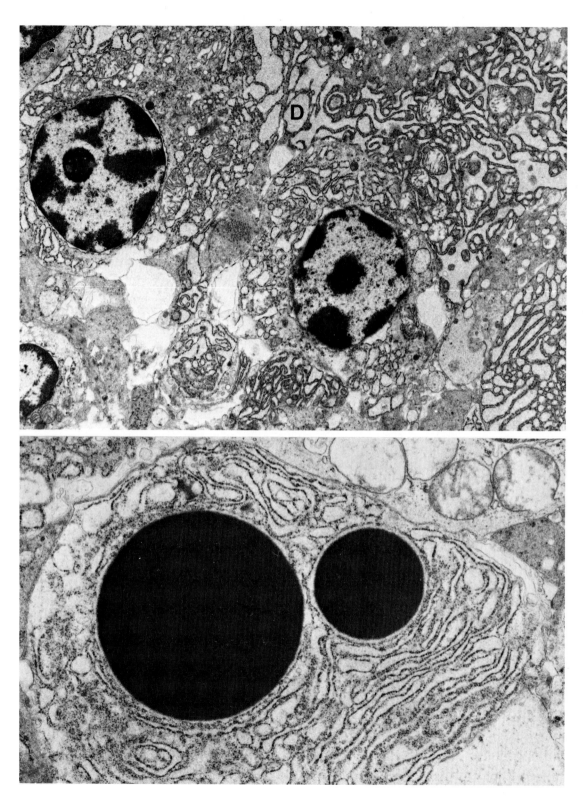

192

morphology described above, a few immature cells of the plasmacytic series may also be found. In these cells the cytoplasm contains scant rough endoplasmic reticulum and chromatin aggregates are smaller and less peripheral in location. The nucleolus is more prominent.

Plasmacytoma

The localized or solitary plasmacytoma may be a harbinger of more widespread malignant disease or it can be benign. The solitary benign plasmacytoma is a rather rare tumour whose ultrastructural features have rarely been documented: only one human case has been studied with the electron microscope (Schweers *et al.*, 1976), and we (Ghadially, Lowes and Mesfin, 1977) have described the appearance of a canine plasmacytoma.

These studies and previous light microscopic studies indicate that in a majority of the cells of the solitary plasmacytoma the characteristic clock-face pattern of heterochromatin aggregates is preserved (i.e. fair-sized chromatin aggregates can be seen adjacent to the nuclear envelope) (*Figure 164*). The nucleolus is round and not too prominent. The rough endoplasmic reticulum is abundant but is often vesiculated. An unusual finding in the canine plasmacytoma we studied was the occurrence of glycogen deposits in the rough endoplasmic reticulum. Numerous intracytoplasmic filaments were also present in some of the tumour cells.

Multiple myeloma

This designation includes neoplasms which may be quite aggressive and fast-growing (*Figure 165*) and others which are indolent and slow-growing (*Figure 166*). In the former instance little or no chromatin aggregation is evident and the nucleus has a homogeneous appearance, while in the latter instance small chromatin aggregates are found dispersed in the nucleus and/or abutting the nuclear envelope. The nucleoli range from moderate-sized to quite large, and at times multiple nucleoli are also seen.*

It seems likely that if most of the cells have a homogeneous nucleus, one is looking at a neoplastic process, for while one can disregard a few as perhaps representing plasmablasts in reactive hyperplasia, one cannot explain away large numbers in this manner.

However, at this point it is useful to correlate the state of development and arrangement of the rough endoplasmic reticulum (i.e. cytoplasmic differentiation) with the degree of nuclear differentiation as evidenced by the state of heterochromatin in the nucleus. In the normal plasma cell series there is synchronous differentiation of these two features. That is to say, as the plasma cell matures, the heterochromatin masses increase in size and move to the periphery of the nucleus; the amount of rough endoplasmic reticulum also increases in step with nuclear

*The size of the nucleolus is not a good indicator of the degree of malignancy or rate of growth in this type of neoplasm. A large nucleolus in this case probably reflects more active secretory protein (immunoglobulin) synthesis.

Figure 162 *A group of plasma cells found in tissue adjacent to a bronchial carcinoma. Note the moderate to marked dilatation (D) of the cisternae of the rough endoplasmic reticulum. The characteristic clock-face pattern of heterochromatin aggregates is well demonstrated in the nuclei. Specimen was fixed in glutaraldehyde followed by osmium; sections were stained with uranium and lead. Compare with Figure 161. See also Figures 3 and 4. ×7000*

Figure 163 *A plasma cell found in tissue adjacent to a bronchial carcinoma. Same case as Figure 162. Two Russell bodies are seen lying in the dilated cisternae of the rough endoplasmic reticulum. The latter point is difficult to appreciate at this low magnification. ×22 000*

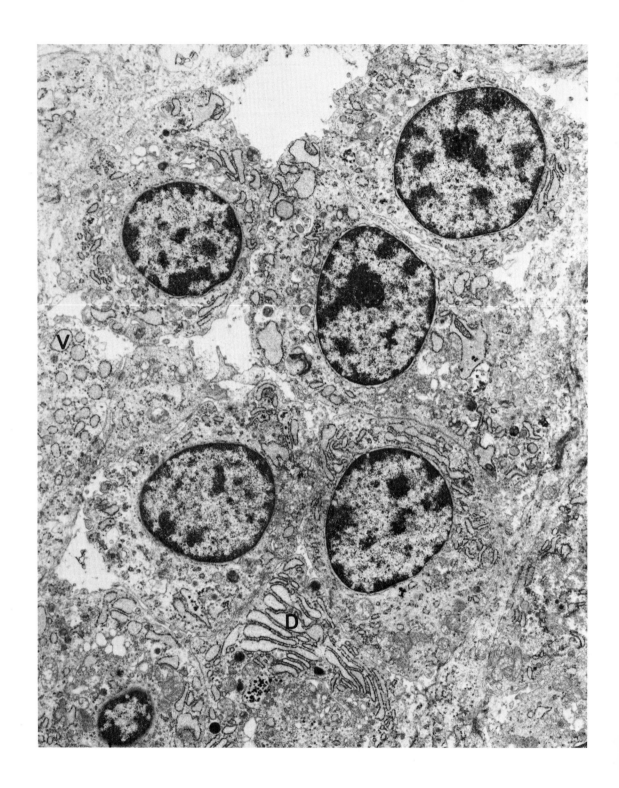

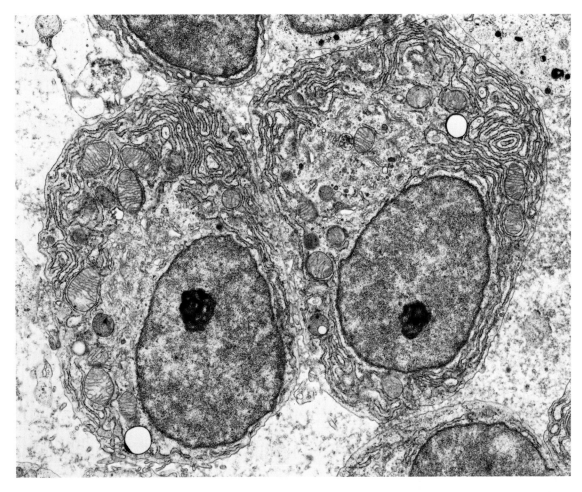

Figure 165 *Plasma cells from a case of multiple myeloma. Fixed in osmium (cacodylate buffer), stained with uranium and lead. Note loss of characteristic cart-wheel pattern in the nucleus. The rough endoplasmic reticulum, although fairly well developed, is not quite as abundant as in normal or reactive plasma cells. The Golgi zone is quite prominent but no more so than that seen in Figure 161. The mitochondria are quite large. ×18 000 (From Ghadially, 1975)*

◀ Figure 164 *Canine plasmacytoma. This surgically excised tumour (2.5 cm in diameter) was sliced and fixed in neutral buffered formalin by a veterinarian. Upon receipt 3 days later small pieces were fixed in osmium (phosphate buffer). Despite this treatment there is fairly good preservation of morphological details. This low-power electron micrograph shows neoplastic plasma cells with dilated (D) and vesiculated (V) rough endoplasmic reticulum. The characteristic clock-face pattern is apparent in most of the nuclei, but the heterochromatin aggregates are perhaps a bit smaller than in normal plasma cells. ×10 000 (From Ghadially, Lowes and Mesfin, 1977)*

195

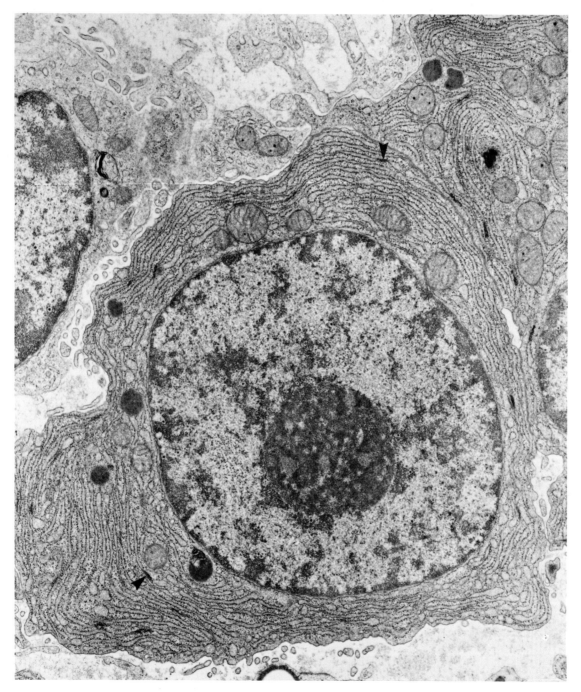

196

differentiation. In the neoplastic state there is asynchrony, for one often finds fairly well-developed rough endoplasmic reticulum in a cell where heterochromatin aggregation is poor or absent (*Figures 165 and 166*).

This idea of nuclear–cytoplasmic asynchrony has been evolved into a grading system by Graham and Bernier (1975). This seems to be quite an impressive technique, for they found asynchrony in 33 of 34 patients with proven myeloma or macroglobulinaemia but in none of the 22 patients with reactive plasmacytosis. In 2 cases response to chemotherapy was associated with reduction in the degree of nuclear–cytoplasmic asynchrony.

Yet another point which helps to distinguish the neoplastic plasma cell from the reactive plasms cell is the mitochondria. In multiple myeloma they are often atypical and enlarged; sometimes to a point where they deserve the appellation 'giant mitochondria'. Quite bizarre-shaped mitochondria are also at times encountered.

In the non-neoplastic plasma cell one also finds quite a degree of mitochondrial pleomorphism but this is never as severe or bizarre as that seen in some myelomas. With increasing anaplasia and malignancy the amount of rough endoplasmic reticulum tends to diminish in amount, but this does not cause confusion, because at this point the malignancy of the process is hardly in doubt.

Acute plasma cell leukaemia

In this condition (*Figures 167* and *168*), which might be regarded as a higher level of malignancy and aggressive behaviour than multiple myeloma, the plasma cells (Klein *et al.*, 1977) show large irregular nuclei often composed of two or three lobes.* The amount of rough endoplasmic reticulum is markedly reduced in amount, and mitochondrial atypia is also quite severe. Intracytoplasmic filaments are also evident.

Some other points of interest

Russell bodies and crystalline inclusions

We noted earlier the occurence of Russel bodies in reactive plasma cells. This probably denotes obstruction and stagnation of secretion in the cisternae of the rough endoplasmic reticulum and subsequent condensation of the secretory product. (For a critique on intracisternal dense granules, including Russell bodies, see Ghadially, 1975). Under such circumstances, on rare occasions, crystalline inclusions may

*Rare binucleate forms may be found in the normal state. Multinucleate and binucleate forms are seen somewhat more frequently in myeloma but are of much more frequent occurence in acute plasma cell leukaemia (Graham and Bernier, 1975; Klein *et al.*, 1977)

Figure 166 *Multiple myeloma. Fixed in glutaraldehyde, post-fixed in osmium and double-stained with uranium and lead. Clinically this was not a very aggressive condition. Immunfluorescence studies lead to the conclusion that this is a 'non-producer'; nevertheless, the rough endoplasmic reticulum is remarkably well developed and the nucleolus is prominent. The nucleus is not quite as 'homogeneous-looking' as that found in highly aggressive versions of multiple myeloma, but, on the other hand, the chromatin aggregates are not as large as those seen in normal and reactive plasma cells. At higher magnifications the linear densities (arrowheads) seen along the rough endoplasmic reticulum turn out to be elongated myelin figures. This is perhaps largely but not entirely a glutaraldehyde artefact. (A. Senoo, unpublished electron micrograph)*

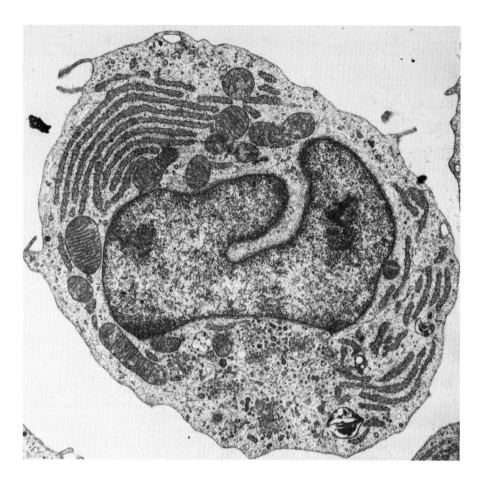

Figure 167 *Plasma cell leukaemia. Leukaemic cell from peripheral blood. The irregularly shaped nucleus with two nucleoli and little attempt at heterochromatin aggregation bears little resemblance to the normal nucleus of the plasma cell. The stacks of rough endoplasmic reticulum and the hof, however, are reminiscent of plasma cells. Note also the pleomorphic enlarged mitochondria. ×13 000 (From Klein et al., 1977)*

also form within the cisternae. Neither of these phenomena (Russell bodies and crystalline inclusions) is of much diagnostic value, for such features are seen in myeloma and also in reactive plasma cells. According to Sanel and Lepore (1968), such crystals in plasma cells '. . .have been invariably associated with dysproteinemia (i.e. cryoglobulinemia, macroglobulinemia of Waldenstrom's disease, or the hyperglobulinemia of multiple myeloma, plasmacytoma or hyperimmune states).'

Immunoglobulin production

There is general agreement that there is no discernible relationship between the type and the amount of immunoglobulin(s) or fragments thereof (e.g. Bence-

Jones protein) produced and the morphology of the rough endoplasmic reticulum (Brecher *et al.*, 1964; Zucker-Franklin, 1964). Mancilla and Davis (1977) studied two cases of non-secretory multiple myeloma and found that in one case no immunoglobulin could be detected in the cells by immunohistological methods, even though the cells contained a modest amount of rough endoplasmic reticulum. In the other case the cells contained intracytoplasmic immunoglobulins and there was abundant rough endoplasmic reticulum. The former, they suggest, might be called a 'non-producer' rather than a 'non-secretor' of immunoglobin(s).

The lack of correlation between the amount of rough endoplasmic reticulum and the production of immunoglobulins is also evidence by the case (Senoo,

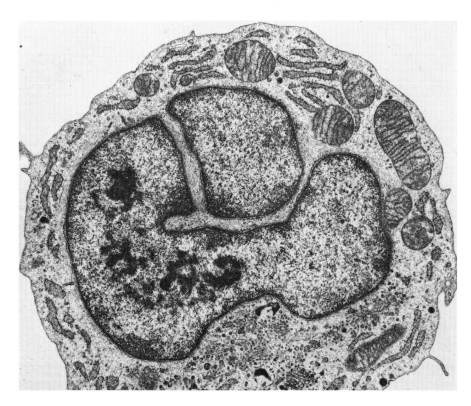

Figure 168 *Plasma cell leukaemia. Leukaemic cell from peripheral blood, showing a lobulated nucleus, scant rough endoplasmic reticulum, enlarged mitochondria and intracytoplasmic filaments, (mainly in the juxtanuclear position), but they are difficult to discern at this low magnification. ×13 000 (From Klein et al., 1977)*

personal communication) shown in *Figure 166*. It seems likely that non-producers produce some other proteins or altered immunoglobulins, so different that they do not react with the antisera employed.

An interesting observation made by Graham and Bernier (1975) in a non-secretor (plasma cell contained λ chains) was that the Golgi complex appeared defective. Such an anomaly would offer a satisfying explanation of the lack of ability to secret the product synthesized by the cell, but then one expects the cisternae of the rough endoplasmic reticulum to be dilated and vesiculated. A closer look at the Golgi complex of more non-secretors is necessary before arriving at such a conclusion.

At the moment, on ultrastructural grounds alone, one cannot distinguish between non-producers, non-secretors and secretors or guess whether light or heavy chains are being produced, but one can go a long way towards deciding whether one is looking at a neoplastic or non-neoplastic proliferation of plasma cells.

References

BRECHER, G., TANAKA, Y., MALMGREM, R. A. and FAHEY, J. L. (1964). Morphology and protein synthesis in multiple myeloma and macroglobulinemia. *Ann. N. Y. Acad. Sci.*, 113, 642

FISHER, E. R. and ZAWADZKI, Z. (1970). Ultrastructural features of plasma cells in patients with paraproteinemias. *Am. J. Clin. Path.*, 54, 779

GHADIALLY, F. N. (1975). *Ultrastructural Pathology of the Cell.* London: Butterworths

GHADIALLY, F. N., LOWES, N. R. and MESFIN, G. M. (1977). Atypical glycogen deposits in a plasmacytoma: An ultrastructural study. *J. Path.*, 122, 157

GRAHAM, R. C. and BERNIER, G. M. (1975). The bone marrow in multiple myeloma: correlation of plasma cell ultrastructure and clinical state. *Medicine,* **54,** 225

KLEIN, B., LEWINSKI, U., SHABTAI, S., FREIDIN, N. and DJALDETTI, M. (1977). Transmission and scanning electron microscopy study on plasma cell leukemia. *Blut,* **35,** 11

MALDONADO, J. E., BROWN, A. L., BAYRD, E. D. and PEASE, G. L. (1966). Ultrastructure of the myeloma cell. *Cancer,* **19,** 1613

MANCILLA, R. and DAVIS, G. L. (1977). Nonsecretory multiple myeloma. *Am. J. Med.,* **63,** 1015

OSSERMAN, E. F. (1971). Plasma cell dyscrasias. In: *Cecil-Loeb Textbook of Medicine,* 13th edn, ed. P. B. Beeson and W. McDermott., p. 1575. Philadelphia: Saunders

SANEL, F. T. and LEPORE, M. J. (1968). Granular and crystalline deposits in perinuclear and ergastroplasmic **cisternae of human lamina, propria cells.** *Expl Molec. Path.,* **9,** 110

SCHWEERS, C. A., SHAW, M. T., NORDQUIST, R. E., ROSE, D. D. and KELL, T. (1976). Solitary cecal plasmacytoma. *Cancer,* **37,** 2220

SNAPPER, I. and KAHN, A. I. (1964). Multiple myeloma. *Semin. Hematol.,* **1,** 87

WALDENSTROM, J. (1970). *Diagnosis and Treatment of Multiple Myeloma.* New York: Grune and Stratton

ZUCKER-FRANKLIN, D. (1964). Structural features of cells associated with the paraproteinemias. *Semin. Hematol.,* **1,** 165

15
Distinguishing erythroleukaemia from other disorders of the erythropoietic system

Glycogen is a normal cytoplasmic inclusion found in many cell types, but no glycogen is discernible in routine electron microscopic preparations* of cells of the erythropoietic series from normal humans (Gibb and Stowell, 1949; Wislocki, Rheingold and Dempsey, 1949; Wintrobe, 1967). A point of some diagnostic importance is that quite substantial deposits of glycogen are readily found in erythroblasts (normoblasts), reticulocytes and erythrocytes in cases of erythroleukaemia (*Figures 169* and *170*).

However, only the clone of neoplastic erythropoietic cells contains glycogen, for side by side quite normal glycogen-free erythrocytes and their precursors are also seen. The occurrence of this phenomenon was reported by Skinnider and Ghadially in 1973. Since then we have found this to be true in four other cases of erythroleukaemia, but we have not found erythrocytes containing glycogen in the bone marrow and/or peripheral blood specimens from over 500 patients with various other haematological disorders.

Only time will tell whether the occurrence of glycogen in the erythropoietic cells is unique to erythroleukaemia, but at least it does seem to be a sufficiently rare finding to be of some diagnostic value.

The results of past light microscopic studies do not help much but they are interesting, because they point to other possible situations where glycogen may occur in erythroid cells. PAS-positive material was first noted in erythroblasts from cases of thalassaemia major, but these inclusions were resistant to diastase digestion; hence, they were considered to be composed of mucoprotein or neutral polysaccharides rather than glycogen (Astaldi *et al.*, 1954). Since then various workers (Baldini *et al.*, 1959; Hayhoe

and Quaglino, 1960; Quaglino and Hayhoe, 1960) have found a PAS-positive reaction in erythroid cells in cases of erythraemic myelosis, erythroleukaemia and refractory sideroblastic anaemia but others have failed to do so (Astaldi *et al.*, 1954), and much uncertainty regarding the nature of the PAS-positive material has also been expressed (Baldini *et al.*, 1959).

We have not studied a case of thalassaemia major, so we are unable to comment on the situation in this condition, but we have studied twelve cases of sideroblastic anaemia and in none of these did we find glycogen.

References

ACKERMAN, G. A. (1973). Ultrastructural localization of glycogen in erythrocytes and developing erythrocyte cells in normal human bone marrow. *Z. Zellforsch. Mikrosk. Anat.*, **140**, 433

ASTALDI, G., RONDANELLI, E. G., BERNARDELLI, E. and STROSSELLI, E. (1954). An abnormal substance present in the erythroblasts of thalassaemia major: cytochemical investigations. *Acta Haematol.*, **12**, 145

BALDINI, M., FUDENBERG, H. H., FUKUTAKE, K. and DAMESHEK, W. (1959). The anaemia of the Di Guglielmo syndrome. *Blood*, **14**, 334

GIBB, R. P. and STOWELL, R. E. (1949). Glycogen in human blood cells. *Blood*, **4**, 569

HAYHOE, F. G. and QUAGLINO, D. (1960). Refractory sideroblastic anemia and erythemic myelosis: Possible relationship and cytochemical observations. *Br. J. Haematol.*, **6**, 381

QUAGLINO, D. and HAYHOE, F. G. J. (1960). Periodic acid-Schiff positivity in erythroblasts with special reference to Di Guglielmo's disease. *Br. J. Haematol.*, **6**, 26

SKINNIDER, L. F. and GHADIALLY, F. N. (1973). Glycogen in erythroid cells. *Archs Path.*, **95**, 139

WINTROBE, M. M. (1967). *Clinical Haematology*. 6th edn, p. 106. Philadelphia: Lea and Febiger

WISLOCKI, G. B., RHEINGOLD, J. J. and DEMPSEY, E. W. (1949). The occurrence of the periodic acid-Schiff reaction in various normal cells of blood and connective tissue. *Blood*, **4**, 562

*However, a few particles of glycogen (monoparticulate glycogen or beta glycogen) are demonstrable in normal erythroid cells by the periodic acid—thiosemicarbazide—silver proteinate reaction (Ackerman, 1973).

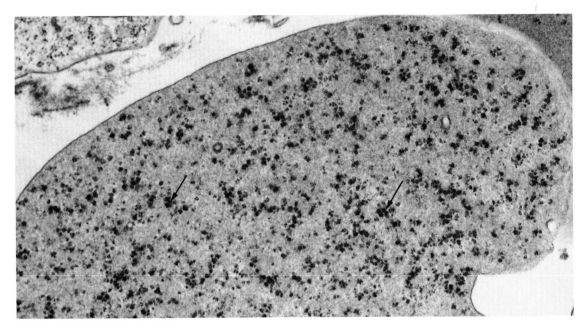

Figure 169   *Erythroleukaemia. Mature erythrocyte with monoparticulate glycogen (arrows) in its cytoplasm. ×36 000 (From Ghadially, 1975)*

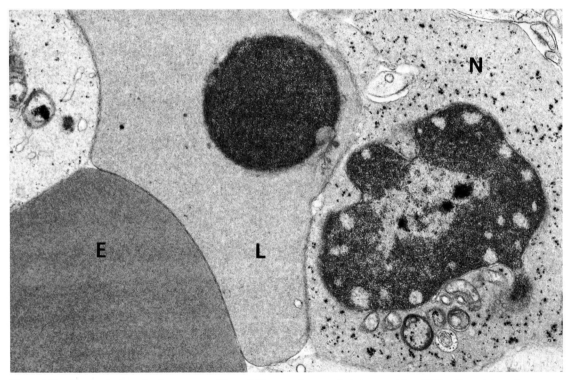

Figure 170   *Erythroleukaemia. Same case as Figure 169. This illustration demonstrates the occurrence of a dual population of erythroid cells in erythroleukaemia. A glycogen-laden normoblast (N) is adjacent to a glycogen-free late normoblast (L) and erythrocyte (E) of normal morphology. ×19 000 (From Skinnider and Ghadially, 1973)*

Part 4

Ultrastructural features of some tumours

16
Tumours of steroid-secreting cells

Steroid-secreting cells occur in the testis, ovary and adrenals. They are characterized by: (1) mitochondria with tubular and/or vesicular cristae; (2) an abundance of smooth endoplasmic reticulum; and (3) a few to many lipid droplets. Collectively these features distinguish the steroid-secreting cells and their tumours from various others where, as a rule, we have mitochondria with lamellar cristae and generally little smooth endoplasmic reticulum.*

These differences are of diagnostic import. For example, Gyorkey *et al.* (1975) report the case of a 54-year-old man with a metastatic growth in the liver which was diagnosed as a carcinoma of steroid-secreting cells on the basis of ultrastructural morphology. At surgical exploration the primary growth was found in the right adrenal.

In the text that follows, verbal descriptions of the steroid-secreting cells and tumours of the testis, ovary and adrenal are presented, but only the adrenocortical adenomas are illustrated, for this is adequate to demonstrate the diagnostic features by which one distinguishes tumours of the steroid-secreting cells from other neoplasms. On the basis of ultrastructural morphology alone, it is usually not possible to distinguish different types of steroid-secreting tumours from one another, but there are some small differences which one should be aware of.

However, before we do this a brief note on how to recognize various types of mitochondrial cristae is essential. It is not always easy to decide whether the cristae in a given mitochondrion are lamellar or tubular. Lamellae cut longitudinally or transversely present an appearance similar to a tubule cut longi-

tudinally. Generally, the gap between the membranes of lamellar cristae is quite narrow and slitlike, while that in the tubular cristae is somewhat wider. However, even when one sees this wider gap, one wonders whether this is 'genuine' or due to a slight influx of water (a phenomenon referred to as intracristal swelling; see Chapter 4). Thus, it is only when one sees some circular profiles (besides the ones described above) acceptable as transverse sections through tubules that one can entertain the idea that tubular cristae are present. Needless to say, vesicles cut in any plane produce circular profiles. Therefore, if only such profiles are present, then one might surmize that vesicular cristae are present; generally, such cristae are seen budding off the inner membrane of the mitochondrion. Such difficulties have led some authors to use the term 'tubulovesicular cristae', which seems an acceptable solution to this dilemma.

Testis

The Leydig cells of the testis produce androgenic steroids, principally testosterone. They are well endowed with smooth endoplasmic reticulum, a few lipid droplets (there are marked species variations in this feature) and mitochondria with tubular, and a few lamellar, cristae. The Sertoli cell also has well-developed smooth endoplasmic reticulum at the cell base, but whether it secretes steroid hormones or not is not known. Reports on Leydig cell tumours show that they contain abundant smooth endoplasmic reticulum at times forming whorls, oval mitochondria with tubular cristae, lipid droplets and Reinke crystals (Cervos–Navarro, Tonutti and Bayer, 1964; Beals, Pierce and Schroeder, 1965; Murakami, Gohara and Yoshida, 1967; Kay *et al.*, 1975). There appears to be only one report on the ultrastructure of a Sertoli cell tumour; here, too, the cells were well endowed with smooth endoplasmic reticulum (Able and Lee, 1969).

*Cell types which have abundant rough endoplasmic reticulum usually have little smooth endoplasmic reticulum, and vice versa (Fawcett, 1967). An exception to this is the hepatocyte, where both forms of endoplasmic reticulum are fairly well represented and continuities between the two can be demonstrated. It is interesting to note that an occasional tubular crista is seen among the lamellar cristae in hepatocyte mitochondria.

Ovary

The lutein cells differentiate from the granulosa cells and theca interna cells. The latter two have a fair amount of rough endoplasmic reticulum but little or no smooth endoplasmic reticulum. The mitochondria are elongated and have lamellar cristae, but occasional tubular cristae may be found, particularly in the theca interna cells. Lipid droplets are scant. It is the lutein cell which is actively engaged in progesterone production. This cell has abundant smooth endoplasmic reticulum, a small amount of rough endoplasmic reticulum and numerous lipid droplets. The mitochondria vary from small and spherical to elongated. They have vesicular and tubular cristae. On reviewing the papers on this topic (Björkman, 1962; MacAulay, Weliky and Schulz, 1967; Gondos, 1969; Gondos and Monroe, 1971; Bjersing, Frankendal and Angström, 1973; Garcia-Bunuel and Brandes, 1976), it is clear that luteomas usually show the expected characteristics of steroid-secreting cells.

Adrenals

The adrenal cortex is composed of: (1) The zona glomerulosa (secretes the mineralocorticoids deoxycorticosterone and aldosterone), where the cells contain a few short cisternae or vesicles of rough endoplasmic reticulum, extensive well-developed smooth endoplasmic reticulum in the form of a network of branching and anastamosing tubules and lipid droplets, which may be large and spherical or crenated. The mitochondria are elongated (sometimes called 'sarcotubular' type of mitochondria) and have lamellar cristae. (2) The zona fasciculata (secretes the glucocorticoids, cortisone and cortisol or corticosterone). The rough endoplasmic reticulum is more prominent here than in the zona glomerulosa. It often occurs as stacks of cisternae. The smooth endoplasmic reticulum is also abundant, and lipid droplets are present. The mitochondria are round or oval, and contain tubular and vesicular cristae; this is in sharp contrast to the long mitochondria with lamellar cristae found in the zona glomerulosa. (3) The zona reticularis shows features similar to that found in the zona fasciculata, except that the mitochondria are more elongated and contain vesicular and lamellar cristae. This zone is characterized by the presence of numerous quite large lipofuscin granules.

The significance and function of lipid droplets in the adrenal cortical cells has long been debated, as also has the role of the smooth endoplasmic reticulum and mitchondria.

Cell fractionation studies show that cholesterol from the blood or synthesized in the adrenal gland from acetate (there are species differences here) is stored in the lipid droplets. The first step in steroidogenesis occurs in the mitochondria (cholesterol to pregnonolone). The enzyme necessary for the conversion of pregnenolone to progesterone and the enzymes which convert progesterone to 17-hydroxyprogesterone or 11-deoxycorticosterone and 17-hydroxyprogesterone to 11-deoxycortisol occur in the smooth endoplasmic reticulum. The final steps of conversion of 11-deoxycorticosterone to costicosterone and 11-deoxycortisol to cortisol occurs in the mitochondria. This, then, is the biochemical 'reason' for the abundant smooth endoplasmic reticulum and the mitochondria with a different morphology found in the steroid-secreting cells.

Electron microscopy can offer little assistance in distinguishing adrenal cortical hyperplasia (diffuse or nodular) from adenoma or carcinoma, if this has proved difficult to establish by gross or light microscopic appearances. The only features that are of any value at the ultrastructural level are nucleolar enlargement and an abundance of polyribosomes lying free in the cytoplasm, for this is the sign of a fast-growing lesion and, hence, in the proper context this would favour the idea that the lesion was malignant.

As a rule, it is not possible to state with any degree of confidence what hormone(s) the tumour is producing and the clinical syndrome present on the basis of ultrastructural features alone. Even so, there are some morphological differences worthy of thought and study.

The hyperplastic and neoplastic lesions of the adrenal cortex comprise a group which might be: (1) non-functioning and produce no hormonal disturbances, or they may produce: (2) Conn's syndrome (secretory product, aldosterone); (3) Cushing's syndrome (secretory product, glucocorticoids); (4) adrenogenital syndrome or adrenal virilization (secretory product, dehydroepiandrosterone or testosterone); and (5) adrenal feminization (secretory product, oestrogens).

Black adenoma and non-functioning adenoma

The black adenoma (also nodular hyperplasia associated with gross blackening of the adrenal) is distinguished by an abundance of lipofuscin granules.* It is not as rare as once imagined and it is almost invariably non-functioning and symptomless. (Usually it is an incidental finding at autopsy.) However, on very rare occasions, it has produced Cushing's syndrome (MacKay, 1969; Bahu, Battifora and Shambaugh, 1974). A fair amount of lipofuscin pigment was present in a virilizing tumour described by Fisher and Danowski (1973); this tumour is referred to in the literature as an example of black adenoma despite the fact that Fisher and Danowski state that it was golden yellow in colour. Prominent lipofuscin granules have been seen in quite a few other reports of virilizing tumours (for references see Aiba *et al.*, 1978), and some have been reddish-brown in colour. Since prominent lipofuscin granules are a feature of the zona reticularis, the black adenoma is thought to be derived from this region of the adrenal cortex.

The black adenoma is not the only variety of non-functioning adrenocortical adenoma. Tannenbaum (1973) describes a few where the ultrastructural morphology was not that of steroid-secreting cells. Neither smooth endoplasmic reticulum nor lipid droplets were prominent and the mitochondria had lamellar cristae like mitochondria in other organs and tumours.

Conn's syndrome

Lipid droplets in varying amounts are seen in many adrenal tumours; they can be electron-lucent or electron-dense. The droplets can be rounded or crenated in outline. Varying degrees of extraction during tissue processing produce different morphological patterns (see, for example, illustrations in Tannenbaum, 1973). This, of course, is not unique for the adrenals; this phenomenon is seen in many different sites (for illustrations of this see Ghadially, 1975). Looking at the illustrations in the literature and *Figures 171–174*, one gets the impression that by and large the aldosterone-producing lesions of the adrenal (usually hyperplasia of the zona glomerulosa or adenoma containing cells resembling those found in the zona glomerulosa and fasciculata) are better endowed with lipid droplets than other varieties of adrenocortical hyperplasia or neoplasia, but, of course, this is not invariably so (Cervos-Navarro *et al.*, 1965; Propst, 1965; Reidbord and Fisher, 1969; Tannenbaum, 1973; Kovacs *et al.*,

1974; Gorgas, Böck and Wuketich, 1976; Kay, 1976). Both smooth and rough endoplasmic reticulum are present in varying amounts (as in the zona glomerulosa). Most of the mitochondria are quite long and have lamellar cristae, although one can find a few round or oval mitochondria with tubular cristae (as in the zona fasciculata). Lipid droplets may be found in some of the mitochondria.

It should be noted that this is not specific for an aldosteronoma or even adrenocortical tumours, for such droplets have been seen in the normal adrenal cortex (see, for example, Ghadially, 1975) and can, in fact, be found in the steroid-secreting cells of the testis and ovary also.

Cushing's syndrome

The ultrastructural features (*Figure 175*) seen in the hyperplastic (diffuse or nodular) or neoplastic (adenoma or carcinoma) adrenal cortex in Cushing's syndrome are well documented (Reidbord and Fisher, 1968; MacKay, 1969; Macadam, 1970; Mitschke, Saeger and Breustedt, 1973; Tannenbaum, 1973; Bahu, Battifora and Shambaugh, 1974; Mitschke and Saeger, 1975; Kay, 1976; Kano and Sato, 1977). In such instances we find that the cells are singularly well endowed with smooth endoplasmic reticulum, and some of the best examples of mitochondria with tubular cristae are also seen in this condition (Cushing's syndrome). Such mitochondria are usually round or oval, but a few elongated mitochondria with lamellar cristae are also often present. Indeed, the mitochondria are quite pleomorphic, and some excellent examples of giant mitochondria with various configurations of cristae are also seen in this condition.

The prominent smooth endoplasmic reticulum may sometimes present as a ramifying network of tubules or tubules arranged in stacks and whorls. However, often it is vesiculated (*Figure 175*), so that one finds innumerable smooth-walled vesicles and quite large vacuoles in the cell. Whether this is a genuine *in vivo* difference or an artefact is difficult to say, for the smooth endoplasmic reticulum is known to be a delicate structure difficult to preserve* and the tubular system readily suffers vesiculation if subject to anoxia or delayed or improper fixation. A moderate number of lipid droplets, usually quite electron-dense, is a common feature. A few lipofuscin

*Lipofuscin, the 'wear and tear' pigment represents the end product of lysosomal activity. Lipofuscin granules are, hence, classified as residual bodies.

*This varies from cell type to cell type. For example, the smooth endoplasmic reticulum in the hepatocyte is more 'robust' than that in the adrenal cortical cells.

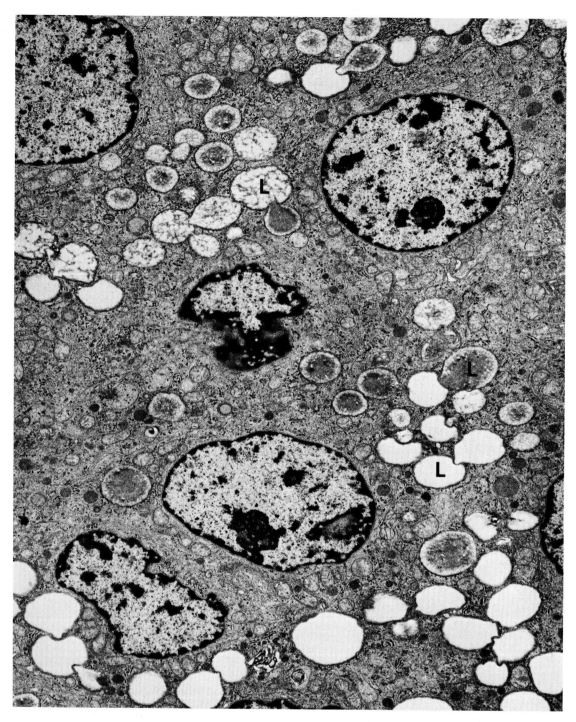

Figure 171   *Adrenal cortical adenoma from a case of*
Conn's syndrome. Note the numerous lipid droplets (L),
showing various degrees of extraction. ×8000 *(From a*
block of tissue supplied by Dr T. K. Shnitka)

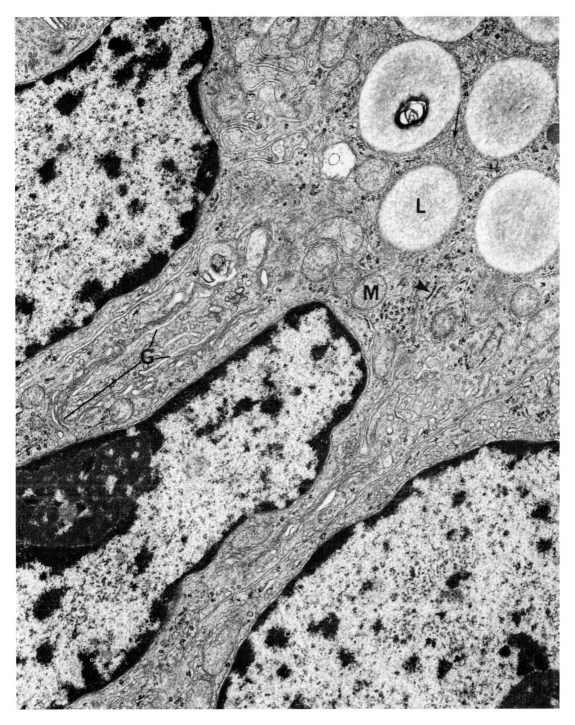

Figure 172 *Conn's syndrome. Same tissue as in Figure 171. The cells contain lipid droplets (L), rough endoplasmic reticulum (arrowhead), smooth endoplasmic reticulum (arrow), which is difficult to discern at this magnification, mitochondria (M) and a well-developed Golgi complex (G). ×21 000 (From a block of tissue supplied by Dr T. K. Schnitka)*

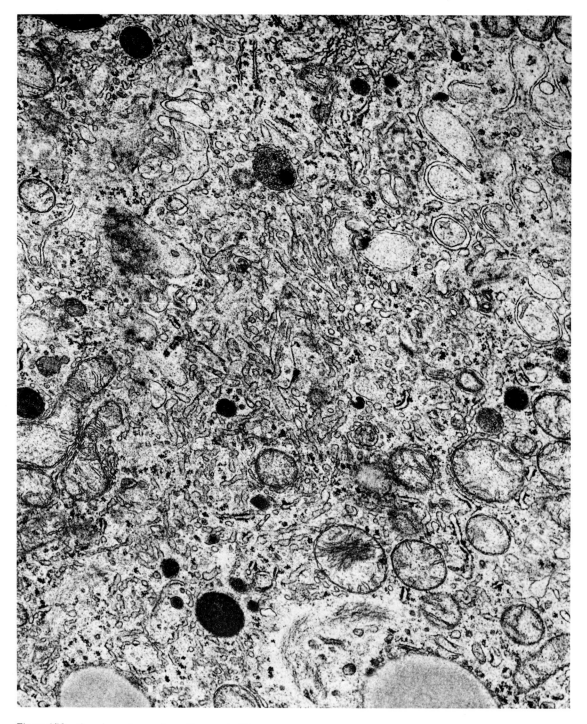

Figure 173   *Conn's syndrome. Same tissue as in Figures 171 and 172. Note the abundant smooth endoplasmic reticulum in this cell. ×25 000 (From a block of tissue supplied by Dr T. K. Shnitka)*

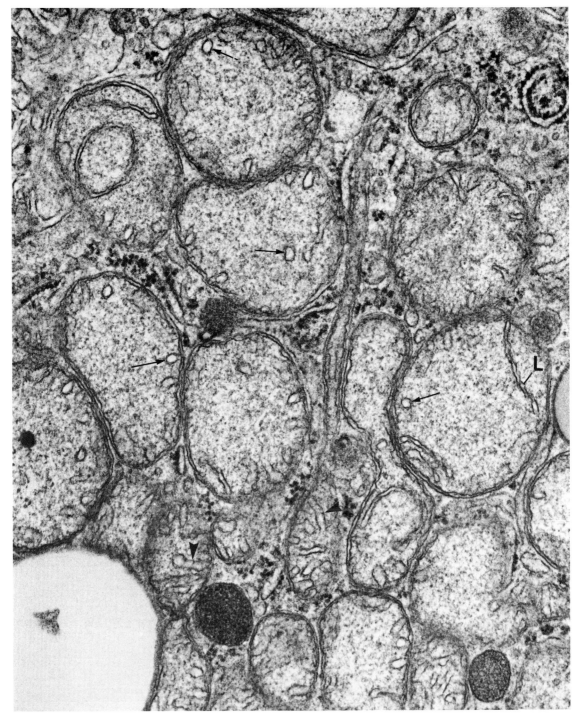

Figure 174 *Conn's syndrome. Same tissue as in Figures 171–173. A variety of cristal profiles are seen in the mitochondria. First we have cristae which present as quite long segments of paired membranes with a narrow interval between them; these are acceptable as lamellar cristae (L). Next we see short lengths of paired membranes with a wider gap between them; these are acceptable as longitudinal sections through tubular cristae (arrowheads). Finally we see numerous circular profiles (arrows) which represent transverse sections through tubular cristae or sections through vesicular cristae. ×59 000 (From a block of tissue supplied by Dr T. K. Schnitka)*

211

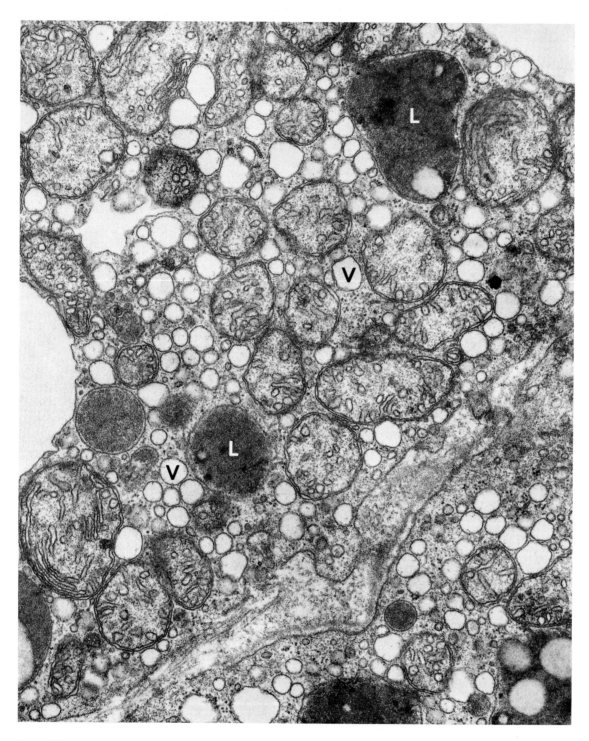

Figure 175   *Cushing's syndrome. Nodular hyperplasia of the adrenal cortex. Note mitochondria with tubulovesicular cristae, vesiculated smooth endoplasmic reticulum (V) and lysosomes or lipofuscin granules (L). ×32 000 (Ghadially and Larsen, unpublished electron micrograph)*

granules are also present. On the basis of the above-mentioned morphological features, it is thought that the adrenocortical hyperplasia or neoplasia producing Cushing's syndrome stems from the zona fasiculata and zona reticularis.

Virilization and adrenogenital syndrome

This syndrome is usually produced by a hyperplasia or adenoma; ultrastructurally the tissue resembles that in the zona reticularis (Fisher and Danowski, 1973; Tannenbaum, 1973; Akhtar, Gosalbez and Young, 1974; Aiba *et al.*, 1978; Huhtaniemi *et al.*, 1978). However, cases of virilizing adrenocortical carcinoma has also been recorded (Yokoyama, 1975; Valente *et al.*, 1978). These lesions are well endowed with smooth endoplasmic reticulum and some rough endoplasmic reticulum is also present. The mitochondria vary from rounded to moderately elongated, and contain tubular and vesicular cristae.

Feminizing adrenocortical tumour

Only one ultrastructural study of this type of adreno-cortical tumour seems to have been published (Mitschke, Saeger and Breustedt, 1978). The status of this particular tumour (benign or malignant) is not clear, but as a rule feminization is caused by an adrenocortical carcinoma rather than an adenoma. The illustrations presented in their paper (Mitschke, Saeger and Breustedt, 1978) show an unusually large number of mitochondria, some vesiculated smooth endoplasmic reticulum and a few lipid droplets. The authors state that most of the mitochondria had lamellar cristae but occasional tubular cristae were also seen. Some cells were well endowed with smooth endoplasmic reticulum and also contained some rough endoplasmic reticulum. Lysosomes and lipofuscin granules were rare and the basal lamina appeared intact.

References

ABLE, M. E. and LEE, J. C. (1969). Ultrastructure of a Sertoli-cell adenoma of the testis. *Cancer*, 23, 481

AIBA, M., KAMEYA, T., SUZUKI, H., NAKAMURA, H., MIZUNO, Y. and KANNO, T. (1978). Enzyme histochemical and electron microscopic study of a virilizing adrenocortical adenoma. *Acta Path. Jap.*, 28, 615

AKHTAR, M., GOSALBEZ, T. and YOUNG, I. (1974). Ultrastructural study of adrenogen-producing adrenocortical adenoma. *Cancer*, 34, 322

BAHU, R. M., BATTIFORA, H. and SHAMBAUGH, G. (1974). Functional black adenoma of the adrenal gland. *Archs Path.*, 98, 139

BEALS, T. F., PIERCE, G. B., Jr. and SCHROEDER, C. F. (1965). The ultrastructure of human testicular tumors. I. Interstitial cell tumours. *J. Urol.*, 93, 64

BJERSING, L., FRANKENDAL, B. and ANGSTRÖM, T. (1973). Studies on feminizing ovarian mesenchymoma (granulosa cell tumor). I. Aspiration biopsy cytology, histology and ultrastructure. *Cancer*, 32, 1360

BJÖRKMAN, N. (1962). A study of the ultrastructure of the granulosa cells of the rat ovary. *Acta Anat.*, 51, 115

CERVÓS-NAVARRO, J., TONUTTI, E. and BAYER, J. M. (1964). Electronenmikroskopische Untersuchung einen androgenbildenden Leydigzelltumors. *Endokrinologie*, 47, 23

CERVÓS-NAVARRO, J., TONUTTI, E., GARCIA-ALVAREZ, F., BAYER, J. M. and FRITZ, H. W. (1965). Electronen-mikroskopische Befunde an zwei Connschen Adenomen der Nebennierenrinde. *Endokrinologie*, 49, 35

FAWCETT, D. W. (1967). *An Atlas of Fine Structure: The Cell, its Organelles and Inclusions.* Philadelphia: Saunders

FISHER, E. R. and DANOWSKI, T. S. (1973). Ultrastructural study of virilizing adrenocortical adenoma. *Am. J. Clin. Path.*, 59, 480

GARCIA-BUNUEL, R. and BRANDES, D. (1976). Luteoma of pregnancy: Ultrastructural features. *Hum. Path.*, 7, 205

GHADIALLY, F. N. (1975). *Ultrastructural Pathology of the Cell.* London: Butterworths

GONDOS, B. (1969). Ultrastructure of a metastatic granulosa-theca cell tumor. *Cancer*, 24, 954

GONDOS, B. and MONROE, S. A. (1971). Cystic granulosa cell tumor with massive hemoperitoneum. Light and electron microscopic study. *Obstet. Gynec.*, 38, 683

GORGAS' K., BÖCK, P. and WUKETICH, S. (1976). Fine structure of a virilizing adrenocortical adenoma. *Beitr. Path.*, 159, 371

GYORKEY, F., MIN, K.-W., KRISKO, I. and GYORKEY, P. (1975). The usefulness of electron microscopy in the diagnosis of human tumours. *Hum. Path.*, 6, 421

HUHTANIEMI, I., KAHRI, A. I., PELKONEN, R., SALMENPERA, M., SIVULA, A. and VIHKO, R. (1978). Ultrastructural and steroidogenic characteristics of an androgen-producing adrenocortical tumour. *Clin. Endocr.*, 8, 305

KANO, K. and SATO, S. (1977). Fine structure of adrenal adenomata causing Cushing's syndrome. *Virchows Arch. Path. Anat. Histol.*, 374, 157

KAY, S. (1976). Hyperplasia and neoplasia of the adrenal gland. *Path. Ann.*, 11, 103

KAY, S., FU, Y-S., KOONTZ, W. W. and CHEN, A. T. L. (1975). Interstitial-cell tumor of the testis: Tissue culture and ultrastructural studies. *Am. J. Clin. Path.*, 63, 366

KOVACS, K., HORVATH, E., DELARUE, N. C. and LAIDLAW, J. C. (1974). Ultrastructural features of an aldosterone-secreting adrenocortical adenoma. *Hormone Res.*, 5, 47

MACADAM, R. F. (1970). Fine structure of a functional adrenal cortical adenoma. *Cancer,* **26,** 1300

MACAULAY, M. A., WELIKY, I. and SCHULZ, R. A. (1967). Ultrastructure of a biosynthetically active granulosa cell tumor. *Lab. Invest.,* **17,** 562

MACKAY, A. (1969). Atlas of human adrenal cortex ultrastructures. In: *Functional Pathology of the Human Adrenal Gland,* ed. T. Symington, pp. 347–489. Baltimore: Williams and Wilkins

MITSCHKE, H. and SAEGER, W. (1975). Ultrastructural pathology of the adrenal glands in Cushing's syndrome. *Curr. Topics Path.,* **60,** 113

MITSCHKE, H., SAEGER, W. and BREUSTEDT, H.-J. (1973). Ultrastruktur der Nebennierenrindentumoren beim Cushing-Syndrom. *Virchows Arch. Path. Anat. Histol.,* **360,** 253

MITSCHKE, H., SAEGER, W. and BREUSTEDT, H.-J. (1978). Feminizing adrenocortical tumor. *Virchows Arch. Path. Anat. Histol.,* **377,** 301

MURAKAMI, M., GOHARA, S. and YOSHIDA, Y. (1967). Electronenmikrokopische beobachtung bei einem Leydigzelltumor eines Erwachenen. *Endokrinologie,* **52,** 335

PROPST, A. (1965). Elektronenmikroskopie der Nebennierenrinde beim primären Hyperaldosteronismus. *Beitr. Path.,* **131,** 1

REIDBORD, H. and FISHER, E. R. (1968). Electron microscopic study of adrenal cortical hyperplasia in Cushing's syndrome. *Archs. Path.,* **86,** 419

REIDBORD, H. and FISHER, E. R. (1969). Aldosteronoma and nonfunctioning adrenal cortical adenoma. Comparative ultrastructural study. *Archs. Path.,* **88,** 155

TANNENBAUM, M. (1973). Ultrastructural pathology of the adrenal cortex. *Path. Ann.,* **8,** 109

VALENTE, M., PENNELLI, N., SEGATO, P., BEVILACQUA, L. and THIENE, G. (1978). Androgen producing adrenocortical carcinoma. *Virchows Arch. Path. Anat. Histol.,* **378,** 91

YOKOYAMA, M. (1975). Electron microscopic observation of adrenocortical tumors. In: *Morphology and Function of Adrenal Cortex,* ed. E., Kumamoto, N. Sasano and H. Tsuchiyama, pp. 31–53. Nankodo [in Japanese]

17
Acinic cell carcinoma

Secretory cells may be classified according to the physicochemical property of their secretory product. Since secretory granules usually have a characteristic ultrastructural morphology, it is possible to identify these cells and their tumours.

In Chapter 6 we dealt with mucus-secreting cells and mucous adenocarcinoma. Here we deal with acinic cells and their neoplasms, characterized by a serous or zymogenic secretion (zymogen granules) which is rich in protein. As one would expect, such cells are well endowed with rough endoplasmic reticulum. Acinic cells are found in mixed salivary glands and the exocrine pancreas, but before dealing with acinic cell carcinoma from these sites it is essential to examine the morphology of zymogen granules.

Morphology of zymogen granules

In glutaraldehyde-fixed material* (post-fixed with osmium and sections double stained with uranium and lead) zymogen granules have a homogeneous electron-dense appearance; a few paler granules with a particulate substructure are also seen. These are probably immature granules. The size of zymogen granules varies from about 0.25 μm to 0.5 μm, but in tumours the average diameter is somewhat smaller and there is also much greater variation in size. These granules are so dense that the closely applied ensheathing membrane is often difficult to discern, but

*Formaldehyde fixation also appears to be adequate for maintaining the morphology and electron density of zymogen granules. Johannessen (1977) reports a case of acinic cell carcinoma of the pancreas, which was diagnosed as such by one pathologist, but the diagnosis was changed to insulinoma by another pathologist. Electron microscopy of tumour tissue retrieved from a paraffin block showed characteristic electron-dense zymogen granules and abundant rough endoplasmic reticulum which unequivocally established the diagnosis of acinic cell carcinoma.

in granules that are not so dense this membrane is easily seen.

Osmium fixation does not preserve zymogen granules adequately. The granules in such preparations can be quite pale or only moderately dense. Diagnostic confusion is likely to stem from such morphological alterations, particularly if only a few granules are present, as in a relatively undifferentiated tumour or distant metastasis. Studies on the normal serous cells of the parotid gland show that there is a rapid loss of enzymatic protein (up to 70 per cent) from the zymogen granules during osmium fixation but not when glutaraldehyde is the primary fixative (Amsterdam and Schramm, 1966). The same phenomenon has been demonstrated by Erlandson and Tandler (1972) in cases of acinic cell carcinoma of the parotid gland. They found that with osmium fixation '...the secretory granules were irregular in outline, and their contents extracted to various degrees' and they also state that '...the delimiting membrane of the granules was often disrupted and showed a tendency to curl into miniature scrolls at broken ends'.

The level of preservation of zymogen granules appears to depend not only on the method of fixation, but also upon various other factors such as: (1) delay in fixation; (2) anoxia; and (3) biology and developmental history of the tumour. Such points must be kept in mind when assessing secretory granules in tumours.

Acinic cell carcinoma of salivary glands

Acinic cell carcinomas of the salivary gland (*Figures 176—178*) occur almost exclusively in the parotid gland (Abrams *et al.*, 1965; Evans and Cruickshank, 1970). They comprise about 1—3 per cent of all parotid gland tumours (Thackray and Lucas, 1974). Although the frequency of occurrence of acinic cell

215

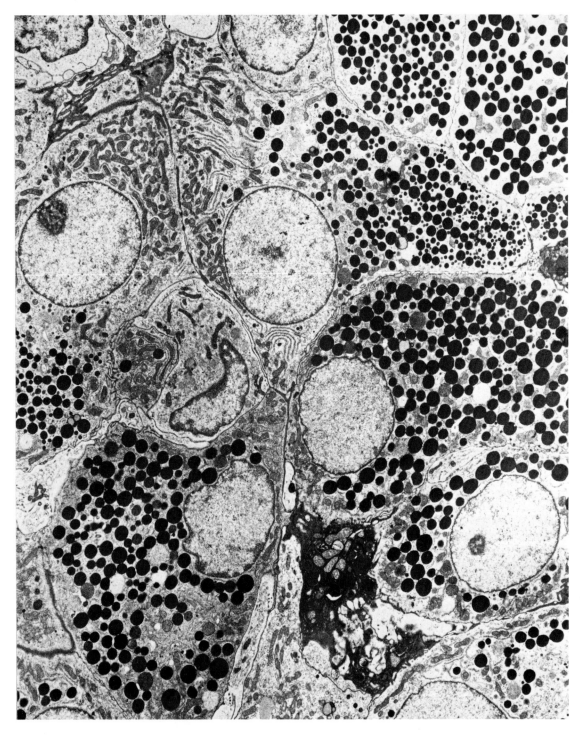

Figure 176   *Acinic cell carcinoma, showing cells containing
characteristic electron-dense zymogen granules.* ×5000 *(R.
A. Erlandson, unpublished electron micrograph)*

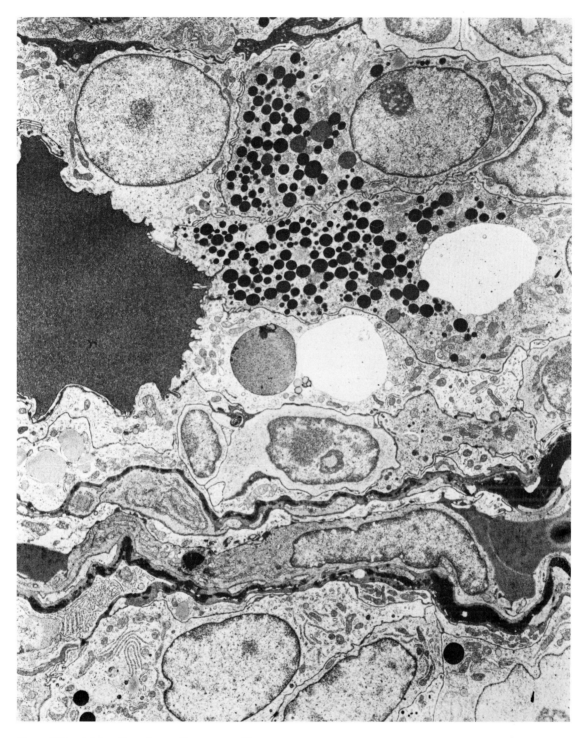

Figure 177   *Acinic cell carcinoma. Same case as Figure 176, showing tumour cells containing secretory granules and various others, such as undifferentiated tumour cells, lymphocytes and connective tissue elements. A capillary is seen running across the lower third of the picture. ×6000 (From Erlandson and Tandler, 1972)*

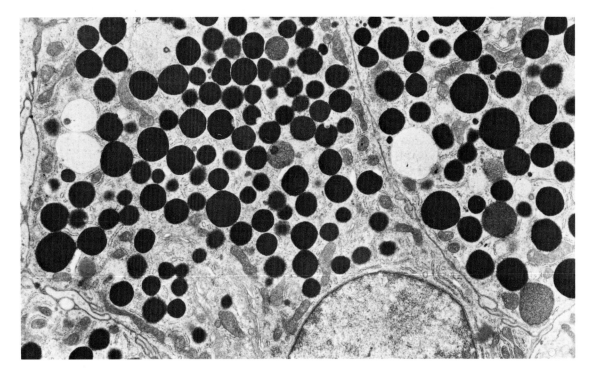

Figure 178 *Acinic cell carcinoma. Same case as Figures
176 and 177. Tumour cells showing secretory granules
and vacuoles of unknown nature.* ×8500 *(From Erlandson
and Tandler, 1972)*

carcinoma from the minor salivary glands is low,*
they have been reported in most locations where
similar glands occur, including the lung (Fechner,
Beatinek and Askew, 1972) and larynx (Crissman
and Rosenblatt, 1978). The latter case is of interest,
because on light microscopy (primary tumour in
larynx and secondary deposits that developed later)
the tumour was diagnosed as an oncocytic adenocarcinoma but on electron microscopy the neoplasm
was clearly an acinic cell carcinoma.

*It works out at about 0.4 per cent if one adds up the cases
reported by Chaudhry, Vickers and Gorlin (1961) and
Spiro *et al.* (1973).
†This appears paradoxical, but the same is evident also in the
normal pancreas. One may speculate that this appearance
may be due to the plane of sectioning, sometimes passing
through granule-rich areas and at other times through areas
rich in rough endoplasmic reticulum, or as an alternative one
may suggest that as the granules accumulate, the rough
endoplasmic reticulum regresses.

Acinic cell carcinoma has only recently been
recognized as a distinct type of low-grade malignant
neoplasm of salivary glands (Hirtzler *et al.*, 1969).
Only a few reports on the ultrastructure of these
tumours has been published (Echevarria, 1967;
Hirtzler *et al.*, 1969; Erlandson and Tandler, 1972;
Batsakis, Wozniak and Regezi, 1977; Sidhu and
Forrester, 1977; Crissman and Rosenblatt, 1978).
The main diagnostic feature is the occurrence of
zymogen granules and prominent rough endoplasmic
reticulum. There seems to be an inverse relationship
between these two features, for rough endoplasmic
reticulum is prominent in cells that do not contain
many granules, but when granules are plentiful, the
rough endoplasmic reticulum is sparse.† Two basic
cell types have been noted: (1) the zymogen granule-
containing cell resembling serous cells of salivary
glands; and (2) smaller cuboidal cells without granules which form duct-like structures. Views regarding
the histogenesis of this tumour include origin from:
(1) altered acinic cells; (2) terminal duct cells; and
(3) the reserve cells of the intercalated ducts.

Acinic cell carcinoma of exocrine pancreas

Human pancreatic cancer ranks fourth as a cause of cancer death (Pledger, Bates and Saffiotti, 1975) but only about 11 per cent of these are acinic cell tumours (Webb, 1977). Virtually all acinic cell tumours of the pancreas are carcinomas, although a rare adenoma is known to occur. Acinic cell carcinomas may occur in a pure form or may contain a mixture of acinar and ductal elements. Ultrastructurally the cells of these neoplasms are characterized by typical zymogen granules and also abundant rough endoplasmic reticulum in cells that are not too loaded with granules. Thus, they bear a striking resemblance to pancreatic acinar cells. These tumours have also been produced in various experimental animals (see Bockman *et al.*, 1978). The origin of these tumours in animals, including man, is thought to be from either altered acinic cells or duct cells.

References

ABRAMS, S., CORNYN, J., SCOFIELD, H. H. and HANSEN, L. S. (1965). Acinic cell adenocarcinoma of the major salivary glands: A clinicopathological study of 77 cases. *Cancer,* **18,** 1145

AMSTERDAM, A. and SCHRAMM, M. (1966). Rapid release of the zymogen granule protein by osmium tetroxide and its retention during fixation by glutaraldehyde. *J. Cell Biol.,* **29,** 199

BATSAKIS, J. G., WOZNIAK, K. J. and REGEZI, J. A. (1977). Acinous cell carcinoma: a histogenic hypothesis. *J. Oral Surg.,* **35,** 904

BOCKMAN, D. E., BLACK, O., MILLS, L. R. and WEBSTER, P. D. (1978). Origin of tubular complexes developing during induction of pancreatic adenocarcinoma by 7, 12-dimethybenz(*a*)anthracene. *Am. J. Path.,* **90,** 645

CHAUDHRY, A. P., VICKERS, R. A. and GORLIN, R. J. (1961). Intraoral minor salivary gland tumours. *Oral Surg.,* **14,** 1194

CRISSMAN, J. D. and ROSENBLATT, A. (1978). Acinous cell carcinoma of the larynx. *Archs. Path. Lab. Med.,* **102,** 233

ECHEVARRIA, R. A. (1967). Ultrastructure of the acinic cell carcinoma and clear cell carcinoma of the parotid gland. *Cancer,* **20,** 563

ERLANDSON, R. A. and TANDLER, B. (1972). Ultrastructure of acinic cell carcinoma of the parotid gland. *Archs. Path.,* **93,** 130

EVANS, R. W. and CRUICKSHANK, A. H. (1970). *Epithelial Tumours of the Salivary Glands,* pp. 98–119. Philadelphia: Saunders

FECHNER, R. E., BENTINCK, B. R. and ASKEW, J. B. (1972). Acinic cell tumor of lung. *Cancer,* **29,** 501

HIRTZLER, R., OBERMAN, B., KULES, M. and LJUBESIC, N. (1969). Acinuszelladenocarcinome der Spëicheldrüsen Bericht über 4 Fälle mit elektronemikroskopischer Bearbeitung von 2 Geschwülsten. *Arch. Ohr-.Nas.-u. KehlkHeilk.,* **195,** 68

JOHANNESSEN, J. V. (1977). Use of paraffin material for electron microscopy. *Path. Ann.,* **12,** 189

PLEDGER, R. A., BATES, R. R. and SAFFIOTTI, U. (1975). Introduction: National Cancer Institute Pancreatic Carcinogenesis Program. *Cancer Res.,* **35,** 2226

SIDHU, G. S. and FORRESTER, E. M. (1977). Acinic cell carcinoma; long-term survival after pulmonary metastases. *Cancer,* **40,** 756

SPIRO, R. H., KOSS, L. G., HAJDU, S. I. and STRONG, E. W. (1973). Tumors of minor salivary origin. *Cancer,* **31,** 117

THACKRAY, A. C. and LUCAS, R. B. (1974). Tumors of the major salivary glands. In: *Atlas of Tumor Pathology,* Fascicle 10, Series 2, pp. 81–90. Washington D.C., Armed Forces Institute of Pathology

WEBB, J. N. (1977). Acinar cell neoplasms of the exocrine pancreas. *J. Clin. Path.,* **30,** 103

18
Clear cell tumour of the lung (sugar tumour)

The sugar tumour is included in this work primarily because of its unusual ultrastructural morphology (*Figures 179* and *180*), but there are also some practical diagnostic implications.

At a casual glance, or if one is unfamiliar with this rare tumour, there is some danger that this benign tumour may be mistaken for metastatic clear cell carcinoma of the kidney and the patient subjected to needless stress and elaborate investigations to find a non-existent primary.

The sugar tumour usually presents as a 'coin lesion' in the peripheral part of the lung. It is well demarcated but not encapsulated. Liebow and Castleman (1963, 1971) were the first to describe this tumour

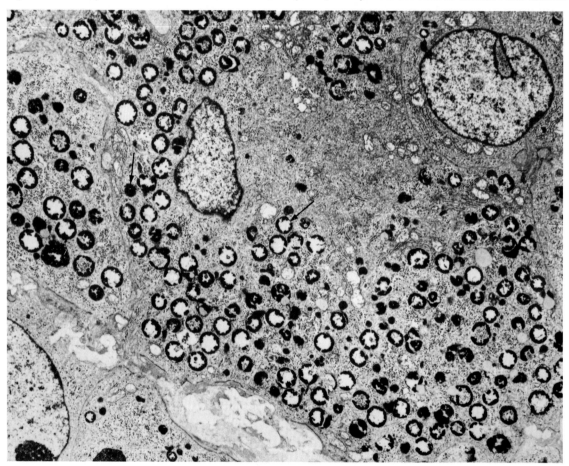

Figure 179   *Sugar tumour. Note the large number of bodies (arrows) containing glycogen. The central clear area is due to a leaching out of glycogen during tissue preparation. ×4750 (From Becker and Soifer, 1971)*

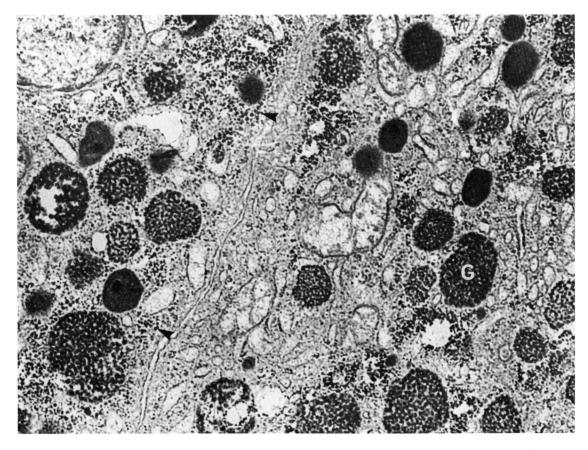

Figure 180   *Sugar tumour. High-power view showing glycogen-laden bodies (G). Note also the abundance of glycogen particles (arrowheads) in the cytoplasmic matrix.* ×14 000 *(From Becker and Soifer, 1971)*

and, according to them, the histological features of this tumour include: (1) large amounts of glycogen in the cytoplasm (probably also glycogen inclusions in the nucleus); (2) absence of lipid and haemosiderin in the tumour; (3) paucity of mitoses; (4) thin-walled, slit-like, vasculature; and (5) absence of haemorrhage and necrosis. However, Sale and Kulander (1976) have now recorded a case where there was extensive haemorrhage and necrosis. Both light and electron microscopic studies have failed to establish the histogenesis of this tumour. The ideas expressed about this include origin from: (1) Kultschitzky cell (Becker and Soifer, 1971); and (2) smooth muscle or pericyte (Hoch *et al.*, 1974).

Ultrastructural examination (Becker and Soifer, 1971; Hoch *et al.*, 1974) reveals massive amounts of

monoparticulate and rosette forms of glycogen in the cytoplasm of the tumour cells. However, the remarkable feature here is that much of the glycogen occurs in single membrane bound vacuoles.* This is reminiscent of the situation seen in Pompe's disease (Type II glycogenesis), where glycogen accumulates in lysosomes (mainly in the liver but also in various

*The occurrence of glycogen in single membrane bound vacuoles, usually but not invariably of a lysosomal nature, is not quite such a rare phenomenon as is commonly imagined (for details about this see Ghadially, 1975). What makes the sugar tumour so remarkable is that such large numbers of presumably lysosomal bodies containing glycogen are found. The only really analogous situation to this is Pompe's disease.

221

other organs). Here it is well known that a genetic defect leading to the absence or deficiency of a single lysosomal enzyme, acid glucosidase (acid maltase), necessary for the breakdown of glycogen to glucose produces accumulations of glycogen in lysosomes. A theory that one can therefore propose is that the somatic mutation which presumably leads to the production of the sugar tumour also encompasses another defect — viz. an inability to produce acid maltase, and, hence, glycogen accumulates in the lysosomes of this tumour.

In diabetic animals (rats and mice) there is an excess of intracytoplasmic glycogen in kidney tubules, and some glycogen is also found in lysosomes (Orci and Stauffacher, 1971). It is thought that this may be due to a relative enzyme deficiency engendered by excessive amounts of glycogen taken in by the lysosomes. One can argue that a similar situation perhaps develops in the sugar tumour also.

Be that as it may, the finding of such large numbers of single membrane bound bodies containing glycogen has been noted in this but in no other tumour. Therefore, this is a feature of diagnostic value which should permit distinction between this and other clear cell tumours when the situation is in doubt, as is the case when extensive haemorrhage and necrosis occurs in the sugar tumour (Sale and Kulander, 1976).

References

BECKER, N. H. and SOIFER, I. (1971). Benign clear cell tumor ('sugar tumor') of the lung. *Cancer,* **27**, 712

GHADIALLY, F. N. (1975). *Ultrastructural Pathology of the Cell.* London: Butterworths

HOCH, W. S., PATCHEFSKY, A. S., TAKEDA, M. and GORDON, G. (1974). Benign clear cell tumor of the lung. An ultrastructural study. *Cancer,* **33**, 1328

LIEBOW, A. A. and CASTLEMAN, B. (1963). Benign 'clear cell tumors' of the lung. *Am. J. Path.,* **43**, 13a (abstract)

LIEBOW, A. A. and CASTLEMAN, B. (1971). Benign clear cell ('sugar') tumors of the lung. *Yale J. Biol. Med.,* **43**, 213

NAKAYAMA, I., TSUDA, N., MUTA, H., FUJII, H., TSUJI, K., MATSUO, T. and TAKAHARA, O. (1975). Fine structural comparison of Ewing's sarcoma with neuroblastoma. *Acta Path. Jap.,* **25**, 251

ORCI, L. and STAUFFACHER, W. (1971). Glycogenosomes in renal tubular cells of diabetic animals. *J. Ultrastruct. Res.,* **36**, 499

SALE, G. E. and KULANDER, B. G. (1976). Benign clear cell tumor of lung with necrosis. *Cancer,* **37**, 2355

19
Juxtaglomerular cell tumour (renin-secreting kidney tumour)

The juxtaglomerular cell tumour, also called the 'renin-secreting tumour' of the kidney, is a rare lesion; only a few cases have been reported (Robertson *et al.*, 1967; Kihara *et al.*, 1968; Kihara, 1969; Eddy and Sanchez, 1971; Bonnin, Hodge and Lumbers, 1972; Conn *et al.*, 1972; Phillips and Mukherjee, 1972; Brown *et al.*, 1973; Orjavik *et al.*, 1975).

All tumours reported so far have been small in size (8—40 mm in diameter), benign and located in the cortex of the kidney. With the light microscope the tumour is seen to be composed of polygonal cells arranged in clusters or surrounding thin-walled blood vessels. Hence, the tumour was first described as a 'renin-secreting haemangiopericytoma'. However, according to Phillips and Mukherjee (1972), this tumour does not show the characteristic reticulin pattern of haemangiopericytoma, where one sees proliferating tumour cells outside the reticulin sheath of blood vessels.

These tumours also contain numerous mast cells (25 per cent in the case reported by Phillips and Mukherjee, 1972). Thus, the presence of granulated cells at light microscopy is not in itself diagnostic of the juxtaglomerular cell tumour, and electron microscopy is essential to distinguish these cells with certainty.

The juxtaglomerular cells in these tumours (*Figures 181* and *182*) are characterized by numerous rhomboidal, polygonal and rounded granules. There is abundant rough endoplasmic reticulum and the cisternae are dilated but the granules are not located here. Small granules about 0.2 μm long are seen in Golgi vacuoles while larger ones up to 1.5 μm long are found in the cytoplasmic matrix.

Various developmental stages of these granules are seen in the tumour cells and they resemble those found in normal human juxtaglomerular cells (Barajas, 1966; Biava and West, 1966a, b, c). Thus, these granules may present as rounded bodies with a homogeneous or granular electron-dense content or they may be rhomboidal in shape and amorphous or show a crystalline lattice with a spacing of 6—10 nm. The rounded form is thought to represent the mature specific granule, because an abundance of these in the juxtaglomerular tumour has been associated with high renin levels (Bonnin *et al.*, 1977). A crystalline lattice has only rarely been demonstrated in the granules of the tumour cells. This may have been due to less than optimum tissue preservation.

The morphological differences between mast cells and juxtaglomerular cells were confused until electron microscopy revealed the structural features of their granules (Thiery, 1963; Barajas, 1966; Biava and West, 1966b). Mast cells are easily distinguished from juxtaglomerular cells on the basis of ultrastructural morphology of the granules. Mast cell granules are quite pleomorphic; they may be homogeneous or granular or contain cylindrical lamellar formations which produce a scroll-like pattern. Mast cell granules are never rhomboidal in shape like the juxtaglomerular cell granules. Spherical electron-dense granules are at times seen in mast cells and they bear some resemblance to the spherical granules in juxtaglomerular cells, but a closer look at such granules and accompanying granules (*Figures 183*) soon reveals the laminated membranous pattern characteristic of mast cell granules.

Such distinctions are important, for while mast cells are rarely seen in the normal kidney (Janes and McDonald, 1948), substantial numbers are found in various pathological states, including certain tumours, notably hamartomas. They tend to be more numerous in primary rather than secondary neoplasms (Pavone-Macaluso, 1960).

It is well known that the juxtaglomerular cell is one of the important sites of renin synthesis. It is therefore not surprising to find that: (1) renin has been demonstrated in this tumour; (2) there is an increased plasma renin activity; and (3) there is an increased plasma renin concentration in patients bearing this tumour. Ultrastructural studies have

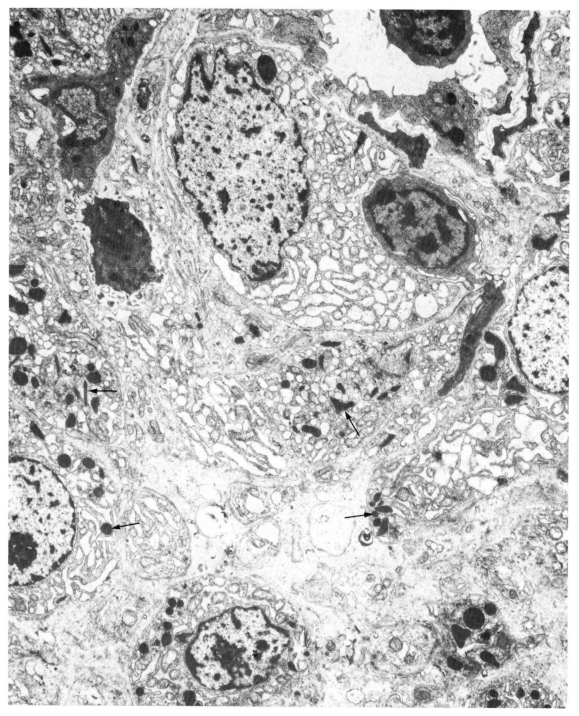

Figure 181 *Juxtaglomerular cell tumour. The tumour cells contain abundant rough endoplasmic reticulum and pleomorphic secretory granules (arrows). ×5500 (Dr T. M. Mukherjee, unpublished electron micrograph)*

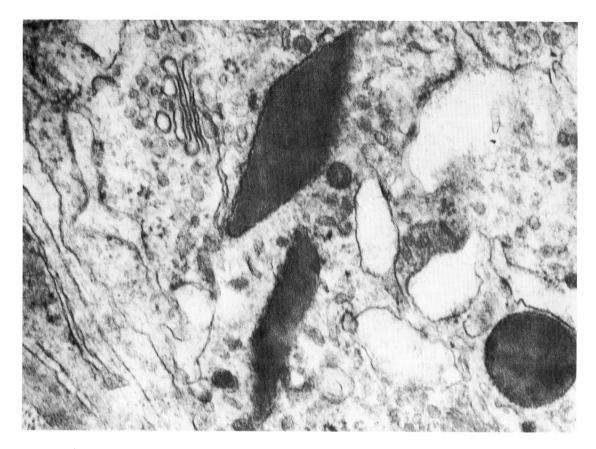

Figure 182 *Juxtaglomerular cell tumour. Same case as Figure 181. A high-power view of the secretory granules.* × 70 000 *(Dr T. M. Mukherjee, unpublished electron micrograph)*

clearly established that the renin-secreting tumour of the kidney is a juxtaglomerular cell tumour; the mast cell infiltration is no doubt a secondary phenomenon.

References

BARAJAS, L. (1966). The development and ultrastructure of the juxtaglomerular cell granule. *J. Ultrastruct. Res.,* **15**, 400

BIAVA, C. and WEST, M. (1966a). Fine structure of normal human juxtaglomerular cells. I. General structure and intercellular relationships. *Am. J. Path.,* **49**, 679

BIAVA, C. and WEST, M. (1966b). Fine structure of normal human juxtaglomerular cells. II. Specific and non-specific cytoplasmic granules. *Am. J. Path.,* **49**, 955

BIAVA, C. and WEST, M. (1966c). Fine morphology of human juxtaglomerular cells in patients with benign essential hypertension. *Lab. Invest.,* **15**, 1902

BONNIN, J. M., CAIN, M. D., JOSE, J. S., MUKHERJEE, T. M., PERRETT, L. V., SCROOP, G. C. and SEYMOUR, A. E. (1977). Hypertension due to a renin-secreting tumour localised by segmental renal vein sampling. *Aust. N. Z. J. Med.,* **7**, 630

BONNIN, J. M., HODGE, R. L. and LUMBERS, E. R. (1972). A renin secreting renal tumor associated with hypertension. *Aust. N. Z. J. Med.,* **2**, 178

BROWN, J. J., FRASER, R., LEVER, A. F., MORTON, J. J., ROBERTSON, J. I. S., TREE, M., BELL, P. R. F., DAVIDSON, J. K. and RUTHVEN, I. S. (1973). Hypertension and secondary hyperaldosteronism associated with a renin-secreting renal juxtaglomerular cell tumour. *Lancet,* ii, 1228

CONN, J. W., COHEN, E. L., LUCAS, C. P., McDONALD, W. J., MAYOR, G. H., BLOUGH, W. M., EVELAND, W. C., BOOKSTEIN, J. J. and LAPIDES, J. (1972). Primary reninism. *Archs intern. Med.,* **130**, 682

EDDY, R. L. and SANCHEZ, S. A. (1971). Renin secreting renal neoplasm and hypertension with hypokalemia. *Ann. Int. Med.,* **75**, 725

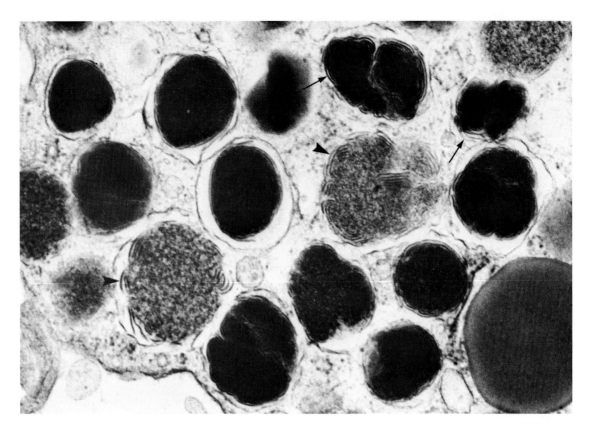

Figure 183   *Human mast cell. Mast cell granules are very
pleomorphic. It would take numerous illustrations to depict
these morphological variations. The mast cell granules shown
in this illustration were chosen to illustrate the point that at
times some of the granules are rounded and electron-dense
and, hence, resemble some of the granules seen in juxtaglomerular cells and their tumours. However, closer
examination usually reveals membranous formations in their
interior, a point which is more easily discerned at the
periphery of the granules (arrows) and in granules that are
not too electron-dense (arrowheads). ×59 000*

JANES, J. and McDONALD, J. R. (1948). Mast cells. Their
    distribution in various human tissues. *Archs Path.*, **45**,
    622

KIHARA, I. (1969). Pathology of the juxtaglomerular cells
    and juxtaglomerular cell tumour. *Jap. J. Clin. Med.*, **27**,
    1251

KIHARA, I., KITAMURA, S., HOSHINO, T., SEIDA, H.
    and WATANABE, T. (1968). A hitherto unreported
    vascular tumor of the kidney: A proposal of 'juxta-
    glomerular cell tumor'. *Acta Path. Jap.*, **18**, 197

ORJAVIK, O. S., AAS, M, FAUCHALD, P., HOVIG, T.,
    OYSTESE, B., BRODWALL, E. K. and FLATMARK, A.
    (1975). Renin-secreting renal tumour with severe hyper-
    tension. *Acta Med. Scand.*, **197**, 329

PAVONE-MACALUSO, M. (1960). Tissue mast cells in renal
    disease. *Acta Path. Microbiol. Scand.*, **50**, 337

PHILLIPS, G. and MUKHERJEE, T. M. (1972). A juxta-
    glomerular cell tumour: Light and electron microscopic
    studies of a renin-secreting kidney tumour containing
    both juxtaglomerular cells and mast cells. *Pathology*, **4**,
    193

ROBERTSON, P. W., KLIDJIAN, A., HARDING, L. K. and
    WALTERS, G. (1967). Hypertension due to a renin-
    secreting renal tumour. *Am. J. Med.*, **43**, 963

THIERY, J. P. (1963). Electron microscopic study of the
    maturation and excretion of mast cell granules. *J.
    Microsc.*, **2**, 549

20
Alveolar cell carcinoma

Alveolar cell carcinoma is a tumour of granular pneumocytes (also called 'great alveolar cell', 'septal cell' and 'Type II epithelial cell'). Ultrastructural studies (Adamson, Senior and Merrill, 1969; Coalson *et al.*, 1970; Lupulescu and Boyd, 1972; Nash, Langlinais and Greenwald, 1972; Levin, 1973; Mollo, Canese and Campobasso, 1973; Bonikos, Hendrickson and Bensch, 1977) have played a key role in establishing this tumour as an entity distinct and different from other pulmonary neoplasms. This tumour shows various histological patterns; hence, electron microscopy is essential for unequivocal diagnosis (Mollo, Canese and Campobasso, 1973).

The granular pneumocyte is a secretory cell which contributes to the surfactant layer essential for lowering surface tension and stabilizing the size of the alveolus. The ultrastructural diagnosis of alveolar cell carcinoma rests on the fact that both normal (*Figures 184–186*) and neoplastic granular pneumocytes (*Figures 187* and *188*) contain secretory granules of characteristic morphology. These comprise single membrane bound bodies containing whorled osmiophilic membranes. Hence, they are best referred to as 'myelinoid bodies' (Ghadially, 1975) or myelinosomes, but they are frequently referred to by various other names also, such as 'cytosomes', 'multilamellar bodies', 'lamellar bodies' and 'osmiophilic lamellar bodies'.

Numerous studies on normal granular pneumocytes attest to the fact that these myelinosomes contain acid phosphatase and that they evolve from multivesicular bodies with an electron-lucent or electron-dense matrix (Campiche *et al.*, 1963; Balis and Conen, 1964; Hatasa and Nakamura, 1965; Balis, Delivoria and Conen, 1966; Sorokin, 1966; Goldenberg, Buckingham and Sommers, 1967, 1969; Kuhn, 1968; Goldfisher, Kikkawa and Hoffman, 1968; Corrin, Clark and Spencer, 1969; Vijeyaratnam and Corrin, 1972).

The probable sequence of events seems to be as follows. The light variety of multivesicular body is converted to the dense variety. Next a few osmiophilic membranes (myelinoid membranes) appear in the matrix of the dense multivesicular body. As the amount of membranous material increases, the number of vesicles in the body diminishes until the fully mature myelinoid body packed with stacks or whorls of electron-dense membranes (myelin figures) is formed. This then moves to the surface of the cell and its contents are discharged like any other merocrine secretion.

The precise manner in which the multivesicular bodies form in the great alveolar cells is not clear, but it is thought that vesicles containing the secretory material are pinched off from the rough endoplasmic reticulum and after their probable passage through the Golgi complex a cluster of vesicles is encompassed within a single limiting membrane, to form the multivesicular body.

Such steps in the evolution of the myelinoid bodies from multivesicular bodies are not depicted in the many ultrastructural studies on alveolar cell carcinoma, nor are myelinoid bodies with stacked osmiophilic membranes evident, as in the normal state. Virtually the only configuration seen is that of whorled membranes (*Figures 187* and *188*). However, electron-dense bodies thought to contain lipid are seen and it has been suggested that myelinoid bodies are derived from these structures.

A more detailed analysis of this situation is needed, for it may well be that the pathway of production of the myelinoid body is different in the neoplastic cell and this may be helpful in distinguishing alveolar cell carcinoma from florid reactive acinar metaplastic proliferations with atypia. At the moment the distinction rests on cytological manifestations of neoplasia at the light microscopic level and the irregularity of size and shape of the nucleus and nucleolus found in alveolar cell carcinoma. Other distinguishing points include groups of cells forming papillae and cells with malignant nuclear features covering relatively normal or unscarred alveolar

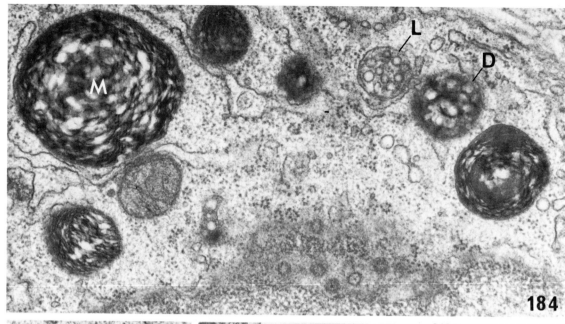

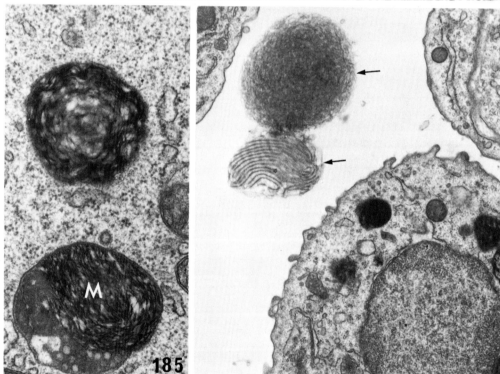

Figures 184–186 *Granular pneumocytes from a newborn rat. (From Ghadially, 1975).*
Figure 184 Some of the stages of evolution of a myelinoid body (M) from light (L) and dark (D) multivesiculated bodies are seen in this electron micrograph. ×43 000. Figure 185 A body with vesicles and dense membranes (M) is seen *in company with another presumably more mature form containing mainly laminated dense membranes. ×42 000.*
Figure 186 Low-power view showing a granular pneumocyte with myelinoid bodies (M) and alveolar space containing discharged secretory material (arrows). ×18 000

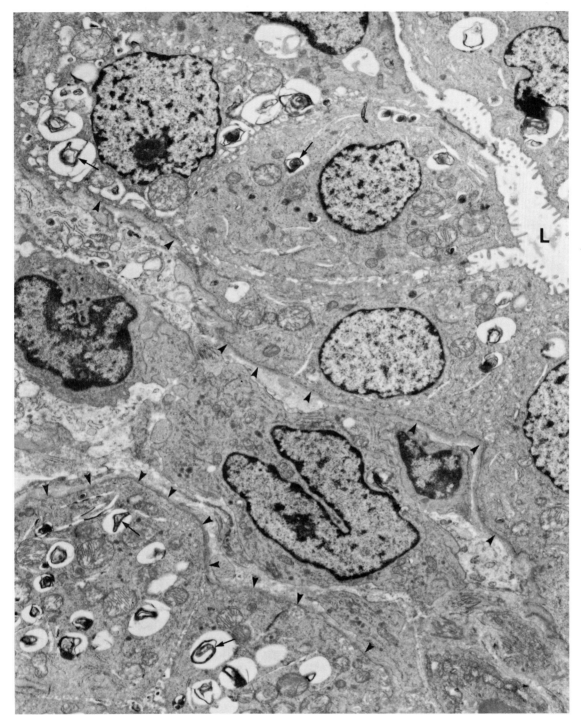

Figure 187 *Alveolar cell carcinoma. Parts of two tumour acini are depicted here. Basal laminae (arrowheads) demarcate these from the connective tissue elements. Characteristic secretory granules (myelinoid bodies) (arrows) are* *seen in the tumour cells. Note also the intercellular lumen (L) bounded by the microvillar surface of the tumour cells. × 7000 (F. Mollo, unpublished electron micrograph)*

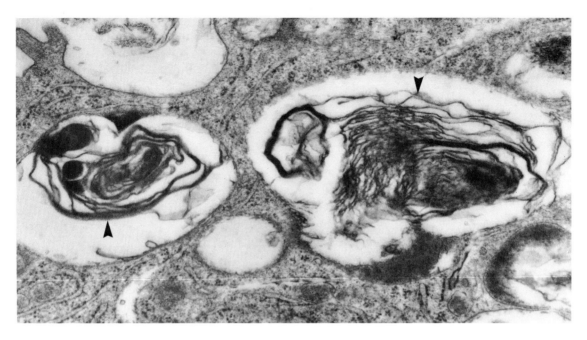

Figure 188 *High-power view of laminated dense membranes (arrowheads) seen in myelinoid bodies. ×33 000 (F. Mollo, unpublished electron micrograph)*

septa. Features such as this are unlikely to be seen in a reactive or hyperplastic proliferation of granular pneumocytes (Bonikos, Hendrickson and Bensch, 1977).

Distinguishing alveolar cell carcinoma from other types of neoplasia rests on the demonstration of the myelinoid bodies which are the characteristic secretory granules of the granular pneumocyte. However, this tumour shares with other adenocarcinomas features such as: (1) cells arranged in alveolar and tubular formations; (2) abundance of microvilli; and (3) intercellular lumina bounded by cells united by tight junctions and desmosomes (Mollo, Canese and Campobasso, 1973).

Despite the evidence provided by electron microscopic studies (Adamson, Senior and Merrill, 1969; Coalson *et al.*, 1970; Lupulescu and Boyd, 1972; Nash, Langlinais and Greenwald, 1972; Levin, 1973; Mollo, Canese and Campobasso, 1973), there has been a reluctance to accept alveolar cell carcinoma as an entity (Bedrossian *et al.*, 1975; Greenberg, Smith and Spjut, 1975). There are at least four other lines of evidence which should surely dispel doubts about this matter. These may be summarized as follows: (1) The propensity of carcinoma (including alveolar cell carcinoma) to arise in areas of pulmonary

scarring and atypical hyperplasia (containing granular pneumocytes) is well known (Raeburn and Spencer, 1953; Beaver and Shapiro, 1956; Berkheiser, 1959; Fox and Risdon, 1968; Haddad and Massaro, 1968; Gerami and Cole, 1969; Fraire and Greenberg, 1973; Bookman, Urowitz and Mitchell, 1974), as also is the propensity for granular pneumocytes to proliferate as a result of alveolar injury and repair in both man (Littler *et al.*, 1969; Farr, Harley and Hennigar, 1970; Bachofen and Weibel, 1974; Bonikos, Bensch and Northway, 1976) and experimental animals (Faulkner and Esterly, 1971; Adamson and Bowden, 1972; Kaufman, 1972; Gould and Miller, 1975; Bonikos, Bensch and Northway, 1976). (2) Studies on spontaneously occurring tumours such as pulmonary adematosis of sheep (including Jaagsiekte) (Bonne, 1939) and experimentally produced pulmonary adenomatous hyperplasia in the guinea-pig, where granular pneumocytes occur (Torikata *et al.*, 1975). (3) Alveolar cell carcinoma produced by various chemical carcinogens which also derive from granular pneumocytes (e.g. Levin, 1973). (4) Long-term organ culture studies (up to 5 months) of alveolar cell carcinoma by Bonikos, Hendrickson and Bensch (1977) which yielded a population of cells with the ultrastructural characteristics of granular pneumocytes. (5) The proliferation of granular pneumocytes found in dogs exposed to cigarette smoke for up to 5 years (Frasca *et al.*, 1974).

The difficulty of confidently identifying alveolar cell carcinoma at the light microscopic level has resulted in a lumping together of alveolar cell carcinoma with bronchiolar carcinoma under the title 'bronchiolo-alveolar carcinoma'. It seems likely that the biological behaviour of these tumours will in the future be better defined as a result of the increasing use of the electron microscope for diagnostic purposes and hopefully this will lead to improved therapy. So characteristic is the ultrastructural morphology of the granular pneumocyte that it can be identified not only in the primary in the lung, but also in extrapulmonary metastatic deposits by electron microscopy of tissue or cytological preparations (Coalson *et al.*, 1970; Woyke, Domagala and Olszweski, 1972; Johnston and Frable, 1976).

References

ADAMSON, I. Y. R. and BOWDEN, D. H. (1972). Intracellular localization of surfactant synthesis in lung explants. *Fed. Proc.*, **31**, 608A

ADAMSON, J. S., SENIOR, R. M. and MERRILL, T. (1969). Alveolar cell carcinoma. *Am. Rev. Respir. Dis.*, **100**, 550

BACHOFEN, M. and WEIBEL, R. R. (1974). Basic pattern of tissue repair in human lungs following unspecific injury. *Chest*, **65**, 14 (Suppl.)

BALIS, J. U. and CONEN, P. E. (1964). The role of alveolar inclusion bodies in the developing lung. *Lab. Invest.*, **13**, 1215

BALIS, J. U., DELIVORIA, M. and CONEN, P. E. (1966). Maturation of postnatal human lung and the idiopathic respiratory distress syndrome. *Lab. Invest.*, **15**, 530

BEAVER, D. L. and SHAPIRO, J. L. (1956). A consideration of chronic pulmonary parenchymal inflammation and alveolar cell carcinoma with regard to a possible etiologic relationship. *Am. J. Med.*, **21**, 879

BEDROSSIAN, C. W. M., WEILBAECHER, D. G., BENTINCK, D. C. and GREENBERG, S. D. (1975). Ultrastructure of human bronchiolo-alveolar cell carcinoma. *Cancer*, **36**, 1399

BERKHEISER, S. W. (1959). Bronchiolar proliferation and metaplasia associated with bronchiectasis, pulmonary infarcts and anthracosis. *Cancer*, **12**, 499

BONIKOS, D. S., BENSCH, K. G. and NORTHWAY, W. H., Jr. (1976). Oxygen toxicity in the newborn. The effect of chronic continuous 100% O_2 exposure on the lungs of newborn mice. *Am. J. Path.*, **85**, 632

BONIKOS, D. S., HENDRICKSON, M. and BENSCH, K. G. (1977). Pulmonary alveolar cell carcinoma. Fine structural and in vitro study of a case and critical review of this entity. *Am. J. Surg. Path.*, **1**, 93

BONNE, C. (1939). Morphological resemblance of pulmonary adenomatosis (Jaagsiekte) in sheep and certain cases of cancer of the lung in man. *Am. J. Cancer*, **35**, 491

BOOKMAN, A. A. M., UROWITZ, M. B. and MITCHELL, R. I. (1974). Alveolar cell carcinoma in progressive systemic sclerosis. *J. Rheumatol.*, **1**, 466

CAMPICHE, M. A., GAUTIER, A., HERNANDEZ, E. I. and REYMOND, A. (1963). An electron microscopy study of the fetal development of human lung. *Pediatrics*, **32**, 976

COALSON, J. J., MOHR, J. A., PIRTLE, J. K., DEE, A. L. and RHOADS, E. R. (1970). Electron microscopy of neoplasms of the lung with special emphasis on the alveolar cell carcinoma. *Am. Rev. Respir. Dis.*, **101**, 181

CORRIN, B., CLARK, A. E. and SPENCER, H. (1969). Ultrastructural localization of acid phosphatase in the rat lung. *J. Anat.*, **104**, 65

FARR, G. H., HARLEY, R. A. and HENNIGAR, G. R. (1970). Desquamative interstitial pneumonia. An electron microscopic study. *Am. J. Path.*, **60**, 347

FAULKNER, C. S. and ESTERLY, J. R. (1971). Ultrastructural changes in alveolar epithelium in response to Freund's adjuvant. *Am. J. Path.*, **64**, 559

FOX, B. and RISDON, R. A. (1968). Carcinoma of the lung and diffuse interstitial pulmonary fibrosis. *J. Clin. Path.*, **21**, 486

FRAIRE, A. E. and GREENBERG, S. D. (1973). Carcinoma and diffuse interstitial fibrosis of lung. *Cancer*, **31**, 1078

FRASCA, J. M., AUERBACH, O., PARKS, V. R. and JAMIESON, J. D. (1974). Alveolar cell hyperplasia in the lungs of smoking dogs. *Expl Molec. Path.*, **21**, 300

GERAMI, S. and COLE, F. H. (1969). Coexisiting carcinoma of the lung and pulmonary tuberculosis. *Ann. Thorac. Surg.*, **7**, 317

GHADIALLY, F. N. (1975). *Ultrastructural Pathology of the Cell.* London: Butterworths

GOLDENBERG, V. E., BUCKINGHAM, S. and SOMMERS, S. C. (1967). Pulmonary alveolar lesions in vagotomized rats. *Lab. Invest.*, **16**, 693

GOLDENBERG, V. E., BUCKINGHAM, S. and SOMMERS, S. C. (1969). Pilocarpine stimulation of granular pneumocyte secretion. *Lab. Invest.*, **20**, 147

GOLDFISCHER, S., KIKKAWA, Y. and HOFFMAN, L. (1968). The demonstration of acid hydrolase activities in the inclusion bodies of type II alveolar cells and other lysosomes in the rabbit lung. *J. Histochem. Cytochem.*, **16**, 102

GOULD, V. E. and MILLER, J. (1975). Sclerosing alveolitis induced by cyclophosphamide. Ultrastructural observations on alveolar injury and repair. *Am. J. Path.*, **81**, 513

GREENBERG, S. D., SMITH, M. N. and SPJUT, H. J. (1975). Bronchiolo-alveolar carcinoma — Cell of origin. *Am. J. Clin. Path.*, **63**, 153

HADDAD, R. and MASSARO, D. (1968). Idiopathic diffuse interstitial pulmonary fibrosis (fibrosing alveolitis) atypical epithelial proliferation and lung cancer. *Am. J. Med.*, **45**, 211

HATASA, K. and NAKAMURA, T. (1965). Electron microscopic observations of lung alveolar epithelial cells of normal young mice, with special reference to formation and secretion of osmiophilic lamellar bodies. *Z. Zellforsch. Mikrosk. Anat.*, **68**, 266

JOHNSTON, W. W. and FRABLE, W. J. (1976). The cyto-pathology of the respiratory tract. *Am. J. Path.,* **84,** 372

KAUFMAN, S. L. (1972). Alterations in cell proliferation in mouse lung following urethane exposure. *Am. J. Path.,* **68,** 317

KUHN, C. (1968). Cytochemistry of pulmonary alveolar epithelial cells. *Am. J. Path.,* **53,** 809

LEVIN, S. (1973). The pathogenesis of alveolar cell carcinoma induced by dibutylnitrosamine in buffalo rats. Abstr. 96, Sixty-fourth Annual Meeting, *Proceedings of the American Association of Cancer Research,* p. 24

LITTLER, W. A., KAY, J. M., HASLETON, P. S. and HEATH, D. (1969). Busulphan lung. *Thorax,* **24,** 639

LUPULESCU, A. and BOYD, C. B. (1972). Lung cancer — A transmission and scanning electron microscopic study. *Cancer,* **29,** 1530

MOLLO, F., CANESE, M. G. and CAMPOBASSO, O. (1973). Human peripheral lung tumours: light and electron microscopic correlation. *Br. J. Cancer,* **27,** 173

NASH, G., LANGLINAIS, P. C. and GREENWALD, K. A. (1972). Alveolar cell carcinoma — Does it exist? *Cancer,* **29,** 322

RAEBURN, C. and SPENCER, H. (1953). A study of the origin and development of lung cancer. *Thorax,* **8,** 1

SOROKIN, S. P. (1966). A morphologic and cytochemical study on the great alveolar cell. *J. Histochem. Cytochem.,* **14,** 884

TORIKATA, C., TAKEUCHI, H., YAMAGUCHI, H. and KAGEYAMA, K. (1975). Histopathological studies on experimentally induced pulmonary adenomatosis in guinea-pig lungs. *Acta Path. Jap.,* **25,** 555

VIJEYARATNAM, G. S. and CORRIN, B. (1972). Pulmonary histiocytosis simulating desquamative interstitial pneumonia in rats receiving oral iprindole. *J. Path.,* **108,** 105

WOYKE, S., DOMAGALA, W. and OLSZEWSKI, W. (1972). Alveolar cell carcinoma of the lung: An ultrastructural study of the cancer cells detected in the pleural fluid. *Acta Cytol.,* **16,** 63

21
Alveolar soft part sarcoma

Alveolar soft part sarcoma was first described by Christopherson, Foote and Stewart in 1952, but its histogenesis still remains a matter of speculation. This tumour has been looked upon as a malignant variant of: (1) granular cell myoblastoma; (2) non-chromaffin paraganglioma; (3) a neural neoplasm; and (4) rhabdomyosarcoma (Christopherson, Foote and Stewart, 1952; Fisher, 1956; Marshall and Horn, 1961; Karnauchow and Magner, 1963).

The distinguishing feature of this tumour is the occurrence of crystals within the tumour cells (*Figures 189–192*). This phenomenon, first noted by Masson (1956), has since been confirmed by light and electron microscopic studies (Shipkey *et al.*, 1964; Fisher and

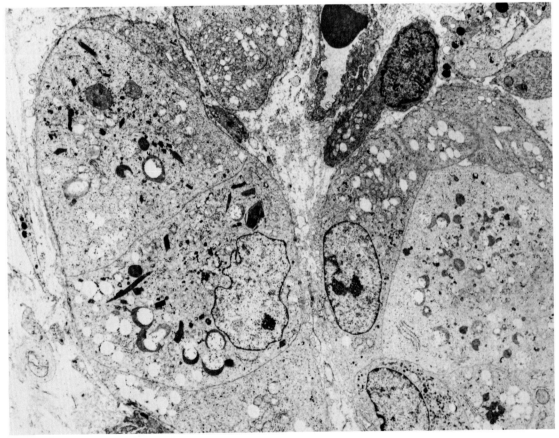

Figure 189 *Alveolar soft part sarcoma. A low-power view showing the alveolar arrangement of cells found in this type of neoplasm. A lumen is not seen in these alveoli but it was demonstrable in other parts of this tumour. ×2750 (J. V. Johannessen, unpublished electron micrograph)*

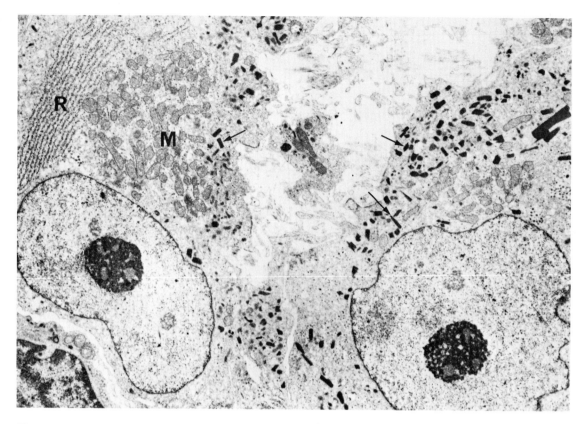

Figure 190 *Alveolar soft part sarcoma. Same case as Figure 189. Note the innumerable small crystals (arrows), rough endoplasmic reticulum (R) and numerous mitochondria* *(M). ×6500 (J. V. Johannessen, unpublished electron micrograph)*

Reidbord, 1971). These crystals are PAS-positive and resistant to diastase digestion. Shipkey *et al.* (1964) state that the crystals present as 'rhomboid, rod-like or spiked forms, singly, stacked like cordwood or in sheaf-life arrangement'.

With the electron microscope the crystals show a periodic pattern of 'lines' set 10 nm apart (*Figure 192*). In other planes of sectioning the 'lines' are seen to be composed of irregularly outlined 'points' (Shipkey *et al.*, 1964). A square grid pattern may also at times be seen (Fisher and Reidbord, 1971). Delayed fixation leads to a loss of the periodic crystalline pattern and also loss of material from the smooth membrane bound spaces within which the crystals lie.

Fisher and Reidbord (1971) find a resemblance between the crystals of alveolar soft part sarcoma and the rods* found in nemaline myopathy (Price *et al.*, 1965; Goldstein, Schroeter and Sass, 1977) and rhabdomyoma (Tandler *et al.*, 1970). They therefore

regard 'the alveolar soft part sarcoma as a distinct type of rhabdomyosarcoma'.

However, it is difficult to accept this view, because filaments have not been reported to occur in these tumours and because Z lines and rods are not membrane bound at any stage of their development, whereas many of the crystals in alveolar soft part sarcoma are.

Crystalline inclusions are proteinaceous in nature, so one may speculate that such secretions transported from the rough endoplasmic reticulum to the Golgi complex crystallized in the Golgi vacuoles, or that the crystals develop in the rough endoplasmic reticulum which later becomes degranulated.

The former hypothesis appears more attractive, for in some cells the crystals are seen in the juxtanuclear region, and the Golgi complex is well developed

*Rods are derived from the Z lines; both have a crystalline structure.

234

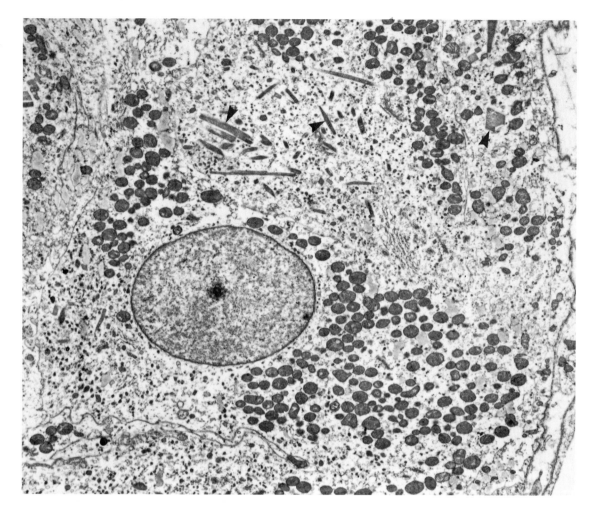

Figure 191   *Alveolar soft part sarcoma. Low-power electron micrograph showing tumour cells containing crystals (arrowheads) which, depending on the plane of section, present as sharp spicules, rhomboids and various polygonal forms. Note also the numerous mitochondria. ×6250 (From Shipkey et al., 1964)*

in the tumour cells. The rough endoplasmic reticulum is also well represented in many but not all cells but an external lamina surrounding individual cells is not evident. Such findings argue against a neurogenic or a myogenic origin, the collective features being closer to a fibroblast than any other cell.

The only other feature of interest is an abundance of mitochondria in many tumour cells. This plus the crystals gives the cytoplasm a granular eosinophilic appearance (Chapter 9).

As mentioned earlier, the histogenesis of this tumour remains obscure and so does the chemical composition of the crystals. Their presence, however, is helpful in establishing the diagnosis of this tumour.

235

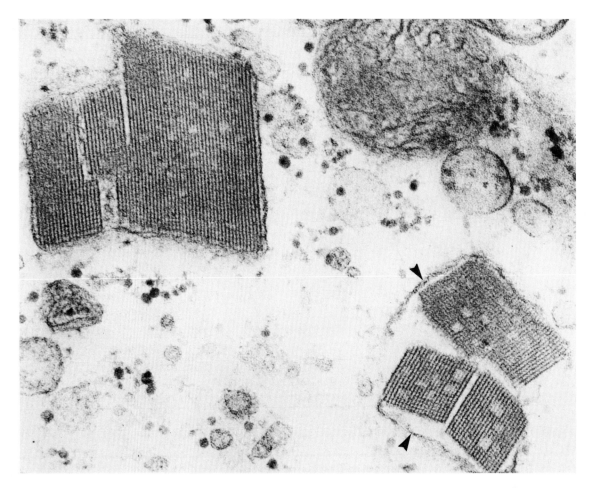

Figure 192   *Alveolar soft part sarcoma. High-power view of crystals demonstrating a periodic pattern of 10 nm. Note also the membrane (arrowheads) surrounding the* crystals. ×*100 000 (F. H. Shipkey, unpublished electron micrograph)*

References

CHRISTOPHERSON, W. M., FOOTE, F. W., Jr. and STEWART, F. W. (1952). Alveolar soft-part sarcomas: structurally characteristic tumors of uncertain histogenesis. *Cancer,* **5,** 100

FISHER, E. R. (1956). Histochemical observations on an alveolar soft-part sarcoma with reference to histogenesis. *Am. J. Path.,* **32,** 721

FISHER, E. R. and REIDBORD, H. (1971). Electron microscopic evidence suggesting the myogenous derivation of the so-called alveolar soft part sarcoma. *Cancer,* **27,** 150

GOLDSTEIN, M. A., SCHROETER, J. P. and SASS, R. L. (1977). Optical diffraction of the Z lattice in Canine cardiac muscle. *J. Cell Biol.,* **75,** 818

KARNAUCHOW, P. N. and MAGNER, D. (1963). The histogenesis of alveolar soft part sarcoma. *J. Path. Bact.,* **86,** 169

MARSHALL, R. B. and HORN, R. C., Jr. (1961). Non-chromaffin paraganglioma. A comparative study. *Cancer,* **14,** 779

MASSON, P. (1956). *Tumeurs humaines; Histologie, Diagnostics et Techniques.* 2nd edn, p. 213. Paris: Librairie Maloine

PRICE, H. M., GORDON, G. B., PEARSON, C. M., MUNSAT, T. L. and BLUMBERG, J. M. (1965). New evidence for excessive accumulation of Z-band material in nemaline myopathy. *Proc. Natl. Acad. Sci. U.S.A.,* **54,** 1398

SHIPKEY, F. H., LIEBERMAN, P. H., FOOTE, F. W., Jr. and STEWART, F. W. (1964). Ultrastructure of alveolar soft part sarcoma. *Cancer,* **17,** 821

TANDLER, B., ROSSI, E. P., STEIN, M. and MATT, M. M. (1970). Rhabdomyoma of the lip. Light and electron microscopical observations. *Archs Path.,* **89,** 118

22
Histiocytosis X

Electron microscopy can be of considerable value in establishing the diagnosis of a group of conditions now collectively referred to as 'histiocytosis X' (Hand–Schuller–Christian disease, Letterer–Siwe disease and eosinophilic granuloma). Thus, for example, Morales *et al.* (1969) report a case of a tumour composed of large compact cell aggregates admixed with eosinophils, lymphocytes and a few plasma cells. On the basis of light microscopy of paraffin sections, the diagnostic possibilities included, amelanotic melanoma, undifferentiated carcinoma and eosinophilic granuloma. Electron microscopic examination ruled out melanoma because of the absence of melanosomes and carcinoma because of the absence of desmosomes and tonofilaments. However, numerous characteristic granules similar to those found in Langerhans cells were found in the histiocytic cells and so the diagnosis of eosinophilic granuloma was unequivocally established.

Ultrastructural studies have now shown that Langerhans cells with their characteristic granules (*Figure 193*) are of wider distribution than had once been imagined. Hence, a brief review of the subject is presented.

The intraepidermal gold chloride-positive dendritic cells described by Langerhans (1868) were at one time regarded either as intraepidermal neural elements (see Niebauer, 1968) or as effete melanocytes (Masson, 1948, 1951; Billingham and Medawar, 1953; Billingham and Silvers, 1960). Ultrastructurally this cell is characterized by the presence of cytoplasmic granules which present rod-shaped, flask-shaped or tennis-racket-shaped and circular profiles* in sectioned material. The rod-shaped structure or the handle of the racket shows a median striated

*Some authors imagine that the Langerhans cell granules are tubular structures. For example, Carr (1973) states that these are 'curious cytoplasmic inclusions, elongated and probably tubular with an electon-dense core'. This naive assumption cannot possibly explain the various profiles presented by this organelle, or the absence of circular profiles acceptable (on the basis of size and internal structure) as transverse sections through these alleged 'tubules'.

line. Three-dimensional reconstruction of these granules by Wolff (1967) and Sagebiel and Reed (1968) show that they are basically discoid bodies (straight, curved or cup-shaped) with a focal vesicular expansion situated usually but not invariably at the margin of the disc. The stippled line represents sections through paracrystalline nets or lattices with a periodicity of 9 nm.

Since Langerhans cell granules (also called 'Birbeck granules') have at times been seen in continuity with the cell membrane, it is thought that they are produced here and represent a unique variety of endocytosis or that they are 'secretory' granules arising from the Golgi discharging their contents on to the cell surface. It is the former hypothesis which is now generally accepted (Hashimoto, 1970).

Langerhans cells characterized by the presence of these specific granules have now been found in various squamous epithelia such as cutaneous, ungual, gingival, buccal, glossal and cervical of man and experimental animals (Birbeck, Breathnach and Everall, 1961; Breathnach, 1964, 1965; Schroeder and Theilade, 1966; Hackemann, Grubb and Hill, 1968; Hashimoto, 1970, 1971; Hutchens, Sagebiel and Clarke, 1971). Occasionally, melanin granules have been demonstrated in Langerhans cells (Breathnach and Wyllie, 1965) but they take the form of compound melanosomes as seen in keratinocytes and melanophages, so there is no reason to believe that melanosome formation and melanin synthesis occur here as in melanocytes. In achromic skin, such as that found in vitiligo, pinta, the halo of halo naevus, the forelock area of human skin in piebaldism and the white areas of skin from recessively spotted black and white guinea-pigs, there is said to be an increase in the number of Langerhans cells and a diminution or absence of melanocytes (for references see Rodriguez *et al.*, 1971). This suggests a close relationship between melanocytes and Langerhans cells, but it is now difficult to accept that Langerhans cells are derived from melanocytes or that these two share a common lineage, because these granules or cells containing these granules have been seen not only in

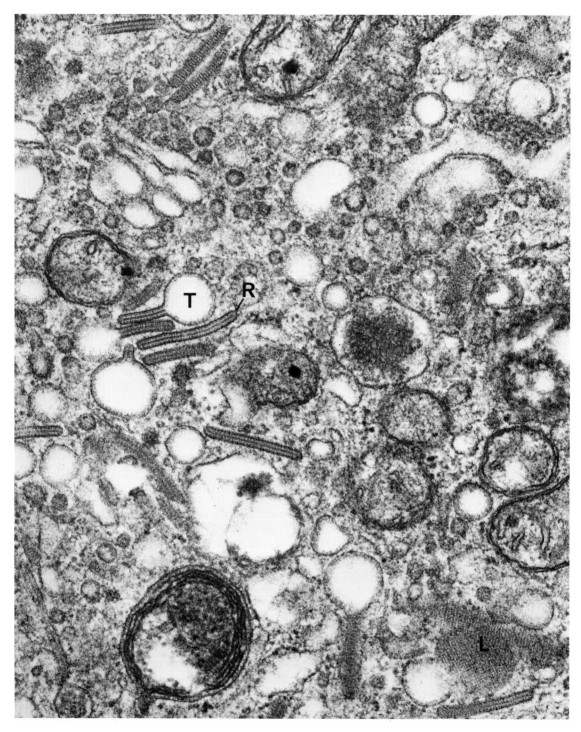

Figure 193   *Langerhans cell from human epidermis, showing granules presenting rod-shaped (R) and tennis-racket-shaped (T) profiles. The discoid shape of the granules and the paracrystalline lattice (L) is better appreciated in tangential cuts through these structures. ×60 000 (From Ghadially, 1975)*

238

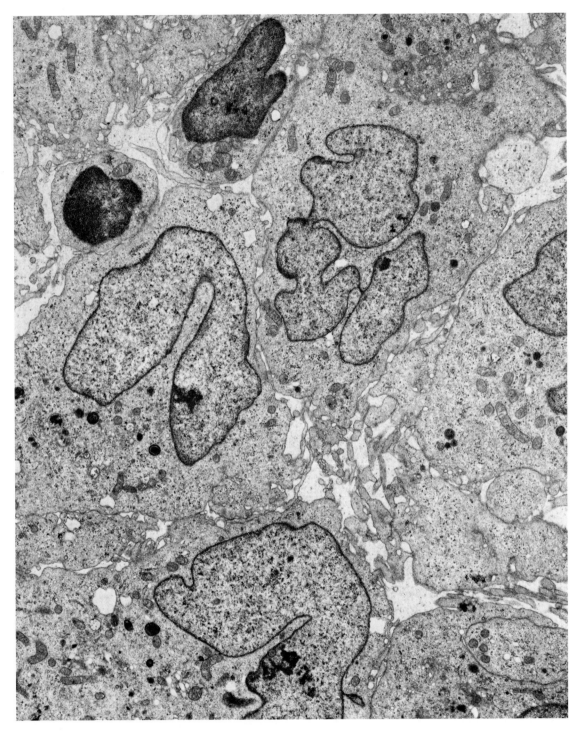

Figure 194 *'Histiocytosis X'. A lymph node from a child with Hand—Schuller—Christian disease, showing histiocytic cells with contorted nuclei. At higher magnifications (Figure 195) some of these cells were found to contain characteristic granules. ×8000 (From a block of tissue supplied by Dr M. Imamura)*

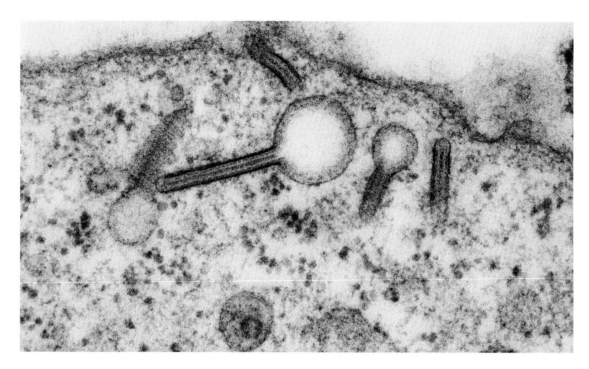

Figure 195　*'Histiocytosis X'. Same case as Figure 194.*
High-power view showing the characteristic racket-shaped
profile of the granules. ✕*94 000 (From a block of tissue*
supplied by Dr M. Imamura)

the epidermis, but also in: (1) the dermis (Zelickson, 1967; Küstala and Mustakallio, 1968); (2) the histiocytes from cases of histiocytosis X (Hand—Schuller—Christian disease, Letterer—Siwe disease and eosinophilic granuloma; *Figures 194 and 195*) (Basset *et al.*, 1965; Turiaf and Basset, 1965; Basset and Nézelof, 1966; Hashimoto and Tarnowski, 1967; Cancilla, Lahey and Carnes, 1967; Gianotti and Caputo, 1969; de Man, 1968; Morales *et al.*, 1969; Shamoto, 1970; Imamura, Sakamoto and Hanazono, 1971; Carrington and Winkelmann, 1972); (3) reticulum cell sarcoma and macrophages of pityriasis rosea (Hashimoto and Tarnowski, 1968); (4) human lymph nodes of dermatopathic lymphadenopathy (Jimbow, Sato and Kukita, 1969); (5) normal lymph nodes of rabbit (Kondo, 1969); (6) hyperplastic lymph nodes of man (Shamoto, Kaplan and Katoh, 1971); (7) thymus of rat (Olah *et al.*, 1968; van Haelst, 1969); (8) monocytic cells from cases of acute monocytic and monomyelocytic leukaemia* (Sanel and Serpick, 1970); and (9) the dermis and

lymphatic vessels during experimentally produced allergic contact dermatitis in man and guinea-pigs (Silberberg, Baer and Rosenthal, 1976).

Thus, it is now thought that the Langerhans cell is not related to melanocytes and that the characteristic granule is a feature of certain histiocytic cells. Since such cells have now been seen crossing the basal lamina by more than one observer, and since such cells have also been observed dividing, Hashimoto and Tarnowski (1968) have proposed that they '... may constitute a self-perpetuating "intraepidermal phagocytic system" to which histiocytes from the dermis are added from time to time'. However, the fact that these cells have now been found in lymph nodes and thymus and seem to be involved in allergic contact hypersensitivity indicates that Langerhans cells are a previously unrecognized cell population of immunological

*Zipper-like junctions and structures resembling Langerhans cell granules developed in these cells during *in vito* experiments to test the phagocytic competence of these cells.

240

importance. Further, the fact that they have now been seen in lymphatics suggests that this might be a circulating population of cells.

Thus, it will be noted from the above that the finding of an occasional Langerhans cell in some site other than the epidermis is not of diagnostic import, but in conjunction with the clinical history and light microscopic findings the demonstration of Langerhans cells in suitable lesions is diagnostic of histiocytosis X.

References

BASSETT, F. and NÉZELOF, C. (1966). Présence en microscopie électronique de structures filamenteuses originales dans les lésions pulmonaires et osseuses de l'histiocytose X. Etat actuel de la question. *Bull Soc. Med. Hôp. Paris,* **117**, 413

BASSET, F., NÉZELOFF, C., MALLET, R. and TURIAF, J. (1965). Nouvelle mise en évidence, par la microscopie electronique, de particules d'allure virale dans une seconde forme clinique de l'histiocytose X, le granulome eosinophile de l'os. *C. R. Hebd. Acad. Sci., Paris,* **261**, 5719

BILLINGHAM, R. E. and MEDAWAR, P. B. (1953). A study of the branched cells of the mammalian epidermis with special reference to the fate of their division products. *Phil. Trans R. Soc.,* **237**, 151

BILLINGHAM, R. E. and SILVERS, W. K. (1969). The melanocytes of mammals. *Q. Rev. Biol.,* **35**, 1

BIRBECK, M. S., BREATHNACH, A. S. and EVERALL, J. D. (1961). An electron microscope study of basal melanocytes and high-lever clear cells (Langerhans cells) in vitiligo. *J. Invest. Derm.,* **37**, 51

BREATHNACH, A. S. (1964). Observations on cytoplasmic organelles in Langerhans cells of human epidermis. *J. Anat.,* **98**, 265

BREATHNACH, A. S. (1965). The cell of Langerhans. *Int. Rev. Cytol.,* **18**, 1

BREATHNACH, A. S. and WYLLIE, L.M.-A. (1965). Melanin in Langerhans cells. *J. Invest. Derm.,* **45**, 401

CANCILLA, P. A., LAHEY, M. E. and CARNES, W. H. (1967). Cutaneous lesions of Letterer—Siwe disease. Electron microscopic study. *Cancer,* **20**, 1986

CARR, I. (1973). The Macrophage. London:Academic Press

CARRINGTON, S. G. and WINKELMANN, R. K. (1972). Electron microscopy of histiocytic diseases of the skin. *Acta Derm-vener., Stockh.,* **52**, 161

de MAN, J. C. H. (1968). Rod-like tubular structures in the cytoplasm of histiocytes in 'histiocytosis X'. *J. Path. Bact.,* **95**, 123

GIANOTTI, F. and CAPUTO, R. (1969). Skin ultrastructure in Hand—Schuller—Christian disease. Report on abnormal Langerhans' cells. *Archs Derm.,* **100**, 342

HACKEMANN, M., GRUBB, C. and HILL, K. R. (1968). The ultrastructure of normal squamous epithelium of the human cervix uteri. *J. Ultrastruct. Res.,* **22**, 443

HASHIMOTO, K. (1970). Lanthanum staining of Langerhans' cell. Communication of Langerhans' cell granules with extracellular space. *Archs Derm.,* **102**, 280

HASHIMOTO, K. (1971). Ultrastructure of the human toenail. I. Proximal nail matrix. *J. Invest. Derm.,* **56**, 235

HASHIMOTO, K. and TARNOWSKI, W. M. (1968). Some new aspects of the Langerhans cell. *Archs Derm.,* **97**, 450

HASHIMOTO, K. and TARNOWSKI, W. M. (1967). Ultrastructural studies of racket-bodies in epidermal Langerhans cells and in histiocytosis-X [abstract]. *Fed. Proc.,* **26**, 370

HUTCHENS, L. H., SAGEBIEL, R. W. and CLARKE, M. A. (1971). Oral epithelial dendritic cells of the rhesus monkey-histologic demonstration, fine structure and quantitative distribution. *J. Invest. Derm.,* **56**, 325

IMAMURA, M., SAKAMOTO, S. and HANAZONO, H. (1971). Malignant histiocytosis: a case of generalized histiocytosis with infiltration of Langerhans' granule-containing histiocytes. *Cancer,* **28**, 467

JIMBOW, K., SATO, S. and KUKITA, A. (1969). Langerhans' cells of the normal human pilosebaceous system. *J. Invest. Derm.,* **52**, 177

KONDO, Y. (1969). Macrophages containing Langerhans cell granules in normal lymph nodes of the rabbit. *Z. Zellforsch. Mikrosk. Anat.,* **98**, 506

KÜSTALA, V. and MUSTAKALLIO, K. (1968). The presence of Langerhans' cells in human dermis with special reference to their potential mesenchymal origin. *Acta Derm. -vener., Stockh.,* **48**, 115

LANGERHANS, P. (1868). Uber die nerven der menschlichen haut. *Virchows Arch. Path Anat. Physiol.,* **44**, 325

MASSON, P. (1948). Pigment cells in Man. In: *The Biology of Melanomas,* ed. R. W. Miner and M. Gordon, p. 15. Special publication of the New York Academy of Sciences, Vol. IV

MASSON, P. (1951). My conception of cellular nevi. *Cancer,* **4**, 9

MORALES, A. R., FINE, G. HORN, R. C. and WATSON, J. H. L. (1969). Langerhans cells in a localized lesion of the eosinophilic granuloma type. *Lab. Invest.,* **20**, 412

NIEBAUER, G. (1968). *Dendritic Cells of Human Skin.* Basel: Karger

OLAH, I., DUNAY, C., ROHLICH, P. and TORO, I. (1968). A special type of cell in the medulla of the rat thymus. *Acta. Biol. Acad. Sci. Hung.,* **19**, 97

RODRIGUEZ, H. A., ALBORES-SAAVEDRA, J., LOZANO M. M. SMITH, M. and FEDER, W. (1971). Langerhans' cells in late pinta. Ultrastructural observations in one case. *Archs Path.,* **91**, 302

SAGEBIEL, R. W. and REED, T. H. (1968). Serial reconstruction of the characteristic granule of the Langerhans cell. *J. Cell Biol.,* **36**, 595

SANEL, F. T. and SERPICK, A. A. (1970). Plasmalemmal and subsurface complexes in human leukemic cells: membrane bounding by zipperlike junctions. *Science, N.Y.,* **168**, 1458

SCHROEDER, H. E. and THEILADE, J. (1966). Electron microscopy of normal human gingival epithelium. *J. Periodont. Res.,* **1**, 95

SHAMOTO, M. (1970). Langerhans cell granule in Letterer—Siwe disease. An electron microscopic study. *Cancer,* **26**, 1102

SHAMOTO, M., KAPLAN, C. and KATOH, A. K. (1971). Langerhans cell granules in human hyperplastic lymph nodes. *Archs Path.,* **92**, 46

SILBERBERG, I., BAER, R. L. and ROSENTHAL, S. A. (1976). The role of Langerhans cells in allergic contact hypersentivity. A review of findings in man and guinea pigs. *J. Invest. Derm.*, **66**, 210

TURIAF, J. and BASSET, F. (1965). Histiocytose 'X' pulmonaire: identification de particules de nature probablement virale dans un fragment pulmonaire prélevé pour biopsie. *Bull. Acad. Natn. Méd.*, **149**, 674

VAN HAELST, U. (1969). Light and electron microscopic study of the normal and pathological thymus of the rat. III. A mesenchymal histiocytic type of cell. *Z. Zellforsch.*, **99**, 198

WOLFF, K. (1967). The fine structure of the Langerhans cell granule. *J. Cell Biol.*, **35**, 468

ZELICKSON, A. S. (1967). Melanocyte, melanin granule and Langerhans cell. In: *Ultrastructure of Normal and Abnormal Skin*, p. 163. Philadelphia: Lea and Febiger

Index

*References to illustrations are italicized. For convenience the page number on which the plate appears is given rather than the plate number itself.